A Global Agenda for Caring

Delores A. Gaut

Editor

National League for Nursing Press • New York
Pub. No. 15-2518

Library of Congress Cataloging-in-Publication Data

A Global agenda for caring / Delores A. Gaut, editor.
    p.   cm.
    "Pub. no. 15-2518."
    Includes bibliographical references.
    ISBN 0-88737-578-2 : $34.95
    1. Nursing—Philosophy—Congresses.   2. Caring—Congresses.
3. Nursing—Psychological aspects—Congresses.   4. Nursing—
organization & administration—congresses.   I. Gaut, Delores A.
    [DNLM: 1. Caregivers—congresses.   2. Ethics, Nursing—congresses.
3. Philosophy, Nursing—congresses.   WY 86 G562 1993]
RT84.5.G56   1993
610.73'01—dc20
DNLM/DLC
for Library of Congress   93-1822
                                                                    CIP

Edited by Maryan Malone. Typeset in Goudy by Publications Development Co. of
Texas. Printed by Northeastern Press. Cover by Lauren Stevens.

Printed in the United States of America

Contents

iii

PART II.   WOMEN, CARING, NURSING

PART III.   ETHICS/RESEARCH METHODOLOGIES

Contributors

Agnes M. Aamodt, PhD, RN, FAAN
Professor Emerita
College of Nursing
University of Arizona
Tucson, Arizona, USA

Siv R. Bäck-Pettersson, RN
Nursing Development Coordinator
Bohus County Council
Gothenburg, Sweden

Rauda Gelazis, PhC, RN
Associate Professor
Ursuline College
Pepper Pike, Ohio, USA

Joan Donoghue, MNSt
Director of Nursing
Mercy Private Hospital
East Melbourne, Victoria, Australia

Christine Duffield, PhD, DNE, MHP,
    RN, FCN (NSW), FCHSE
Head, School of Nursing Therapeutics;
    Director, Centre for Graduate Nurs-
    ing Studies
Associate Professor
University of Technology, Sydney
Sydney, New South Wales, Australia

Joanne R. Duffy, DNSc, RN, CCRN
Director of Critical Care and Cardio-
    vascular Nursing Services
Assistant Professor, Graduate Nursing
    Services
Georgetown University Medical Center
Washington, DC, USA

Margaret Dunlop, DNursSc, MEd, RN
Professor and Head, School of Nursing
Griffith University
Nathan, Queensland, Australia

Payom Euswas, PhD, RN
Faculty of Nursing
Mahidol University
Bangkok, Thailand

Julianna Finn, MSN, RN
Nursing Faculty
Oakland Community College
Union Lake, Michigan, USA

Sara T. Fry, PhD, RN, FAAN
Associate Professor, School of Nursing;
Codirector, Center for Biomedical
    Ethics
University of Maryland at Baltimore
Baltimore, Maryland, USA

Jill Hill, MSc, GradDipEd, RN
Faculty of Health Science
University of Western Sydney
(MacArthur)
Campbelltown, New South Wales,
Australia

Kirsten Pryds Jensen, RN
Nursing Development Coordinator
Danish Labour Inspection
Copenhagen, Denmark
Gothenburg College of Health and
Caring Sciences
Gothenburg, Sweden

Olga Kanitsaki, DipHospNsg and Unit
Mgmt., MEd Studies, RN, RM
School of Nursing, Lincoln Faculty of
Health Sciences
La Trobe University
Melbourne, Victoria, Australia

Janet M. Lakomy, PhD, RN
The University of Texas at Tyler
Tyler, Texas, USA

Madeleine Leininger, PhD, DS, RN,
CTN, LHD, FAAN
Professor of Nursing and Anthropology
Wayne State University
Detroit, Michigan, USA

Debra Woodard Leners, PhD, RN
Assistant Professor
School of Nursing
University of Northern Colorado
Greeley, Colorado, USA

Judy Lumby, DNE, MHPEd, RN,
FCN, FRCNA
Head, School of Nursing Health
Studies
University of Technology, Sydney
Sydney, New South Wales, Australia

Barbara E. Place, DipNEd (MID),
MA, RN, RM
Ballarat University College
Mt. Helen, Victoria, Australia

Gwen Sherwook, PhD, RN
Associate Professor and Assistant Dean
for Educational Outreach

School of Nursing
The University of Texas Health
Science Center at Houston
Houston, Texas, USA

Sandie Soldwisch, PhD, RN
Assistant Professor
School of Nursing
Northern Illinois University
DeKalb, Illinois, USA

Zen Spangler, PhD, RN
Director of Nursing Education and Re-
search
Guthrie/Robert Packer Hospital
Sayre, Pennsylvania, USA

Elizabeth H. Thomlinson, MN, RN
Director, Northern Bachelor of Nursing
Program
The Pas, Manitoba, Canada

Kathleen L. Valentine, PhD, RN
Assistant Professor and
Director of Evaluation
School of Nursing
University of Wisconsin—Eau Claire
Eau Claire, Wisconsin, USA

Toni M. Vezeau, PhD, RN
School of Nursing
University of Colorado
Denver, Colorado, USA

Vera Regina Waldow
School of Nursing
Federal University of Rio Grande do
Sul
Porto Alegre, Brazil

Robin Watts, PhD, MHSc, BA,
DipNEd, RN
Associate Professor
Curtin University of Technology
Perth, Western Australia

Alanna Wells, MS, RN
Director of Inpatient Services
Petaluma Valley Hospital
Petaluma, California, USA

Preface

*T*his publication celebrates a first for the International Association for Human Caring, Inc. The annual Caring Research Conference was held outside of the United States in the land down-under—Australia, the world's largest island and smallest continent. Melbourne was the host city and the conference entitled Human Caring: A Global Agenda was the culmination of combined efforts with the Royal College of Nursing, Australia. The aim of the conference was to provide an international forum to pursue the advancement of knowledge in care and caring from a transcultural nursing perspective, and to develop new insights for nursing practice and health care decisions.

The twenty-five papers included in this book were all accepted for presentation at the conference, and then peer-reviewed prior to inclusion in this publication. The authors, from Australia, Brazil, Canada, Denmark, New Zealand, Sweden, Thailand, and the United States of America, represent the very best in international nursing scholarship focused on the global concerns of nursing, human care, and caring. The book is organized by five major themes:

Cross-cultural human care and caring.

Women, caring, and nursing.

Ethics of caring and research methodologies for the study of caring.

Nursing practice and nursing experiences.

Caring and nursing administration.

The first six papers set the stage for understanding a global, transcultural theory of care and caring. Transcultural nursing focuses on culture care differences and similarities within differing contexts. As these authors demonstrate, culturally based care is a dominant factor to guide nursing care practices. In Chapter 1, "Culture Care Theory: The Comparative Global Theory to Advance Human Care Nursing Knowledge and Practice," Madeleine Leininger presents a theory of culture care that generates knowledge to help nurses appreciate the covert aspects of human care within specific cultural structures and values.

In Chapter 2, "Transcultural Human Care: Its Challenge to and Critique of Professional Nursing Care," Olga Kanitsaki further illustrates the challenge of culture care and suggests that transcultural human care differs significantly from mainstream professional nursing care. The author presents the results of a qualitative research study investigating the health-illness-suffering and care experiences of a sample of "Greek-born" members of Greek-Australian families living in Melbourne, Australia.

Zen Spangler, in Chapter 3, "Generic and Professional Care of Anglo-American and Philippine American Nurses," focuses on the values and care-giving practices of nurses from two cultures. Using the qualitative methodology of ethno-nursing, the findings further support the potency of Leininger's theory of culture care and provide support for the interlinking of professional and generic care in nursing.

In Chapter 4, "Caring in Birthing: Experiences of Professional Nurse and Generic Care," Julianna Finn looks for congruence between finalized descriptions of professional nursing care and generic care as defined in Leininger's theory of culture care. Using phenomenological analysis, the author attempts to discover childbirthing women's lived experiences of professional nursing and generic care/noncare.

Chapter 5, "Education: One Means for Caring for Clients and Nurses in Isolated Northern Settings," by Elizabeth H. Thomlinson, offers a unique approach to caring through education. The author discusses the development of an educational program that would provide clinical skills and cultural education for nurses who provide primary health care to indigenous communities in remote settlements in northern Canada.

In Chapter 6, Rauda Gelazis presents the results of a field study entitled "Care: What It Means to Lithuanian Americans." The author, utilizing ethno-nursing methodology, attempts to address two questions relative to the study group: (1) What are the experiences, expressions, meanings, and patterns of care as influenced by their particular environmental contexts? and (2) Are there any interrelationships among care, well-being, and humor?

The next set of papers focuses on women caring—the language of caring in the context of economic rationalism, and the *conscientization* of women in the caring profession of nursing. In Chapter 7, "In the War Years: Women, Caring, and Economic Rationalism," Margaret Dunlop suggests that, despite our experiences to the contrary, caring is often talked about as if it were a harmonious process. The author suggests that the greatest danger to the caring practices of nurses and nursing lies in the marketing of caring as a commodity, a consumer "good" within a free-market economy where women's work, including nursing, is undervalued. In the language of economic rationalism, caring is discussed as unskilled work requiring only minimal costs. In order to continue to develop knowledge and understanding of caring practices, Dunlop challenges us to recognize the environmental threats to our caring within the structures in which caring is embedded.

In Chapter 8, "Healthworld Theory: A Universal Language of Caring," Jill Hill also warns of the insidious threat to caring from within the nursing profession itself. Nursing interests have sought to acquire status and legitimized power through adopting the empiricist values of language, science, and technique. Within an even wider political discourse of economic rationalism, care is expensive, subjective, and inefficient. Society's philosophic, institutional, and political assumptions about caring are often hidden within the language of power and economics. The author suggests a theoretical framework by which the language of nurse–client interaction can be used to explain the process of caring and increase our understanding of the nurse's function to care.

Robin Watts, in Chapter 9, "Caring: Beyond the Dyad," challenges the reader, through the use of storytelling, to reflect on the potential problems and limitations with the descriptions of caring as currently explicated. The author raises the issue of relationships in the context of caring and asks the reader to identify the knowledge, tact, craft, and wisdom embedded in the stories presented to extend and improve the skill of involvement and the practices that go with care and caring.

The last chapter in this grouping, "Toward Conscientization: A Feminist Course Experience," by Vera Regina Waldow, develops the case for feminist process as a pedagogical strategy with nursing students from Brazil. The author designed a course utilizing Freire's *conscientização*, the process by which human beings, as knowing subjects, perceive and understand the sociocultural reality that shapes their lives and their capacity to take action against oppressive elements of reality. The goal for the course was to achieve consciousness-raising through reflection about the caring environ-ment women can build when exercising their own power and how, through such an environment, they can gain strength for change.

The next set of papers, although at first glance apparently quite unre-lated, when woven together provide a picture of human context and of hu-man responses that are essential for the further development of caring knowledge and caring practices. The ethical, interdisciplinary, and method-ological approaches to human care and caring challenge the reader to dis-cover and create new meanings of human caring that will provide a guide to nursing and personal action.

Sara Frye, in Chapter 11, "The Ethic of Care: Nursing's Excellence for a Troubled World," provides a brief overview of the concept of human caring, several definitions and models of caring, and suggestions for the develop-ment of a practical ethic of human care.

Janet Lakomy's chapter, "The Interdisciplinary Meanings of Human Caring," suggests the necessity for a deep interdisciplinary understanding about the nature and meanings of human caring. Utilizing hermeneutical strategies, the author addresses three questions: (1) What is the meaning of human caring within a selected disciplinary focus? (2) How does one un-derstand the meanings of human caring from a selected interdisciplinary focus?, and (3) How does one access the caring literature?

Chapter 13, by Agnes Aamodt, "Experiencing the Mystery in Cross-Cultural Research on Care," challenges the readers to consider not only ways to think about clinical nursing research, but also ways to use oneself as a cru-cial tool or instrument in collecting, analyzing, and writing about experi-ences. The author weaves her field-work stories and her personal knowing throughout the chapter as she discusses mystery and listening and learning.

Continuing with the theme of storytelling, Toni Vezeau, in Chapter 14, "Use of Narrative in Human Caring Inquiry," discusses the aesthetic method of inquiry called fictional narrative as one approach to exploring human experiences within the framework of human care nursing.

In the last paper in this group, Chapter 15, "Nursing Intuition: The Deep Connection," Debra Woodard Leners chose to study intuition as a way of knowing in the culture of nursing care practice. Utilizing an ethno-graphic design along with metaphorical analysis, the author identifies and describes the language, images, feelings, actions, and processes of intuition identified by a select group of nurses.

The fourth theme focuses on nursing experiences in the context of clini-cal practice. The chapters in this group discuss both patient and nurse re-sponses to experiences of caring. In Chapter 16, "A Qualitative Analysis of Patient Responses to Caring: A Moral and Economic Imperative," Gwen

Sherwood examines the impact of caring through the perspective of the patient. Using Spiegelberg's steps of phenomenology, the author presents eight major themes and elements derived from patient responses to nurses' caring.

In Chapter 17, "'She Dares': An Essential Characteristic of the Excellent Swedish Nurse," Siv R. Bäck-Pettersson and Kirsten Pryds Jensen tell the story of a group of peer-identified excellent nurses who seem to have a "green thumb" for nursing. Through exploratory methodology, the authors present the characteristics and caring moments described by this select group of nurses.

In Chapter 18, "Humanistic Care and Nurses' Experiences," Joan Donoghue presents the results of a study designed to measure the degree to which humanistic care behaviors are enacted in clinical nursing practice in hospital situations. In addition, the study explored the relationship between humanistic care behaviors and nurses' characteristics, attributes, and experiences.

In Chapter 19, "Understanding the Meaning of Chronic Illness: A Prerequisite for Caring," Barbara Place explores the meaning of chronic illness and the strategies persons develop to live with illness. Within this context, the author discusses the need for authentic caring for and about those who live with chronic illness.

Sandie Soldwisch, in Chapter 20, "Care, Caritas, and Ego Development," presents the results of a case study design that examined the correlation of caring as a virtue of adulthood. Utilizing Erikson's epigenetic psychosocial theory as a framework, the author demonstrates the need for education focused on ego development, caring, and caritas—a global perspective of human caring.

The last paper in this section, Chapter 21, "The Actualized Caring Moment: A Grounded Theory of Caring in Nursing Practice," by Payom Euswas, is a grounded theory approach to identify and authenticate those aspects of nursing practice that best typify caring. The study attempts to uncover the human experience of caring and being cared for from the perspectives of nurses and patients.

The closing section of the book focuses on caring related to issues of concern to nursing administration. The four papers focus on an essential question for nursing in any care system: At what cost caring?

In Chapter 22, "Utilization of Research on Caring: Development of a Nurse Compensation System," Kathleen Valentine discusses how research on caring and participatory decision-making processes were used as the basis for the development of a nurse compensation system within one organization.

In Chapter 23, "Shared Governance: A Model of Caring in Practice," Alanna Wells utilizes caring theory to support the administrative structure of shared governance. The author suggests that a shared governance model embodies caring action and provides a model for administrative caring.

In Chapter 24, "Caring Behaviors of Nurse Managers: Relationships to Staff Nurse Satisfaction and Retention," Joanne Duffy examines nurse manager caring behaviors and the relationship of those caring behaviors to staff nurse satisfaction and retention. The author attempts to demonstrate a positive relationship between nurse manager caring behaviors and job satisfaction and an inverse relationship between caring behaviors and staff nurse turnover.

The last paper, Chapter 25, "Caring Nurse Managers: Have They a Future in Today's Health Care System?", by Judy Lumby and Christine Duffield focuses on the climate and culture within which nurse managers develop decision-making skills. The authors explore the dissonance faced by nurse managers as they attempt to make decisions based on caring in care systems that are increasingly controlled by business principles.

A very special thank-you to all of the authors and peer reviewers (listed below) for the excellent scholarship and furthering of caring knowledge. In addition, I would like to express my appreciation to the Royal College of Nursing, Australia, and the many nurses who participated in the coordination of the Fourteenth Annual Caring Research Conference.

This publication would not have been possible without the encouragement and assistance of the editors from the National League for Nursing Press, Sally Barhydt and Allan Graubard. Lastly, I would like to thank all of the readers who have purchased this book. A percentage of the proceeds from the sale of this book is returned to the International Association for Human Caring, Inc., and provides financial support for continuing the annual research conferences and furthers the goals of developing and expanding caring knowledge and research for the profession of nursing.

Delores A. Gaut, RN, PhD
President, IAHC, Inc.

IAHC, INC. PEER REVIEWERS

Agnes Aamodt, PhD, RN, FAAN
Professor Emerita
University of Arizona College of
   Nursing
2330 W. Wagonwheels
Tucson, AZ 15745

Anne Boykin, PhD, RN
Dean, College of Nursing
Florida Atlantic University
Boca Raton, FL 33431

Joyceen S. Boyle, Phd, RN
Professor and Chair
Medical College of Georgia School
  of Nursing
1446 Harper St.
Augusta, GA 30912

Carolyn L. Brown, PhD, RN
Assistant Professor
Florida Atlantic University
College of Nursing
Boca Raton, FL 33431

Linda Brown, PhD, RN
Assistant Professor, Research
University of Washington School
  of Nursing
2717 11th Ave. East
Seattle, WA 98102

Linda Dietrich, MS, RN
Clinical Nurse Specialist
Bess Kaiser Medical Center
5055 N. Greeley Ave.
Portland, OR 97217

Kathryn G. Gardner, MSN, RN
Director of Nursing Research
Rochester General Hospital
Rochester, NY 14621

Cheryl Demerath Learn, PhC, RN
Lecturer
University of New Mexico College
  of Nursing
Albuquerque, NM 87131

Madeleine Leininger, PhD, RN,
  FAAN
Professor
Wayne State University College of
  Nursing
Detroit, MI 48202

Ruth M. Neil, PhD, RN
Assistant Professor
University of Colorado School of
  Nursing
4200 E. 9th Ave.
Box C-288
Denver, CO 80262

Marilyn A. Ray, PhD, RN
Christine E. Lynn Eminent Scholar
  Endowed Chair in Nursing
Florida Atlantic University
Boca Raton, FL 33431

Francelyn Reeder, PhD, RN
Assistant Professor
University of Colorado HSC
School of Nursing
Denver, CO 80222

Sister M. Simone Roach, PhD, RN
Researcher/Lecturer
2661 Kingston Rd.
Scarborough, Ontario, Canada
  M1M 1M3

Gwen Sherwood, PhD, RN
Assistant Dean for Educational
  Outreach
University of Texas—Houston
School of Nursing
Houston, TX 77030

Sue A. Thomas, EdD, RN
Professor, Department of Nursing
Sonoma State University
Rohnert Park, CA 94928

Kathleen L. Valentine, PhD, RN
Director of Evaluation
University of Wisconsin—Eau
    Claire
Eau Claire, WI 54702

Robin J. Watts, PhD, RN
Head, School of Nursing
Curtin University of Technology
GPO Box 11987
Perth, WA 6001
Australia

Anna Frades Z. Wenger, PhD, RN
Associate Professor and
Director, Transcultural and
International Nursing Center
Nell Hodgson Woodruff
School of Nursing
Emory University
Atlanta, GA 30322

Foreword

Global perspectives of human care and caring have created a challenge for nurse scholars and clinicians worldwide. There is an increased momentum among nurses to establish connectedness with nurses in other countries, to share knowledge, and, by actively pursuing the advancement of the knowledge of caring, to develop new insights for health care. Nurses throughout the world recognize that the call to focus on human caring as a global agenda has become an imperative.

Believing that human caring is a global agenda, the Royal College of Nursing, Australia, entered into a cosponsorship with the International Association for Human Caring (IAHC) for the Fourteenth Annual Caring Research Conference. Held in Melbourne, Australia, in July 1992, the conference was the culmination of four years of planning efforts. Its theme was "Human Caring: A Global Agenda."

For the first time, the conference was held outside the United States. Nurses from fourteen countries attended, the largest representation of nations since the inception of the annual conferences. This book is a reflection of the conference's international character. Its purpose is to enhance our knowledge of human caring from a variety of perspectives.

It was significant that Australia was selected as the first country to host the conference outside the United States and to participate in the process of establishing a greater global awareness of caring as the essence of nursing. Since its inception in 1949, the Royal College of Nursing, Australia (RCNA), as a national organization, has fostered professional excellence in nursing and has had a major impact in influencing the advancement of nursing in Australia. The RCNA, in conjunction with the IAHC, has recognized the need to further expand nursing's global connectedness in order to advance the knowledge of human care and caring. June Cochrane, former Executive Director of the RCNA, and Barbara E. Place, former chair of the Australian Planning Committee, were the primary nurse leaders who initially supported the hosting of the conference in Australia and fostered its international planning and development. Katherine McInerney, current Executive Director of the RCNA, also played a significant role in the further development of the conference. Australian nurses from a variety of higher education institutions responded affirmatively to the hosting of the conference in the Southern Hemisphere.

During the past decade, an increasing number of nursing faculty and clinicians from countries throughout the world,—including Australia, Brazil, Canada, Denmark, Finland, Iceland, New Zealand, Sweden, Thailand, and the United States—have become interested in studying care and caring from philosophical, epistemological, economic, administrative, educational, and practice perspectives. As we anticipate the challenges of health care in the future, we can expect that caring will be increasingly recognized as the essence of nursing and that the need to further develop an international forum for the purpose of sharing our scholarly efforts will become more intense. This book adds to an expanding body of international knowledge of human care and caring, with contributions by nurse scholars from five continents.

The historic 1992 conference fostered the systematic study of caring, the development of theoretical models of caring, the significance of caring in relation to patient outcomes, and the examination of caring from health policy perspectives and in comparative contexts.

Caring is a global agenda. The contributions in this book challenge us to reaffirm and sustain a global connectedness that will help to realize the full potential of studying caring worldwide.

Sue A. Thomas, RN, EdD
International Coordinator
Fourteenth Annual Caring Research Conference
Professor of Nursing
Sonoma State University
Rohnert Park, California
USA

Introduction

Human Caring: A Global Agenda" was the theme for the Fourteenth Annual Caring Research Conference, held in Melbourne, Australia in July 1992. This theme is a reflection of the sharing of knowledge and the collaboration among nurses in different countries, as they seek to advance health care through the study of human caring.

The Royal College of Nursing, Australia, was delighted to join with the International Association for Human Caring in cohosting this annual research conference, the first one held outside the United States. The opportunity to enhance a drawing together of nurses from all parts of the world was seen to be a valuable objective by both organizations.

The Royal College of Nursing, Australia, is a national organization of nurses striving for professional excellence in nursing practice, for the benefit of the health of the community.

Prior to 1949, Australian nurses traveled overseas to gain further education. In 1949, the College was established by nurses; beginning in 1950, the College became a provider of higher education courses for nurses within Australia. In the late 1970s, the College's teaching role was transferred to the general education sector.

Since its formation in 1949, the College has functioned as a professional organization. Through its professional leadership, the College has involved its members in influencing the quality of health care in the community and the advancement of nursing in Australia.

The College fulfills its mission by providing nursing leadership in nursing, health, and community services. Its diverse activities and projects include nursing and health care policy analysis and development, distance education, research, publications, and networks.

The International Association for Human Caring (IAHC) serves as a scholarly forum to advance knowledge in care and caring. In 1978, the National Research Care Conference was conceived and initiated in the United States by Dr. Madeleine Leininger. The annual conference was designed so that scholars could share ideas, research, and theories of care and caring. The philosophy of the group is based on the belief that care and caring are the essence of nursing and should be the unique and unifying focus of the profession.

The formal organization of this group was established in 1987. At that time, the Association was renamed the International Association for Human Caring, Inc.

The 1992 conference was the result of four years of planning and collaboration by the Royal College of Nursing, Australia, and the IAHC. The trigger for this collaboration was the sharing of ideas and of an interest in caring between nurses from the United States and Australia. The idea of an international conference cohosted from two sides of the Pacific was conceived to bring the science of caring to greater awareness in the health care community through the exploration of caring's many dimensions.

We believe the debate and discussion generated fulfilled this objective. This publication is one of the outcomes; the ideas carried away by the participants are another. We hope that they will further develop the philosophy and science of caring.

Katherine McInerney
Executive Director
Royal College of Nursing, Australia

Part I

Cross-Cultural Caring

1

Culture Care Theory: The Comparative Global Theory to Advance Human Care Nursing Knowledge and Practice

Madeleine Leininger

In the evolutionary development of the discipline and profession of nursing, nurses are now systematically studying and using human care knowledge as a central and distinct feature of nursing. Of great significance in this trend is the study of human care from a transcultural nursing perspective. The comparative study of human care, to identify culture care commonalities and differences, is leading to a global knowledge from which a sound and worldwide discipline of nursing can emerge. This knowledge is essential if nursing care decisions and actions are to provide culturally sensitive, congruent, and competent care (Leininger, 1978, 1988a, 1988b, 1989, 1991). The study of human caring from a transcultural perspective is also leading to some new and unique insights about care and the nature of nursing in different cultures. Most importantly, global knowledge of comparative care is advancing nursing's distinctive contributions and helping nurses to serve people in meaningful ways. Indeed, transcultural global knowledge of care and practice will significantly transform nursing in beneficial ways.

In the mid-1950s, I identified culture care as a glaring need, a missing dimension of nursing. I began to study care and caring from a transcultural perspective, drawing on nursing and anthropological insights. I was already committed to care as the essence of nursing and as the central and distinct phenomenon that made nursing what it is or should be (Leininger, 1965, 1967, 1970, 1976a, 1981, 1984a). Uniting culture with care within a new conceptual and theoretical frame of reference began to give nursing a much broader and more relevant view of the nature of humans than was possible with the traditional mind–body perspective. Today, culture care has brought forth many new insights about how people live, what they value, and how they set norms for the practice of health care. Increased knowledge of diverse peoples in the world is leading to a wealth of new ideas for culture-specific care and is helping nurses to reexamine past nursing practices in which cultural dimensions were unknown. Most importantly, the culture care movement is stimulating nurse clinicians, teachers, and researchers to expand greatly their view of the care needs of diverse cultures. As they study the meanings and functions of humanistic care in Western and non-Western cultures, these nursing professionals are just beginning to realize the tremendously rich and meaningful knowledge of comparative nursing care that is available.

During the past three decades, a cadre of transcultural nurse specialists and generalists has been committed to research of care knowledge and to making it meaningful to nurses in their teaching and clinical practices. Boyle and Andrews (1989), Leininger (1965, 1970, 1976a, 1976b, 1981, 1984b, 1988a, 1988b, 1991), Horn (1978), Luna (1989), Ray (1981), Wenger (1991), and many others have been active in explicating culture care knowledge. These nurses' focus on transcultural care phenomena has stimulated other nurses, and especially nursing students, to learn about cultural care differences and similarities in client care services. In addition, the work of care theorists such as Aamodt (1978), Gaut (1981), Roach (1987), Valentine (1985), Watson (1985), and others, has helped to advance care knowledge. However, from the beginning, transcultural nurses have always maintained that care is the central focus of nursing and transcultural nursing.

As an envisionary nursing leader, I was committed to transcultural nursing care that would have a global perspective; the body of nursing knowledge and practices that would emerge had to have worldwide relevance rather than a local or parochial scope. I envisioned that, by 1990, nurses would be traveling to all parts of the world and would need to be knowledgeable and skilled in transcultural care and health. This was indeed, during the 1950s, a futuristic view (Leininger, 1970, 1978). Transcultural care knowledge was needed to expand nurses' worldview as well as their need to develop culture-specific care practices for quality-based services. Culture-specific care was predicted to bring client satisfactions, early recovery, or meaningful death experiences. Thus, the transcultural care movement seemed logical and inevitable, but some nurses needed to take leadership roles in the 1950s and make the movement a reality for the year 2000 and beyond. This has occurred, and human care with a global perspective is now an exciting, relevant, and important area of rigorous study.

In this chapter, I identify several factors that have greatly influenced transcultural caring and its relationship to the global view of nursing that is gradually emerging. I take the position that the Theory of Culture Care Diversity and Universality and the use of the Sunrise Model are important means to advance culture care knowledge that will give the discipline and profession of nursing a comparative perspective. I contend that the theory of culture care is important because human care is usually deeply embedded and takes on meanings within the worldview, social structure factors, language, cultural values, and environmental contexts of different cultures (Leininger, 1981, 1988a, 1988b, 1991). The discovery of the fullest dimensions of the meanings and patterns of care must be studied within a holistic culture perspective. The theory generates knowledge that can help nurses appreciate the covert aspects of human care within specific cultural structures and values. Moreover, the theory findings have become valuable means to contrast care in different cultures. From the use of the culture care theory, some of the richest insights about culture care knowledge are identifiable, and nurses can use this knowledge to guide nursing practices. Finally, I argue that the theory is holistic and can be used to study all cultures to discover the multiple factors influencing human care meanings, expressions, and patterns (Leininger, 1991). As the world continues to change to intense multiculturalism, nurses must realize their need for transcultural care knowledge if they are to be effective in their nursing practices with new immigrants, especially those from cultural minorities, and with peoples whom they have never seen or heard about in the past. The focus of the Fourteenth Annual Caring Research Conference—*global culture care* with a comparative stance—is extremely timely, and Australia is a society with many cultures. As transcultural knowledge grows, we will see a major impact on the world's nearly 5 million nurses. They will become committed to the advancement of humanistic and scientific caring in their education and practice endeavors. This outcome is, indeed, most encouraging to think about as it begins to be a reality.

FACTORS INFLUENCING TRANSCULTURAL CARE AS A GLOBAL IMPERATIVE

Several factors that have significantly influenced transculturalism have made the study and practice of comparative global care imperative in nursing. My statement (and the motto of the Transcultural Nursing Society) is that we are living and practicing in *"One world with many cultures."* I also held to the motto, *"The cultural needs of people in the world will be met by nurses prepared in transcultural nursing."* These two mottos were important not only to conceptualize and develop transcultural caring, but also to discover multiple societal and world factors that influence nursing. From my anthropological knowledge, I became fully aware that nurses must realize they are living in *one world* in which human caring needed to be discovered and used in practice. I envisioned that cultures would be closely interacting with one another by the end of this century, and that nurses would be expected to care for people of diverse cultures. Nurses would need to speak several languages, to value cultural diversities, and to develop new care strategies for people who held different values and beliefs. In the 1950s and 1960s, most nurses could not imagine these expectations nor foresee that new, more rapid modes of transportation and communications would link nurses almost instantly with other cultures worldwide, as well as those within their own communities and nations. These ideas about culture care did not gain relevance until the early 1980s; today, they are being fully realized. The growth of the transcultural care movement is an indication that nurses need to look ahead and be prepared for futuristic changes.

The ideal of nursing that maintains humanistic care, and of nurses who are compassionate, empathetic, interested in, and concerned about human beings, must become explicit and deeply valued among individuals and groups from diverse cultures. The belief or assumption that exquisite and meaningful client care leads to health and well-being is important. Moreover, as nurses learn about and interact with many different cultures in the world, the cultural meanings of care in various professional contexts will lead to positive relationships and well-being. The idea that people of different cultural origins could be helped and healed by nurses who understood their care beliefs, values, and practices was as important as the nurses' use of this care knowledge in practice. The idea that nurses could promote caring diversities and still seek universals was fascinating to me. Anthropologically, and from a nursing view, I said in the early 1960s that *homo sapiens* needed care to survive. Neither anthropologists nor nurses took that stance in those days. My belief led to my launching the field of transcultural nursing, with human care as the central focus—an important phenomenon of nursing four decades ago (Leininger, 1970, 1978, 1981, 1989, 1991).

It is important to realize that, after World War II ended, nursing took on a highly intensive technological and task-oriented practice focus. High technology's alliance with medicine became clearly apparent and, with this trend, the "cult of efficiency" for nurses occurred. Especially in hospitals, the focus turned to medical diseases, symptoms, and a host of diagnostic and treatment regimes. As technical–medical tasks were introduced, nursing began to lose its earlier signs of caring and of providing comprehensive care to clients and families. Nurses spent much of their time fulfilling physicians' many medical orders and demands, and carrying out medical treatments. The pretechnology era in which one could identify different modes of caring yielded to the new cultural ethos of high technology and of medical services mandated by patriarchal physicians who were controlling the hospitals and agencies (Ashley, 1976; Leininger, 1970). In the 1950s and 1960s, only a few nurses were concerned with preserving some of the caring ethos and preventing a technological takeover in nursing; most nurses were becoming intrigued with high technology. Thus, beginning in the 1950s, the very heart of nursing was continually threatened by high technology and many other worldwide forces. The caring focus was finally reestablished with new goals and insights in the early 1980s.

Today, change continues at a rapid pace virtually everywhere in the world. Indeed, many global changes have occurred so rapidly and frequently in recent decades that their actual and potential impact on nursing is hard to realize. For example, in the past few years has come the fall of communism, which has led to mass migrations and emigrations of people from Eastern, Central, and Northern Europe. The Persian Gulf War had a major impact on cultural relationships among the members of the United Nations. The struggle of Africans in the Republic of South Africa has made nurses aware of intense cultural changes related to politics, religion, economics, social structure, and worldview. Major changes in South America, Southeast Asia, and other Third World regions have made nurses attentive to the many diverse and rapid cultural changes occurring worldwide and to how people are trying to cope with these changes or survive their effects. In addition to societal changes, there have been disastrous environmental events worldwide—floods, hurricanes, droughts, and fires caused by natural and human forces. In the aftermath of these disasters has come a realization of the demand for *human caring* knowledge, for the understandings and practices that are needed globally for the survival of the human race.

What are some of the specific factors that have led to the urgent need for global human care with a transcultural caring perspective? In recent years, the following factors have become evident worldwide:

1. Sudden collapse, and consequent changes, of several political, economic, and cultural structures and organizations of specific cultures and political geographic entities.

2. Marked increase in worldwide migrations and emigrations in the past decade, amid widespread cries for freedom, new opportunities, or political escape.

3. Increased global or worldwide illnesses such as acquired immune deficiency syndrome (AIDS), drug abuse, tuberculosis, malaria, and a host of sociocultural human conditions that will continue to change over time.

4. Increased intermingling of people from Western and non-Western worlds, often involving conflict of different cultural values, beliefs, and life-styles.

5. Increased cultural identity among people of different cultures, especially those whose cultural identities have been suppressed, devalued, or politically threatened.

6. Increased cultural and racial problems arising from marked differences in values and competition for limited resources.

7. Increased demand by cultural groups to be understood as human beings with rights rather than as "foreigners" or threatening strangers.

8. Increased numbers of clients from diverse cultures who enter health care institutions and agencies or seek home care services from professional staff.

9. Increased spiritual and religious explanations dealing with uncertainty, catastrophes, "horrible crimes," torture experiences, and major losses.

10. Increased consumer demands, especially from cultural minorities who have been "silent" or have received limited hearing or recognition in the past.

11. Increased demand for greater understanding of people from different cultures who speak different languages and may have unique human needs.

12. Increased women's rights and public leadership roles for women in Western and non-Western cultures, even when in conflict with traditional male leadership roles.

13. Increased incidents of cultural clashes, conflicts, and imposition practices and problems between staff and clients and among intercultural staff employees in service and educational settings.

14. Increased misdiagnoses and faulty assessments of clients in health services, because of cultural blindness, cultural ignorance, and cultural imposition practices by health personnel.

15. Increased consumer legal suits, in a context of intercultural conflicts, cultural negligence, and cultural imposition practices.

16. Increased global violence, occurring as a result of intercultural stresses and conflicts.

17. Increased demand for multicultural education in health education and service institutions, and a marked shift away from the largely unicultural focus of the past.

18. Global planning of health care proposals and practices in regional cultural areas, to facilitate cultural, economic, social, and political interests and marketing practices (for example, the European Unification Plan).

19. Increased cultural care health reforms and models, and greater use of qualitative research methods to establish epistemic and ontological data bases for diverse cultures. (Quantitative research methods are predicted to decrease in use during the 21st century.)

As one considers the above current and future cultural factors influencing transculturalism in health care worldwide, one must ask: What dominant concepts, theories, or modes of action will lead to the reduction of cultural conflicts and to peace and human survival? I contend that *human care is culturally constituted and maintained by people and institutions that will prove to be the most powerful and significant influence on people's well-being, health, and survival.* Furthermore, I believe that the world's nearly 5 million professional nurses can have a tremendous impact by providing leadership practices in the humanistic care of people from both diverse and similar cultures. Professional nurses who are knowledgeable of and sensitive to cultural differences and similarities can, by the year 2010, make a significant difference not only in nursing care practices, but in health maintenance, well-being ethos, world peace, and human survival. Nurses who use research-based culture care knowledge will have great impact on the quality of living and of service among people of diverse cultures. Improvement of that quality is the major goal of the future.

With these thoughts and predictions in mind, a brief overview of the major tenets of my theory of culture care is highlighted in the next section. I contend that this theory offers the most holistic and comprehensive means to achieve the above goals. The theory also will help nurses to understand the holistic components that hold (or fail to hold) cultures together, and the importance of worldview, social structure, and environmental context to cultural structures and practices. The reader is encouraged to study more fully the theory of culture care, the use of the ethnonursing research method, and the research findings from the theory, in order to appreciate its potential as an approach to global care. My definitive work, *Culture Care Diversity and Universality: A Theory of Nursing* (Leininger, 1991), will provide these insights.

OVERVIEW OF THE THEORY OF CULTURE CARE

Essentially, with the theory of culture care, I predicted that there would be *diverse and universal* features of human care transculturally—different structural care forms, meanings, expressions, beliefs, values, patterns, and practices related to human care, by people of different cultures and among nurses functioning in different health care systems and environmental contexts (Leininger, 1985, 1988a, 1988b, 1991). I contended that there would be some similarities or "universal" features in caring modalities, which would help nurses to see the humanistic commonalities in human care among many different cultures. Systematic and rigorous studies of human care and of caring meanings and expressions could establish a worldwide body of care knowledge to guide nursing practices and to legitimize nursing as a discipline and a profession. This was an exciting idea to me in the 1950s, when nursing had not yet explicated or systematically studied care phenomena and had not declared the essence and nature of the nursing phenomenon. Instead, nursing was depending on and functioning within a medical ethos, and medical cultural expectations were guiding nursing practices and education. It was clear to me that nursing could never be the same as medicine; it had to delineate its own unique or distinct nursing perspective: human care, with emphases on health and environmental context. Moreover, in those early days of the 1950s, there were formal or well-conceived nursing theories, and no research projects were focused on human care or caring. To me, care was what made nursing distinct and important in client recovery, health, or state of well-being. Indeed, I held tenaciously to the idea that *care is the essence of nursing or what will best characterize nursing from an epistemic and ontological disciplinary perspective* (Leininger, 1970, 1976a, 1978, 1984a, 1991). However, nurses needed to study care systematically and to interpret accurately the meaning and nature of care from peoples' *emic* (local) viewpoint and from nurses' *etic* (outsider) viewpoint. If these steps were achieved, then nurses could provide *the goal of the theory,* which was *culturally congruent nursing care* (Leininger, 1988a, 1988b, 1991).

I also theorized that *generic* (folk, indigenous, or naturalistic) care, the oldest form and expression of human care, had not been studied by nurses. This knowledge dimension was important in making human care meaningful to clients of particular cultures and in linking knowledge with professional care. *Professional nursing care,* as it was learned in nursing schools, provided some different knowledge that was often in sharp contrast with generic care. Bringing *generic* and *professional* care together was important, but it would require consideration of three modes of nursing actions or decisions based on research:

1. Culture care preservation and/or maintenance.
2. Culture care accommodation and/or negotiation.
3. Culture care repatterning and/or restructuring (Leininger, 1988a, 1988b, 1991).

I predicted that, when culture care research-based data were used by nurses, health and well-being among clients would occur. The nursing care would then make sense or would reasonably fit the clients' world, and congruent care would be provided to individuals, families, groups, or communities. Or, if culture care were in operation for dying clients, then culture care would be of great value because nurses would know how best to help them within the context of their values, beliefs, and expectations regarding death. Thus, the major purpose of the theory was to discover human care diversities and universalities in relation to the worldview, social structure, features, ethnohistory, environment, and generic professional care predicted to influence human care and, ultimately, the health or well-being of clients. The goal of the theory was to improve or to establish anew culturally congruent nursing care, which was not being cognitively practiced in most nursing services. The goal was allied with the desire to establish transcultural nursing and formed the future arching framework for all nursing education and service arenas. Transcultural nursing knowledge was desperately needed by

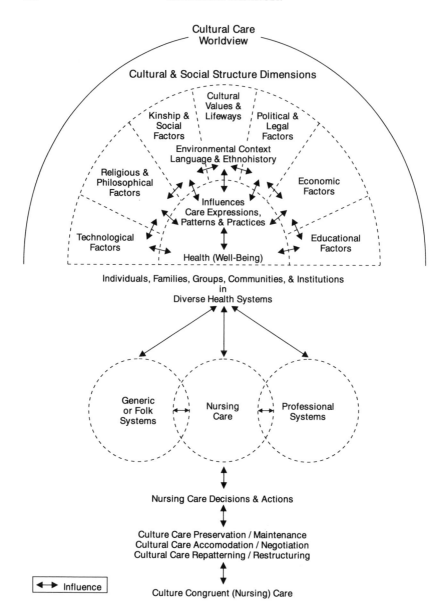

From *Culture Care Diversity and Universality: A Theory for Nursing* by M. Leininger, 1991. New York: National League for Nursing. Reprinted by permission.

Figure 1–1
Leininger's Sunrise Model: The Theory of Culture Care
Diversity and Universality

individual nurses and by the entire discipline of nursing, as a guide for giving quality nursing care now and in the future.

To help nurse theorists conceptualize the important dimensions and the tenets of my theory on the discovery of care, I developed the Sunrise Model (see Figure 1–1). This model has become well-known to many nurses over the past three decades and has been used not only for theoretical applications but also for cultural and holistic nursing care assessments for clients, families, groups, communities, and institutions. The Sunrise Model is like a cognitive map to depict the worldview and social structure (including religion, kinship, political–legal–cultural values, economics, education, and technology) as influencers of human care expressions, and the patterns for the health or well-being of people. The environmental context, language, and ethnohistory were considered very important factors to identify human care needs, patterns, and practices in relation to individuals, families, groups, communities, and institutions. The lower part of the Sunrise Model helps nurses to focus on the generic and professional health practices in relation to nursing. The information gleaned through the ethnonursing research method is valuable for this process as well as for the three modes of nursing care decisions and actions that provide *cultural congruent nursing care* (Leininger, 1991).

Culture Care theory, with the Sunrise Model used as a cognitive map, can guide the nurse researcher toward in-depth knowledge of the cultural diversities and universalities that are relevant to care values. The theory is sufficiently broad to identify the different factors and forces influencing human care, and it emphasizes the use of inductive ethnonursing qualitative methods. When using the theory, the nurse researcher looks for embedded meanings about care, seeks interpretations and explanations about human care and health ways, and, most importantly, remains a learner, gathering information from and confirming findings with the people receiving the care. The nurse researcher must also be ready to discover unknown care aspects that may be difficult for nurses to understand. Much can be learned about human care and ways to promote and maintain wellness through use of the culture care theory.

CARE MEANINGS AND ACTION MODES: COMPARISON OF TWO CULTURES

Although a wealth of in-depth information is obtained from studying individuals and groups within a particular culture, a glimpse of two major cultures in the United States—the Anglo-American middle class, and African Americans—provides an example of culture care expressions, values, and patterns. From my ethnonursing qualitative study of 40 key and 65 general informants over the past decade, the culture care meanings and action modes given below were confirmed and made credible from the Anglo-Americans. The informants identified the following care means and their related action modes (Leininger, 1991, p. 355):

1. To provide *stress alleviation* measures, largely through physical and psychological means.
2. To provide *personalized acts* such as doing special things and giving attention to individuals.
3. To rely on *self-care* modes rather than care by others, in order to become independent and self-reliant.
4. To obtain from health personnel *health instruction and medical facts* that allow expanded self-care.

The italicized words (the major care constructs of the informants) are important to guide nurses' thinking and actions. There were some cultural variations among Anglo-Americans, but these were the dominant themes, patterns, and practices that prevailed over a considerable time span (more than a decade) and are still clearly evident today.

The African American informants (35 key and 60 general) had different meanings and action modes about human caring. They viewed care and caring as follows (Leininger, 1991, p. 357):

1. To show *concern for* "my brothers and sisters" at all times.
2. To demonstrate ways to *be involved with* family members.
3. To give *physical presence* when someone is ill or "under the weather."
4. To give *family support* and maintain family "get-togethers."
5. To use *touching* appropriately and frequently, when well or sick.
6. To rely on *folk home remedies* to communicate caring and to restore health.
7. To rely on "*Jesus to save us*," especially through use of prayers and songs.

Cultural variability among African Americans was observed and spoken about, but these dominant care themes, representing values, patterns, and practices, were clearly evident over a 10-year time span and are still extant today.

These culture care findings, and others from 54 Western and non-Western cultures, are providing new nursing care knowledge that is different from the past medical symptom–disease–treatment focus of nursing practice. These new domains will provide important dimensions for shifting to nursing care practices. They will guide nursing actions and decisions and will become perfected over time. Medical, social, and other knowledge will be used in relation to these major care constructs for the health and well-being of nursing clients.

From almost a lifetime of studying human care in different cultures, I have found that the following statements can be made:

1. There is very rich, meaningful, and still largely universal *emic* information about human care to be gained from cultures.

2. Human care is globally diverse but can be identified as specific to individuals, families, groups, communities, and institutions of a culture.

3. Human care phenomena tend to be imbedded in the worldview, language, social structure, and environmental context of a culture, and discovering them and confirming them with people takes time.

4. Transcultural human care expressions, meanings, and practices tend, worldwide, to be more diverse than universal; nurses must therefore be prepared to deal with diversities.

5. A few human care constructs and expressions exist universally, but they are less frequent than anticipated.

6. Care expressions and patterns can and do contribute significantly to the well-being, health, and recovery of humans, if the knowledge and skills of health providers are evident.

7. The significant knowledge gap that still remains between generic and professional care must be reduced, to achieve congruent care practices.

These statements, which confirm the importance of the theory of culture care over the past three decades, have been endorsed by a number of transcultural nurse researchers (Bodnar & Leininger, 1992; Gates, 1991; Leininger, 1981, 1984b, 1988c, 1991; Luna, 1989; Morgan, 1992; Wenger, 1991), and others.

CONCLUSION

Human care and caring must be conceptualized, studied, and practiced with a transcultural global perspective because they are inextricably and tightly woven together in all cultures. Until recent decades, human care was not systematically and rigorously studied. Caring was vaguely covert and unknown but was still valued linguistically. Now, most care reseachers are beginning to join transcultural nurses, to discover care phenomena. Care, as the essence of nursing and as a central and major domain of nursing knowledge and practice, offers the greatest hope for establishing nursing's distinct discipline and professional contributions to humankind. Much research work lies ahead; there are many cultures and subcultures to be studied indepth. *Emic* and *etic* cultural knowledge is essential to guide nurses in the care they give to clients, but reflections and awareness of cultural variabilities must always be present. Comparative care knowledge and practices from many different cultures are essential if nursing is to gain new insights and a deep appreciation that human care worldwide cannot be viewed as "all alike." Instead, as comparative care knowledge becomes disseminated, nurses will understand more fully why and how societal and worldwide changes influence cultural care diversities and universalities among human groups. The explication of human care in different environmental contexts and from a global transcultural nursing care perspective will remain a future and major focus of all nurses but especially of care researchers. We can expect that other health disciplines will become interested in the use of nursings' research findings as new health care reforms and practices are initiated in the 21st century. The future looks most promising for nurses: they may discover the unknown secrets about human care, but they must also be well-grounded in anthropology if they wish to grasp the world of clients and the nursing culture. As nurses value and study human care with commitment, they will see the full power of care and its tremendously rich and varied ways to serve humanity, which is the real goal and purpose of nursing.

REFERENCES

Aamodt, A. M. (1978). Socio-cultural dimensions of caring in the world of the Papago child and adolescent. In M. Leininger (Ed.), *Transcultural nursing: Concepts, theories, and practices.* New York: Wiley.

Ashley, J. (1976). *Hospital paternalism and the role of the nurse.* New York: Teachers' College Press.

Bodnar, A., & Leininger, M. (1992). Transcultural nursing care values, beliefs, and practices of American (USA) Gypsies. *Journal of Transcultural Nursing, 4*(1), 17–28.

Boyle, J., & Andrews, M. (1989). *Transcultural concepts in nursing care.* Boston: Scott, Foresman/Little, Brown.

Gates, M. (1991). Transcultural comparison of hospital and hospice as caring environments for dying patients. *Journal of Transcultural Nursing, 2* (2), 3–15.

Gaut, D. (1981). Conceptual analysis of caring. In M. Leininger (Ed.), *Caring: An essential human need* (pp. 17–24). Detroit: Wayne State University Press.

Horn, B. (1978). Transcultural nursing and childbearing of the Muckleshoot people. In M. Leininger (Ed.), *Transcultural nursing: Concepts, theories, and practice* (pp. 223–238). New York: Wiley.

Leininger, M. (1965). *Culture care as a central theoretical concept in the discipline and professional of nursing.* Unpublished manuscript, University of Colorado, Denver.

Leininger, M. (1967). The culture concept and its relevance to nursing. *Journal of Nursing Education, 6*(2), 27–39.

Leininger, M. (1970). The culture concept and American culture values in nursing. In *Nursing and anthropology: Two worlds to blend* (pp. 45–52). New York: Wiley.

Leininger, M. (1976a). Caring: The essence and central focus of nursing. *Nursing Research Report, 12*(1), 2, 14.

Leininger, M. (1976b). Towards conceptualization of a transcultural health care system: Concepts and a model. In M. Leininger (Ed.), *Transcultural health care issues and conditions* (pp. 3–22). Philadelphia: Davis.

Leininger, M. (1977). The phenomenon of caring: Caring—the essence and central focus of nursing. *Nursing Research Report, 12*(1), 2–14.

Leininger, M. (1978). *Transcultural nursing: Concepts, theories, and practices.* New York: Wiley.

Leininger, M. (1980). Care: A central focus of nursing and health care services. *Nursing and Health Care, 1*(3), 135–143.

Leininger, M. (1981). *Care: An essential human need.* Thorofare, NJ: Slack.

Leininger, M. (1983). Cultural care: An essential goal for nursing and health care. *Journal of the American Association of Nephrology Nurses and Technicians, 10*(5), 11–17.

Leininger, M. (1984a). *Care: The essence of nursing and health.* Detroit: Wayne State University Press.

Leininger, M. (1984b). Transcultural nursing: An essential knowledge and practice field for today. *The Canadian Nurse, 41*–45.

Leininger, M. (1985). Transcultural care diversity and universality: A theory of nursing. *Nursing and Health Care,* 6(4), 209–212.

Leininger, M. (1987). *Care: Discovery and uses in clinical and community nursing* (pp. 1–30). Detroit: Wayne State University Press.

Leininger, M. (1988a). *Care: The essence of nursing and health.* Detroit: Wayne State University Press.

Leininger, M. (1988b). *Care: An essential human need.* Detroit: Wayne State University Press.

Leininger, M. (1988c). Leininger's theory of nursing: Cultural care diversity and universality. *Nursing Science Quarterly,* 2(4), 11–20.

Leininger, M. (1989). Transcultural nursing: A worldwide necessity to advance nursing knowledge and practice. In J. McCloskey & H. Grace (Eds.), *Nursing issues.* Boston: Little, Brown.

Leininger, M. (1991). *Culture care diversity and universality: A theory of nursing.* New York: National League for Nursing.

Luna, L. (1989). Transcultural nursing care of Arab Muslims. *Journal of Transcultural Nursing,* 1(1), 22–27.

Morgan, M. (1992). Pregnancy and childbirth beliefs and practices of American Hare Krishna devotees within transcultural nursing. *Journal of Transcultural Nursing,* 4(1).

Ray, M. (1981). Philosophical analysis of caring. In M. Leininger (Ed.), *Caring: An essential human need* (pp. 25–36). Thorofare, NJ: Slack.

Roach, S. (1987). *The human act of caring.* Ottawa: Canadian Hospital Association.

Valentine, K. (1985). Advancing care and ethics in health management: An evaluation strategy. In M. Leininger (Ed.), *Care: Discovery and uses in clinical and community nursing.* Detroit: Wayne State University, 151–169.

Watson, J. (1985). *Nursing: Human science and human care: A theory of nursing.* Norwalk, CT: Appleton-Century-Crofts.

Wenger, A. F. (1991). The culture care theory and the Old Order Amish. In M. Leininger (Ed.), *Culture care diversity and universality: A theory of nursing* (pp. 147–178). New York: National League for Nursing.

2

Transcultural Human Care: Its Challenge to and Critique of Professional Nursing Care

Olga Kanitsaki

$\boldsymbol{M}$ainstream professional nursing, as we know it, is about caring for human beings and responding professionally to their health needs. All nurses are expected to know about care and to use care in their practice. However, until recent years, human care per se and its relationship to professional nursing were not systematically investigated by nurses or considered central to or part of nursing education (Leininger, 1984, 1988, 1990). Professional nurses generally assume that all nurses know and understand the essence, nature, expression, and function of care and caring. There is, however, emerging evidence to suggest that, although human care is a universal concept, its nature, content, expression, and practices are not shared by people cross-culturally (transculturally) (Boyle & Andrews, 1989; Giger & Davidhizar, 1991; Kanitsaki, 1983, 1988, 1989; Leininger, 1984, 1988, 1990; Rosenbaum, 1990).

Human care (in particular, transcultural human care) differs significantly from mainstream professional nursing care in that transcultural human care recognizes that health and care (what they are, how they are expressed), health and care needs (and how they are met), perceptions of care and healing, and health and care knowledge and practices (1) are all culturally constructed and (2) are mediated, negotiated, prioritized, and experienced in culturally specific ways (Leininger, 1984, 1988). In short, knowledge of human care and of health and care needs is embedded in culture and takes culture as the key to understanding and to transcultural identification of people's health and care needs.

Professional nursing and its knowledge base have evolved primarily from beliefs, common sense, intuition, and past experiences, and have developed into rules (Gortner, 1980) and practices that reflect a newly formed, composite culture base. This culture base is not shared transculturally. It is dominated by Anglo-American professional nursing culture, and by characteristic Anglo-Australian human care values, beliefs, and practices (Boyle & Andrews, 1989; Giger & Davidhizar, 1991; Kanitsaki, 1983, 1988; Lawler, 1991; Leininger, 1970, 1988, 1990). This essential recognition and difference—the primacy of culture in human care and care practice—not only distinguishes transcultural human care from professional nursing, but also enables it to challenge and critique mainstream nursing as it is constructed and practiced in countries where models of health care are influenced by dominant Anglo-American cultural values.

This chapter presents the results of a qualitative exploratory research study in which I investigated the health–illness–suffering and care experiences of a sample of "Greek-born" members of twelve Greek-Australian families living in Melbourne (Kanitsaki, 1989). These results will be discussed in order to demonstrate:

1. The critical role that transcultural human care research can and must play in the construction and development of professional nursing knowledge and of practice that is responsive to the health and care needs of people of different cultures.

2. The critical importance of transcultural human care as a means of informing and critiquing mainstream professional nursing and challenging it to be relevant and effective in meeting the health and care needs of the culturally diverse populations it serves.

IDENTIFYING HUMAN REALITIES POSED BY CULTURAL DIVERSITY IN HUMAN CARE

Research Method

Grounded theory was chosen as the most appropriate research method for *discovering* the health–illness perceptions, expectations, and lived experiences of the Greek-born families. These families were interacting in Australia's dynamic, multicultural, modern, and technological society—specifically, in Melbourne's sociocultural context.

A primary aim of this study was to discover the meaning, significance, and logic that they gave to their health–illness experiences. Grounded theory's procedures are systematic, but they allow for flexibility and creativity, and they give recognition to the value and power of theoretical sensitivity in building theory. The acceptability of theoretical sensitivity allowed me to use my rich, multidimensional experience as a Greek-born immigrant, transcultural nurse, and member of several ethnic communities. This combination of multidimensional experience and theoretical knowledge gave me insights into the human and social phenomena under investigation that otherwise might have been missed. I found the effect very liberating and facilitative: it aided the development of generative questions and propositions, it guided theoretical sampling, and it enhanced insight for deep data analysis and formulation of abstractions grounded in the data (Glaser, 1978; Strauss, 1987; Strauss & Corbin, 1990).

Because of the complexity, variability, and multidimensionality of the health–illness phenomena and lived experiences of these Greek-born people living within a multicultural society, I felt that this qualitative method could achieve the interactive investigation and abstraction needed. For instance, I found this method most appropriate in examining the logic and meanings they applied to their health–illness perceptions, and the strategies they used to fulfill their health and care needs. In addition, this method allowed discovery of the meaning the families gave to the events that occurred while they were interacting within a dominant Anglo-Australian/American-Australian society, as well as within a patriarchal and biomedicine-dominated health care system.

Sample and Sampling Techniques

The only unchanging and basic criteria for including informants in this study were:

1. The mother and father in the families had to have been born in Greece.

2. The family had to include at least one member who perceived that he or she was sick, and that person had to volunteer to participate in the study.

As data were collected and the first two interviews were transcribed and open-coded, generative questions and propositions led to theoretical sampling. The sampling brought about the inclusion of informants with the following variable characteristics:

1. They had been in Australia for differing lengths of time.

2. They had different medical conditions.

3. They had received medical and/or nursing care in different institutions, community medical facilities, and/or local clinics.

4. They had received care in different sections of the same institution—the emergency room, outpatient department, general ward, intensive care, and so on.

5. They represented various life situations: employed (in a variety of occupations) or unemployed; male or female; divorced or widowed; their children lived at home or their children had left home.

6. They were born in different places in Greece.

7. They had originated from both rural Greece (eleven families) and urban Greece (one family).

8. They had different levels of education (the range was from 2 years in primary school to achievement of a high school certificate).

It is important to reiterate that this study commenced without any preset questions or hypotheses. Theoretical sampling was used to check the emerging theoretical abstractions and framework, not to verify any preconceived hypotheses. Continually, comparisons were made during coding of the data and in the field. As a result, generative questions were raised from the data and, while in the field, I was able to check the relevance and fit of the emerging categories and their relationships. Emerging codes, questions, and propositions were used as conceptual guides as to where to go next to collect data for comparison—which group, subgroup, person, conditions, events, settings, and so on.

I was also very aware of the barriers that my own theoretical sensitivity might have posed for my research. Consequently, I developed and continuously used, during the 7 months of my research project, a process that I called "cognitive surveillance" (Kanitsaki, 1989). Cognitive surveillance enabled me to maintain a balance between the benefits and risks of theoretical sensitivity. Cognitive surveillance can be best described as a continual and acute awareness of possible conceptual barriers. I attempted to overcome it by introspection, reflexivity, and actual checking of all abstractions derived from the data; other Greek community members were peripheral to the research. For example, in addition to theoretical sampling, during the data collection from the informants and the data analysis, I was giving educational seminars on health to diverse groups of Greek-born people. I continued to check and compare emerging conceptual categories and their indicators with these groups, as well as with my family and Greek-born friends.

Access to the informants was gained by using a network sample method. Before I actually commenced the data collection and analysis process, I informed the Greek community in Melbourne, via the ethnic radio, of my intentions to undertake such a research study. Subsequently, access to the informants was through two general channels: ethnic radio, and Greek-Australian and Anglo-Australian friends and acquaintances. Twelve families were accessed and interviewed over a period of 5 months. Interviews were unstructured and were guided by generative questions and emerging propositions. These were utilized to collect dense data and verify ideas and theoretical abstractions in regard to the lived experiences of Greek-born families' health–illness conditions, dimensions, circumstances, strategies for interaction, and consequences of interaction with the health care system. Substantial field notes were compiled.

Each interview took place in a family's own home and was taped with the permission of the informants. Informed consent was verbally obtained. Seeking written consent was, I felt, an unpleasant demonstration of lack of trust between the informants and myself. I had tested the idea by mentioning to some families the desirability of obtaining a signed consent form, but soon abandoned that approach. The pursuit of a written consent was having negative effects, and I needed to promote a warm and trusting relationship between myself and the families concerned. Signing documents was considered unnecessary and suspect by the families—a signal of mistrust. In the

Greek cultural context, trust and warmth were most important to facilitate the free flow and dense collection of meaningful data.

The interviews ranged between 3.5 and 5.5 hours. During the interviews, family members and friends would flow in and out in the interview context and would continue their daily activities in my presence. They would participate, share their similar experiences, argue, clarify points of contention between family and friends, and share cups of Greek coffee, sweets, and, in a number of cases, lunch and/or dinner. Interviews took place at all hours of the day and often lasted until 11:30 P.M.

I obtained verbal permission to collectively publish the results of the study. Strict confidentiality and privacy regarding the informants' identity were promised. I have maintained their anonymity by not revealing any information that could lead to their identification.

Data Analysis

Data collection and data analysis were done simultaneously. The procedure used was nonlinear but rather circular or spiral in nature. During the processes of open, axial, and selective coding, the emerging and emerged abstractions, the categories and their indicators, and the relationships formed were always firmly grounded on the data.

Systematically, data were analyzed sentence-by-sentence in open coding. Codes were developed as they emerged from the data; common and contrasting categories and conceptual indictors were represented. Memos were written, and generative questions, propositions, and conceptual abstractions continued to guide theoretical sampling in a multidimensional way. The process of grounding theory from data collection to finished writing is composed of a set of double-back steps; as one moves forward, one goes back to previous steps (Strauss, 1987). The process is not linear. As Strauss explained: "[T]hrough comparing the data as they were collected [as I was] creating more abstract levels of theoretical connections, theory was gradually built up inductively from the progressive stages of analysis of the data" (p. 39).

The focus was on organizing ideas that emerged from the open coding of data. Abstracted codes and ideas were constantly compared and grouped into categories; saturation was aimed for and was achieved by dense data collection under variable conditions and circumstances. Constant comparison, during analysis, was undertaken among codes, ideational indicators, and categories. As the categories inductively emerged, they were deduced, modified, and differentiated into higher-order categories. Core categories were then further compared with their ideational indicators by building their relationships around the axis of each category. After additional comparisons between categories, dense memoing, and further saturation, these categories were further deduced, and substantive theories were developed. These substantive theories were health, care, protection, and suffering, which, as Strauss (1987) explained, "became automatically a springboard or stepping stone to the development of a grounded formal theory" (p. 79). Ultimately, a grounded theory was conceptualized and deduced by further comparisons and memoing within and between substantive theories.

As noted earlier, data collection and analysis were circular or spiral in nature. As I was moving forward multidirectionally, I was repeatedly going back to previous multidirectional steps in a comparative manner. By using grounded theory as an inductive and deductive process, ultimately a theory was built that was grounded in the data.

UNDERSTANDING THE CULTURAL CONSTRUCTION OF CARE AND CARING: A GREEK EXAMPLE

During analysis of the data, eight structural characteristic cultural categories emerged and were saturated. Subsequently, when these categories and their indicators were compared and contrasted, they were further abstracted to a higher level. Four substantive theories emerged from the data: health, protection, care, and suffering. Further comparative analysis led me to abstract a grounded theory, which I named Familial Cultural Advocacy Theory.

The eight structural characteristic cultural categories, with their particular cultural indicators, supported the four substantive theories. One of those theories, care, is the focus of this chapter.

The eight structural characteristic cultural categories that emerged and were abstracted from the data were: Family (*Oikogenia*), Psychological (*Psychologia*), Ethical/Moral (*Ithiki*), Cognitive (*Gnosis*), Body (*Soma*), Social (*Koinonia*), Economic (*Oikonomia*), and Religious/Spiritual (*Thriskia*). (See Figure 2–1.)

Each of these categories formed a "characteristic formulated value system" that was intricate, complex, and interconnected with the others. The achievement, balance, and maintenance of the value systems were reflective of and influenced by the life goals that the informants were striving for in Australia. The achievement and maintenance of these goals were perceived by the informants and their families as leading to happiness, vitality, and

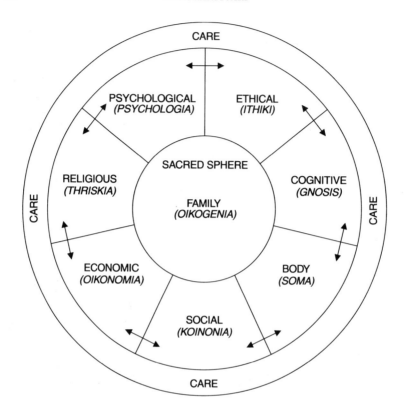

Figure 2–1
Cultural Value Categories of Twelve Greek Families: Life Goals

joy. In turn, happiness, vitality, and joy were perceived as constituting "health," a high-value "treasure" (*thisavros*) as well as an ideal for which to strive. Consequently, care was seen as a lifelong process that is essential for safeguarding and promoting individual and family health.

Significantly, my informants' concepts and definitions of family were closely tied to their notions of health (happiness, vitality, and joy). However, the *achievement of the family's life goals* was what gave rise to happiness, vitality, and joy (Figure 2–2). Thus, the achievement of health was inextricably linked to the families' constant struggle to achieve family life goals, within the sometimes hostile Australian sociocultural context. A failure to achieve

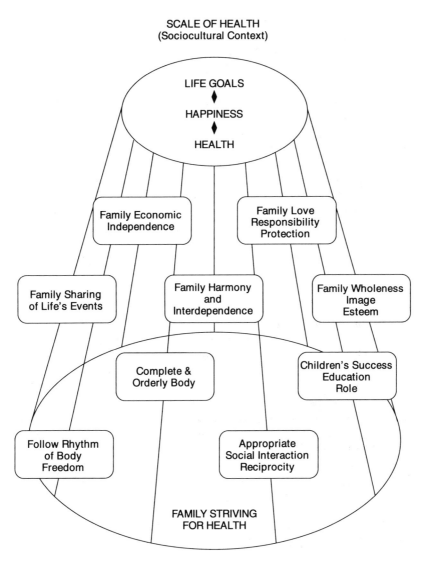

SCALE OF HEALTH
(Sociocultural Context)

LIFE GOALS
♦
HAPPINESS
♦
HEALTH

Family Economic
Independence

Family Love
Responsibility
Protection

Family Sharing
of Life's Events

Family Harmony
and
Interdependence

Family Wholeness
Image
Esteem

Complete &
Orderly Body

Children's Success
Education
Role

Follow Rhythm
of Body
Freedom

Appropriate
Social Interaction
Reciprocity

FAMILY STRIVING
FOR HEALTH

Figure 2–2
Families' Perception of Health

those goals invariably resulted in a failure to achieve health. Some life goals were more important than others, and the most important goal was the maintenance of a unified and harmonious family.

The importance and centrality of *family* in Greek culture emerged as a dominant theme in the study. This theme is also reflected in the research findings of Rosenbaum (1990). Authors such as Storer (1985), Moraitis (1972), Bottomley (1976), Mead (1955), Isaacs (1976), Kanitsaki (1989), and Piperoglou (1988) have also articulated the centrality of family in Greek culture generally.

Analysis of the research data revealed that every member of a Greek family was considered a part of the family whole, not an independent individual; the family's individuality and independence were paramount. Further analysis indicated that my informants valued the freedom and independence of the *family unit* above those of the individual. Within the family sphere, *interdependence* was cultivated and expected, not *individual independence*. (See also Mead, 1955, pp. 73–76.) Even though individual independence in the public sphere (outside the family) was seen as critical and was encouraged and promoted, individuality and personhood remained inextricably linked with the identity of the family as a whole.

Within the family unit, all activities were expected to be shared, and social events were experienced communally. A problem was regarded as the family's problem, not just the individual's. Duties, rights, and obligations were finely balanced and interlocked within the family network. My informants trusted members of their own families, friends, and persons connected through religious relationships. This overriding view emerged: "One trusts those one knows, those whose worth has been tested." Further, there was an expectation that care and assistance would be provided to family members as needed and without being requested. This was a well-established fact of life that had been enculturated in each family member.

Other consistent and interrelated cultural family patterns that emerged from the study and are relevant to this discussion are summarized as follows:

1. Maintenance of group wholeness so that the needs of individuals in the group could be fulfilled for the maximum happiness of the whole.

2. Avoidance of harm to the individual and thus to the group (active prevention of harm, and maximization of happiness, vitality, and joy, identified as health).

All families except one indicated that this particular value system was under threat within the Australian context, and the threat was causing them to have concerns about their own and their children's health. It was evident that their Australian-born children had a different concept of individuality and wished to experience events *alone* and not within a family unit. The children tried to persuade their parents that acting independently of the family did not mean they loved or respected their parents less, but the children's view caused consternation to the parents/families involved.

The families expressed the view that, whatever the strengths and weaknesses of the individual within the family, these were only to be known intimately by the family and remained the concern of the whole family. Whenever the family was threatened (for example, by the acts, behavior, or health status of a member/part of the family group), intricate and interdependent family decision making and action taking became paramount. Here, protection of the individual and/or family became the main concern and was seen as crucial to preventing possible harm to the family and to enhancing the happiness (health) of the family and its individual members.

The more *vulnerable* a member of the family was, or was perceived to be, the more the family would try to assist and protect that person. This response was motivated by love, which was perceived to be the ultimate arbiter of justice among the family members.

Given the meaning and significance of the family within Greek culture, and the great emphasis that is given to interdependence, the principle of *autonomy* in the individualized sense was considered not only of little priority, but quite inappropriate within the family sphere. In fact, claims of autonomy, when expressed without any due consideration for other members of the family, were regarded as insulting to human dignity as well as a cause for shame. In this context, shame was engendered because a claim of autonomy by an individual family member was interpreted as a diminution of love of family and a failure to fulfill responsibilities to the family and to the broader social group of which the family was a part. Claims of autonomy and individuality, as they are understood in Australia and in the nursing profession, were perceived by my informants as the most dangerous and disruptive forces within the finely webbed, interdependent, and balanced structure of their Greek-born families.

Cultural Creation of the Sacred Family Sphere

Significantly, care was perceived by informants as a loving and intense interpersonal life process, an interest in and involvement with other family members, and a lifelong, multidimensional, individual and family caring process aimed at preventing illness and promoting individual members' as well as the family's health. These aims were achieved by a caring process, maintained by all members of the family, that was believed to enhance the achievement of individual and family goals as constructed within their cultural context. All informants believed (with intense emotion) that family care and caring processes were creating and maintaining a "sacred sphere" that reflected "God's family," a sphere in which life chances were promoted and protection from the public/profane sphere was ensured. The family's sacred sphere was seen as safe, meaningful, all-inclusive, and characterized by constant watchfulness of other family members' happiness and health. The sphere was active and intersubjective, and was protected by love. Family members saw the caring sphere as being filled with activities that signified and were symbolic of their love, interest, concern, commitment, and loyalty to each other. This sphere was enhanced within the home by religious acts and icons.

Cultural Creation of the Public of Profane Sphere

The public or profane sphere (of which professional care was seen as a part) was perceived as being dangerous, risky, untrustworthy, deceitful, uncaring, and controlled more by evil than good. Individuals who had no sacred sphere of family to shelter and protect them were considered extremely vulnerable; they were facing many risks that could place them and their goals in danger. Informants saw care as a way of life, an individual and family process that was utilized constantly and was aimed at influencing and enhancing their life chances and health within an Australian context.

The intensity with which care and caring actions were expressed and activated depended on individual family members and their families' perceptions of the "normality" of their daily lives, and on the progress they made toward achieving their life goals. Other factors were family members' perceptions of potential dangers or risks to their life goals within the public sphere—failure in education, failure at work, overwork, assaults to their self-image and self-esteem, or failure in finding an "appropriate" partner for marriage.

Differences in intensity of care and caring behaviors between parents and children were noted. They seemed to depend on whether the family members in question were Greek- or Australian-born, and on whether there had been an attenuation of Greek family value systems by Anglo-Australian values. For instance, Greek-born parents of Australian-born children differed slightly in their perceptions of what changes had occurred in their "normal" life-styles and what threats to the family unit existed. Life events perceived as having the potential to obstruct the achievement of life goals by either an individual and/or the family would activate more intense caring processes than those utilized on a daily basis. For example, a major factor commonly considered by informants as a threat to their health was individual family members' exhibition of excessive individualistic tendencies. Such an exhibition was perceived as having the potential to estrange individual family members (e.g., Australian-born children) from their families (Greek-born parents, uncles, aunts, cousins, and so on) and to remove them from the sacred sphere of the family. They would then be placed firmly in the public sphere, where there were more dangers and risks. Further, the family unit was threatened: its bonds of love and unity were diminished or severed, and family responsibilities and obligations were undermined. Anticipated loss of traditional family value systems engendered powerful caring actions, to prevent further harm. Other factors commonly considered by Greek-born informants as threatening their health and as engendering caring actions included:

- Eating too frequently outside the home.
- Not dressing warmly or attractively.
- Experiencing lowered vitality, overwork, or loss of weight.
- Exhibiting disinterest or mood changes; going to bed too early; sleeping in; and frequently staying out late at night.
- Not mixing with people, or not sharing events with the family.
- Mixing with friends whom the family judged as inappropriate.
- Neglecting education and/or avoiding work.
- Indulging in personal regimentation and not being able to follow body rhythms—for example, going to sleep or resting "when I feel like it."
- Showing tendencies toward illegal behaviors and sexual promiscuity.
- Indicating changes in attitude toward family moral values of respect, responsibility, obligations, and duties.
- Evidencing changed attitudes and increased disrespect toward parents and other family members.
- Deviating from religious beliefs and practices.

Indicators of potential health risks such as those given above would always be sensed and identified by family members, and necessary action would be taken to protect the person exhibiting the health-threatening behaviors. Care had many faces and could be expressed multidimensionally and in varying intensity.

CARE (*PHRONDIDA*):
DOMAINS AND MEANINGS

Care of immediate family (*Oikogenia*), other family members, and friends or social acquaintances was perceived as differing in terms of intensity, extent of expression, and action (*praxis*), as well as in regard to *care-motivating forces*. Care by all families was perceived and described as a lived reality, not as an ideal. Care was expected to be transformed into action. It was perceived as a part of life born out of love (*agape*), and it carried a "natural" obligation of reciprocity arising out of deep and meaningful interpersonal and filial relationships. The nature and meaning of care were expressed and constructed in the following terms (Figure 2–3):

1. Intense interest (*enthiaferon*), sensitivity (*evesthesia*), and action (*praxis*), with regular individual and family multidimensional activities that promoted the individual's and family's life goals and thus contributed toward the achievement of health.

2. Constant intense involvement, with each person finely tuned cognitively and emotionally to anticipate the needs and hopes of the others. An essential characteristic is physical presence—sharing and participating in events such as meals, births, baptisms, marriages, dances, visits, illnesses, funerals, and religious and cultural traditions.

3. Sharing, sensing, anticipating, and identifying threats—individual and/or family fears and weaknesses that endanger life goals and health. The aim here is early detection of threats in order to initiate specific caring actions that will protect the individual and family.

4. Expecting that each individual will perceive dangers, will warn family members of potential problems, and will take protective actions in order to support and promote the life goals of persons within the family network.

5. Standing close by and hovering—observing intensely, collecting information, creating meaning, and discussing the significance of initial indications of a change in an individual's and/or family's behavior that signals a health problem; giving advice (e.g., on self-care), support, and encouragement to family members perceived as being vulnerable.

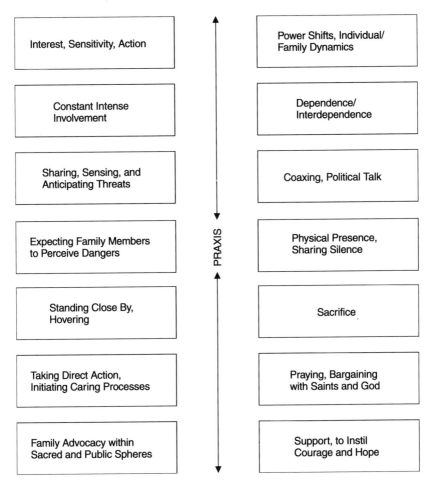

Figure 2–3
Human Care Constructs Emerging from Twelve Greek-Born
Families Living in Melbourne

6. Taking direct action (*praxis*) within the family network—
eliciting and creating appropriate protective, enhancing, and/or
creative caring processes and activities, in order to protect against
the potential loss of individual and/or family goals and thus promote health.

7. Family advocacy, mediation, and action, within both the sacred and public family spheres in "critical" life situations, in order to negotiate and realize the fulfillment of a family member's or the entire family's needs.

8. Power shifts in family/individual dynamics, which involve observing and standing by the ill person and encouraging self-care within the protection of the family unit. The family as a whole is independent of and more powerful than the individual. However, should the family member become more vulnerable to illness, the care activities become more intense, more united, and more directed. When a family member succumbs to illness, family dynamics change; whereas the family previously was more powerful and more independent than the individual, the sick person becomes more powerful and more dependent. The family becomes subordinate to her or his wishes. The more critically ill the person is, the more powerless the family becomes in relation to the individual. His or her wishes and demands, as well as the illness experiences, become embodied in all family members.

9. Acceptance of dependence and interdependence—because human beings who love are interconnected, dependence and interdependence are acceptable and understood.

10. Coaxing (*politiki*), a particular way of persuading a person to do things that are for her or his benefit, by being encouraging and supportive in a meaningful way. During illness states, this particular care construct is constantly and skillfully utilized.

11. Physical presence (*paravriscome, parousia*), a sharing of silence and of the intersubjective unspoken, embodied love, interest, pain, and concern that radiate from and embrace all persons involved. Presence creates a context of meaning related to the past, the present, and the anticipated future. Metaphorically and symbolically, the past, present, and anticipated future meet concurrently at a still moment in time.

12. Sacrifice (*thisia*), which, if needed, might be made to the extent that all other family members may suffer poverty, exhaustion, and hardship for the sake of one member. Often, "extraordinary" actions are taken in order to assist an ill family member; for example, a home may be sold to finance a trip to seek medical assistance in another country where the family believes a cure may be found, or visits may be made to sacred places to petition saints believed to be healers. In my study, two families had visited Eastern European

countries seeking help for a family member from doctors and at churches.

13. Praying, requesting, and bargaining (*tasimo*): for spiritual assistance in healing the family member.

14. Support, hope, courage, and future possibilities, when an illness is considered ominous or life-threatening and calls for culture-specific human courage and hope-instilling behaviors. These responses are to ensure that the person feels strongly interconnected and central to the family's life. Examples include giving to the ill member meaningful, encouraging, and hope-engendering words or information, and/or withholding a poor prognosis; avoiding words or acts that inspire fear, anxiety, or desperation; evading questions asked about impending death; creating hope and courage by describing how the family needs the person, how critical he or she is to the family's happiness and meaning of life, and how happy times together can lie ahead.

Metaphorically speaking, all members of the family share, in body, mind, and soul, the illness experiences of their family member. Care within the family and the home sphere is intensified and continuous, and involves physical presence and immediate response to the care needs of the family member. The sick person would not be confined to bed unless seriously ill, and family members become extremely alarmed. Care intensifies, independence and self-care are discouraged, and the family member is accepted as physically dependent, vulnerable, lacking in strength, and deserving of all family members' and the community's attention.

The sick person's vulnerability becomes a powerful force that controls the family's behaviors. For example, the person is most likely to follow body rhythms: if feeling nauseated, he or she may desire to avoid food. The family, however, may try to persuade the person to eat or to do other things that he or she may not want to do: go to a doctor, take medicine, have a back massage with methylated spirits or with special herbs and ointments, sit up in bed, and so on. Persuading the person to do something against his or her wishes requires devotion, expression of love, concern, hovering about, and the use of "political talk" (*politiki*). At times, it requires the family to collectively and constantly explain in detail, and in a culturally meaningful way, why the person may feel the way he or she does, and to give reasons why certain feelings exist and how they relate to the person's illness. The family simultaneously strives to give hope and courage, to assist in and promote recovery. In short, the greatest challenge for the family in caring for a loved one is to persuade that person to do beneficial things that he or she might not feel like doing.

CARE AND CARING—A POWERFUL CULTURAL AND SYMBOLIC CONSTRUCTION

Motivation Forces

In my study, the motivating forces for care and caring stemmed from whether one was a member of the family ("our family") or a member of the community (other people or other families) (Figure 2–4).

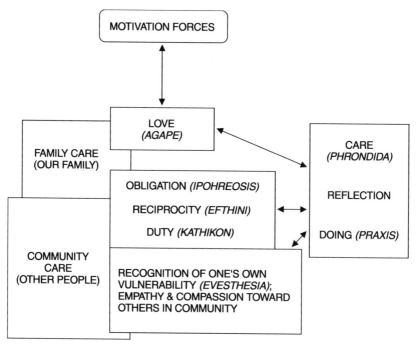

Figure 2–4
Motivation Forces—Moral Dimensions Based on
Meaningful Human Relations

All my informants revealed passionately and clearly that the main motivating forces for family care (*phrondida*) were:

- Love (*agape*)—the eternal source of life, a blessing and gift to humanity. Love is sharing, experiencing togetherness, and creating meaning. It is fearless and full of hope and courage. It endures great suffering and calls for great sacrifices when life crises are experienced by loved ones who "share the same blood."
- Obligation, reciprocity, and/or duty (*ipohreosis, efthini,* and *kathikon*) to each other, based on the type, kind, and meaning of family and other interpersonal relationships. For example, parents are obligated to care for their children, children for their parents, and siblings for each other. All are obligated to reciprocate care to those in the community with whom they have formed social relationships.
- Intense recognition of one's own human vulnerability (*evesthesia*), which engenders strong empathy and motivates caring processes toward others outside the family sphere—persons who live alone, have no family or support system, are isolated, live in poverty, have been abused, and so on, and are identified as deserving care assistance.

These *motivating forces* for the existence and expression of care and caring processes clearly indicate that care and caring are firmly grounded in human and filial relations and in perceptions of human vulnerability and finite existence. Perceptions, beliefs, and practices in regard to care and caring are thus mediated by human interactions and relationships, moral obligations derivative of these, and an awareness of one's own vulnerability and finite life. Care was perceived by my informants as culturally constructed; culturally symbolic, meaningful, and significant; and culturally activated, negotiated, practiced, and evaluated.

Experiencing the Public or Profane (*Koini*) Caring Sphere

My informants' cultural construction of the public sphere viewed the Australian health care context as one that was not bound by love (*agape*), human or filial relationships, or a sense of human vulnerability, but by self-interest and uncontrolled social forces. It was perceived as "unknown," insensitive, dehumanizing, detached from the informants' reality and thus unaware of their vulnerability, and not to be trusted. Without the family's surveillance and protection, the health care context in the public sphere (including hospitals) was considered risky and dangerous.

During illnesses for which professional care was required and the ill person had to be removed from the sacred family sphere, the family embodied the wishes, suffering, anxieties, and fears of the ill person. My informants felt that their ill member was in constant danger and at risk. They perceived that the ill person was decontextualized because he or she was dislocated from their meaningful and protective sacred family sphere. Family members were ready to make any sacrifice, to take any action, and to seek the help of multiple sources in order to protect their ill member and promote his or her healing. The family would be present (at their own insistence) and watchful. They would constantly evaluate the care and healing behaviors exhibited by the professional caregivers, and were ready to take any action necessary to ensure that their family member was not harmed and was receiving the best care possible.

The family's trust of attending health professionals (including nurses) had to be gained. This would only happen when the health professionals accepted and validated the sick person's and family's social and illness reality, and acknowledged that the ultimate responsibility for care lay with the family and not with the professional caregivers. The health professionals had to accept that the family wanted their professional expertise and human support, and their partnership in the care of their family member, but did not see them as the ultimate carers and decision makers.

The responsibility to care and give care, which was deeply felt by all my informants, was clearly nurtured within the Greek family from early childhood. It was a cultural norm to which the informants subscribed, especially during critical illness. In an Australian context, critical illness presented as a source of constant torment for those family members—particularly when hospital rules, regulations, and medical and nursing culture and practices made it difficult for them to be partners in their family member's caring process and in the responsibilities that came with that process.

Juxtaposing Transcultural Human Care and Professional Care

The findings of this small exploratory research study cannot be generalized as holding for all Greek-born persons living in Australia or indeed for other people of different cultural backgrounds. Nevertheless, the study offered an important and substantive example of how one group of people from another culture (within the dominant culture) viewed health and care, and sought to achieve and promote health and care in a way that differs significantly from professional nursing's notions of health and care.

The study provided a strong backdrop against which the deficiencies and ethnocentricity of professional nursing care in multicultural societies like Australia can be distinguished, critiqued, and challenged. This is well-illustrated by the Family Cultural Advocacy Theory, a major grounded theory that emerged from the study's data and is considered briefly in the next section.

FAMILY CULTURAL ADVOCACY COMMUNICATION MODEL

The Family Cultural Advocacy Communication Model was used in response to perceived threats to my informants' "normal" life processes. It was also used by the informants in their attempts to secure a meaningful context and the most appropriate and relevant care for their loved one, either upon admission to a hospital or when they were seeking expert health assistance from health professionals in the community.

Family involvement was particularly important in the area of contextualizing the ill person and the family's illness experiences, expectations of care, and caring practices. Upon admission to a hospital (and thereafter, as the informants' and professional cultural contexts met (Figure 2–5)), the

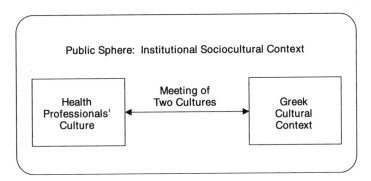

Figure 2–5
Family Cultural Advocacy Communication Model—Phase One:
Meeting of Two Cultures

patient's family actively sought to give to attending nurses and doctors relevant human caring information about their loved one. This was done in an attempt to contextualize the person and to draw the health professionals' attention to their own illness–suffering experiences and to the vulnerability of both the sick person and the family. The family also actively sought scientific information on the intimate details of their loved one's condition and on the possible care and therapeutic choices being considered by the nurses and doctors. My informants clearly indicated that the family's persistence and urgency in seeking and giving information that they perceived as necessary for making sense of what was going on, and as contributing to the sensitive care of their ill member, were sometimes perceived by nursing and medical staff as "demanding," "interfering," and "intensely irritating."

Upon gaining the scientific and professional information needed to make an informed choice, family members would first come together to talk over the situation among themselves, and would then attempt to discuss it with the patient's nurses and doctors. (Their aim was to get the nurses and doctors involved in an intersubjective sharing experience, and to obtain their opinions so as to ensure that all possibilities were considered, and that the best choices were made within a meaningful cultural context.) Each family member would suggest what he or she thought might be the health problem, and what should be done. Intimate details of the patient's signs and symptoms, relevant dates, and activities were shared in precise detail and interpreted in a culturally meaningful way within the broader Australian context, before any final decisions were made.

The family always wanted (and expected) nurses and doctors to collude with them. They sought to have them join in the interdependent relationship of the family and share the illness experience and clinical reality with a view to making the care environment personal, family-like, and safe (a sacred sphere), for the benefit of their family member.

However, the family and the ill member only felt safe if, in addition, nursing and medical staff had embodied the family's anxiety and concern and showed genuine interest and willingness to share the family's and ill member's illness experience without judging them. It was critical for both the family and sick person to feel that they had transmitted to the nursing and medical staff their vulnerability, and thus the moral motivation to care. Once this was perceived to have happened, the family believed that the care would not be compromised.

This phase of negotiation and collusion is clearly identified as the protection and communication phase of the Family Cultural Advocacy Communication Model (see Figure 2–6). If this phase was unfruitful (if, for some reason, nurses and doctors would not collude), then the families would move

Public Sphere:
Health Care Context

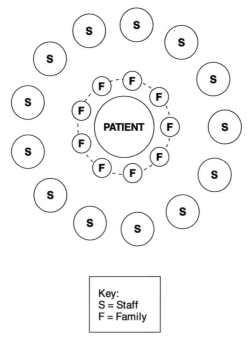

Key:
S = Staff
F = Family

Figure 2–6
**Family Cultural Advocacy Communication Model—Phase Two:
Protection and Communication**

into what may be identified as the aggressive phase of the model. Here, the family members would aggressively demand that they be given the information they required, and that certain behaviors be subscribed to by attending health professionals—for example, that particular actions of care be taken immediately for their loved one. This approach was perceived as necessary because they felt they could not rely on the nursing staff to give *safe care*. At this stage, the families requested, in somewhat aggressive terms, that the patient *not* be told any information about diagnosis or condition (particularly in the case of a cancer diagnosis). The families also attempted constantly to keep surveillance of the health professionals' care, and evaluated their every action and move. Some of the informants had sought other medical opinions, complained vigorously, and used perceived influential community members as advocates. Two families were so unsatisfied with the professional care given to their loved ones that they removed them from the care contexts in question.

When family members felt they had a sympathetic and accepting communication environment and had regained some control over the situation, they would set about once more to negotiate with the nursing and medical staff for the scientific information they required, and would provide the human care knowledge they believed was beneficial for their family member. The synthesis of the scientific information with their lay caring reality was vital for the creation of a meaningful (sacred-sphere) context within which their family member was safe, and from within which they could empower

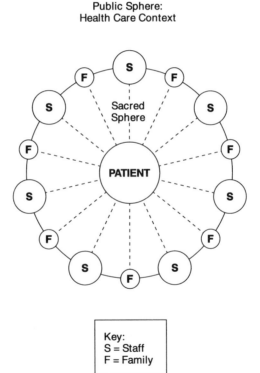

Figure 2–7
Family Cultural Advocacy Communication Model—Phase Three:
Collaborative Communication and Interaction

themselves, regain control and responsibility, make choices, and offer effective support and courage to their family member and to each other. This phase may be identified as the collaborative communication and interaction phase (Figure 2–7).

All three phases of the Family Cultural Advocacy Communication Model (Figure 2–8), while appearing to be discordant with hospital structural norms, ensured the maintenance of the patient's humanity, wholeness, uniqueness, and integrity, and had the protection of the patient's best interests firmly at heart. Once this elaborate advocacy communication process had been completed and a consensus had been reached, the family would collaborate with professional staff in order to safeguard the best care of their family member. The speed with which the respective families passed through the three phases of the model depended, at least partially, on the *cultural sensitivity, knowledge,* and *preparedness* of attending nurses and doctors to act on the families' requests and to respond to the shared illness–suffering experience and care expectations.

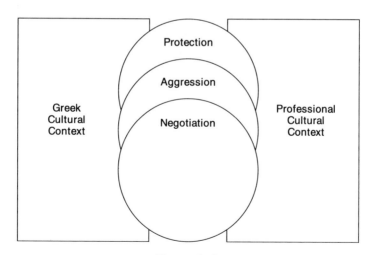

Figure 2–8
The Complete Cultural Advocacy Communication Model

CONCLUSION

Although the example considered here is small, it nevertheless demonstrates the importance of cultural knowledge and potential conflict, both in the delivery of nursing care and in challenging the commonly accepted notions on the profession's ability to deliver holistic care in the absence of such knowledge. In my own view, care that is not culturally informed is at best only mechanistic and, as such, falls far short of the ideals of humanistic, holistic care as it is espoused and aimed for by nursing with a dominant Western worldview.

The diverse human care and caring knowledge and practices revealed by transcultural research clearly challenge professional nursing as it is currently known and practiced in multicultural societies, and place into question its presumed social utility and effectiveness. Whether professional nursing will be able to respond well and effectively to the challenges posed by transcultural human care research will, however, depend not so much on its ability to define human care per se (insofar as this is possible), but on its capacity to identify, reflect critically on, and incorporate the transcultural knowledge of the many, varied, and culturally specific forms care can take.

I would like to suggest that further research undertaken in this area might well be directed at ethnographic research in particular wards or institutions, to observe firsthand the interactions that take place. Such research should not necessarily be restricted to health care systems. It should be conducted within other social systems such as education and law. In this way, further validation of the Family Cultural Advocacy Theory can be achieved.

REFERENCES

Bottomley, G. (1976). Rural Greeks and illness: An anthropologist's viewpoint. *The Medical Journal of Australia, 1*(2), 798–800.

Boyle, S., & Andrews, M. (1989). *Transcultural concepts in nursing care.* Boston: Scott, Foresman/Little, Brown.

Giger, J. N., & Davidhizar, R. E. (1991). *Transcultural nursing: Assessment and intervention.* St. Louis: Mosby.

Glaser, B. (1978). *Theoretical sensitivity: Advances in the methodology of grounded theory.* San Francisco: University of California San Francisco.

Gortner, S. R. (1980). Nursing research out of the past and into the future. *Nursing Research, 29*(4), 204–207.

Isaacs, E. (1976). *Greek children in Sydney.* Canberra: Australian National University Press.

Kanitsaki, O. (1983). Acculturation: A new dimension to nursing. *The Australian Nurses Journal, 13*(5), 42–45, 53.

Kanitsaki, O. (1988). Transcultural nursing: Challenge to change. *Australian Journal of Advanced Nursing, 5*(3), 4–11.

Kanitsaki, O. (1989). *An investigation into the health–illness–suffering experience of a sample of Greek-born members of 12 Greek-Australian families living in Melbourne.* Thesis for partial fulfillment of M.Ed. Studies, Monash University, Melbourne, Australia.

Lawler, J. (1991). *Behind the screens.* Melbourne: Churchill Livingstone.

Leininger, M. (1970). *Nursing and anthropology: Two worlds to blend.* New York: Wiley.

Leininger, M. (1984). *Care: The essence of nursing and health.* Thorofare, NJ: Slack.

Leininger, M. (1988). *Caring: An essential human need.* Thorofare, NJ: Slack.

Leininger, M. (1990). *Ethical and moral dimensions of care.* Detroit: Wayne State University Press.

Mead, M. (1955). *Cultural patterns and technical change.* New York: Mentor.

Moraitis, S. (1972). Medico-social problems in the Greek population in Melbourne: 2. Paediatric problems as seen by the medical practitioner. *The Medical Journal of Australia, 2*(16), 881–883.

Piperoglou, M. V. (1988). The stress of change: The Greek migrant experience. *Australian Family Physician, 17*(6), 453–456.

Rosenbaum, J. (1990). The health meanings and practices of older Greek-Canadian widows. *Journal of Transcultural Nursing, 2*(1), 37–47.

Storer, D. (Ed). (1985). *Ethnic family values in Australia.* Sydney: Prentice-Hall.

Strauss, A. L. (1987). *Qualitative analysis for social scientists.* New York: Cambridge University Press.

Strauss, A., & Corbin, J. (1990). *Basics of qualitative research: Grounded theory procedures and techniques.* Newbury Park, CA: Sage.

3

Generic and Professional Care of Anglo-American and Philippine American Nurses

Zen Spangler

A growing interest in care is inspiring many nurse scholars and researchers to examine and probe the nature, origin, epistemics, and ontology of care (Aamodt, 1979; Benner & Wrubel, 1989; Fry, 1990; Gadow, 1988; Gaut, 1981, 1984; Kelly, 1990; Ray, 1991; Vezeau & Schroeder, 1991). Although nurse leaders claim that care is the essence, dominant domain (Leininger, 1978, 1988, 1991), and moral responsibility (Watson, 1985) of nursing, professional nursing does not hold an exclusive interest or right to this concept. Caring as part of the human complexion has caught the attention of moralists and philosophers (Buber, 1970; Heidegger, 1962) and continues to hold a grip on non-nurse thinkers, scholars, and practitioners (Frankena, 1983; Gaylin, 1979; Mayeroff, 1971; Noddings, 1984). Thus,

This study was supported by the American Nurses Association Ethnic/Racial Minority Fellowship Programs.

47

caring may be paramount to professional nurses, but its value and practice have generic or universal foundation.

Leininger's conceptualization of care from the perspective of culture delineates the generic as well as the professional components of care. Leininger's theory of culture care depicts the influence of the interrelated components of worldview, culture, and social structure dimensions, within the context of language and environment, on individuals', groups', communities', and institutions' care decisions and actions. A major premise of Leininger's theory of culture care is that all cultures of the world have folk or generic ways to express or manifest care, and that some members of the various cultures have been exposed to professional care (Leininger, 1991). Generic care is local, indigenous, and culturally transmitted; professional care is formal, cognitively learned, and usually acquired through educational institutions (Leininger, 1978, 1988, 1991). Leininger asserts that both the folk and professional health care systems are capable of providing care that is beneficial, satisfying, and favorable. Indeed, she suggests that the favorable aspects of generic care may be the epistemic and ontological base of professional nursing care (1991).

This chapter is part of a larger study in which I explored and analyzed the cultural differences in the nursing care values and caregiving practices of Anglo-American and Philippine American nurses (Spangler, 1991). Here, the focus is on expounding the generic and professional roots of the care values and caregiving practices of nurses from two cultures. The purpose is to discover, analyze, and explicate the generic and professional care values and caregiving practices of Anglo-American and Philippine nurses.

RESEARCH DESIGN

Ethnonursing, a qualitative research methodology developed by Leininger (1985, 1990) for the purpose of providing a systematic, rigorous, humanistic, and scientific process of discovering, explicating, and analyzing human care and health phenomena, was the research method used in this study. Ethnonursing interviews and observation–participation–reflection guides were used as the enabling tools to elicit the care values and caregiving practices of the Anglo-American and Philippine nurses.

The informants were twenty-two Anglo-American and twenty-six nurses originally from the Philippines who worked in a 200-bed acute care hospital located in the Northeastern United States. The ten key Philippine and nine key Anglo-American informants worked in the intensive care unit and in one medical–surgical nursing unit. The sixteen Philippine and thirteen Anglo-American general informants worked in the various nursing units of the hospital, including the units where the key informants worked. All informants were knowledgeable bearers of culture but the key informants were chosen because they had worked full-time and had been assigned to their particular nursing units for longer than one year. Tables 3–1 through 3–4 show the demographic characteristics of the informants.

Data collection involving observation–participation–reflection and ethnonursing interviews lasted seven months. As I observed and worked with the key informants, I noted their ways of providing care, the daily activities and routines, special events, unusual occurrences, and their relationships with patients, patients' families, physicians, and each other. The key informants were interviewed twice, for periods lasting between forty-five minutes to one hour; the general informants were interviewed once. Nurses were encouraged to relate their understanding and meaning of care and professional nursing care.

Data analysis was performed utilizing Leininger's four phases of analysis for qualitative data (Leininger, 1990). In phase 1, raw data were analyzed and comparatively studied for their association to generic and professional cultural values and beliefs. In phase 2, all statements and field notes related to factors and conditions that influenced generic and professional caring were coded using Leininger–Templin–Thompson ethnoscript (Leininger, 1990). In phase 3, generic and professional patterns were identified by careful scrutiny of meanings from prevalent and recurrent expressions, observations,

Table 3–1
Key Anglo-American Informants

Code ID	Education	Experience (Years)
KAA01	AD (enrolled in BSN)	6
KAA02	BSN	1
KAA03	AD	1 (3 as LPN)
KAA04	BSN	1
KAA05	Diploma	9
KAA06	BSN	2
KAA07	AD	3
KAA08	BSN	1
KAA09	BSN	1
		Mean = 2.8

Table 3–2
Key Philippine Informants

Code ID	Education	Experience		Visa
		Philippines	U.S.	
KPA01	BSN	2	6	H-1
KPA02	BSN	2	6	H-1
KPA03	BSN	15	7	Permanent
KPA04	BSN	2	3	H-1
KPA05	BSN	0	4	H-1
KPA06	BSN	3	4.5	H-1
KPA07	BSN	5.5	3	H-1
KPA08	BSN	1	6	H-1
KPA09	BSN	2	5	H-1
KPA10	BSN	1.5	4	H-1
		Mean = 3.4	4.85	

Table 3–3
General Anglo-American Informants

Code ID	Education	Experience (Years)
GAA01	Diploma	20
GAA02	AD	10
GAA03	BSN	1
GAA04	AD, BS sociology	2.5
GAA05	BSN	2
GAA06	AD	1
GAA07	BSN	2
GAA08	BSN	1
GAA09	BSN (enrolled in MS)	10
GAA10	BSN	1
GAA11	AD, BS biology	6
GAA12	AD	8
GAA13	Diploma	2
		Mean = 5

Table 3–4
General Philippine Informants*

| Code ID | Education | Experience | | Visa |
		Philippines	U.S.	
KPA01	BSN	4	9	H-1
KPA02	BSN	2	16	U.S. citizen
KPA03	BSN	4	4	H-1
KPA04	BSN	7	1.5	H-1
KPA05	AD (US)	0	12	U.S. citizen
KPA06	BSN	4	2	H-1
KPA07	AD (US)	0	14	U.S. citizen
KPA08	BSN	1	2	H-1
KPA09	BSN	2	4	H-1
KPA10	BSN	3	3	H-1
GPA11	AD (US)	0	3	Permanent
GPA12	BSN	1	15	U.S. citizen
GPA13	BSN	0	5	H-1
GPA14	BSN	1	3	H-1
GPA15	BSN	5	3	Permanent
GPA16	BSN	3	15	U.S. citizen
		Mean = 2.3	7	

* Nurses originally from the Philippines and now practicing in the United States.

and events. In phase 4, abstract themes were derived from broad inductive ratiocination of patterns.

PROFESSIONAL NURSING CARE WITH GENERIC CARE BASE

This study provided strong support for the influence of culture, social structure features, language, and environmental factors on nurses' care values and caregiving practices. Of interest for this chapter was the strong overlap between the generic and professional care values and practices of nurses. Generic and professional nursing care *overlapped*—both were influenced by culture and social structure. The influence of culture on professional nursing care was not surprising because professional education occurs within the context of culture. Anglo-American and Philippine nurses cited professional education and personal/cultural upbringing as the sources of their nursing care values and caregiving practices. It was clear that the predominant societal and cultural values influenced the nurses' generic and professional care values and practices. Figure 3–1 shows a diagrammatic representation of my findings.

Given the influence of culture and social structure on the generic and professional care of the Anglo-American and Philippine nurses, a brief overview of the predominant cultural characteristics of the two groups will help elucidate their nursing care values and caregiving practices.

Anglo-American Culture

Social scientists who have characterized the Anglo-American culture have noted that the values of individualism, self-reliance, and mastery of nature are its substantive makeup. Kluckhohn (1949) characterized American individualism as the dramatization of the individual, in that activities, achievements, and their consequences are personalized. According to Kluckhohn, the term "rugged individualism" represents the romanticized image of a person who has belief in oneself, works hard, takes risks, and achieves great success. The Anglo-American value for individualism was also noted by Leininger (1978), who characterized it as a recognition of the person as singularly special and therefore entitled to recognition and status in the culture. The marked emphasis on each person highlights the attention given to the

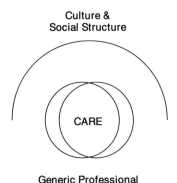

Figure 3–1
The Influence of Culture and Social Structure on
Generic and Professional Care

rights, the welfare, and the privileges of the individual rather than the group. Achieving and doing are celebrated in the value placed on work and success.

The concept of individualism was further articulated by Hsu (1983), who proposed that the basic element of American individualism is self-reliance. He described American self-reliance as an ideal state in which individuals see themselves as their own masters, in control of their own destinies. According to Du Bois (1955), the American middle-class conception of self-reliance and mastery of nature is rooted in the optimistic belief that one can not only attain one's goal through hard work but also can master the mechanical universe. Optimistic outlooks are reflected in phrases such as "If you don't succeed, try, try again," or "Never say die." According to Du Bois, Americans hold dear the belief that material well-being follows success. He noted that America's conquest of its frontiers, its economic development, and its advances in science and technology have convinced Americans of the validity and power of individualism, self-reliance, and mastery of nature.

Philippine Culture

The predominant values of the Filipinos are "other"-directed and are aimed at maintaining harmony and respect. Social scientists who have studied the Philippines have noted the importance of relationships in the structure of values. Cultural value terms such as *bayanihan* (helping one's neighbors), *utang na loob* (debt of obligation), *pakikisama* (smooth interpersonal relationship), and *pakikipagkapwa* (being one with others) were preeminent and expressed one's relationship and commitment to others. The Philippine society was described by Hunt et al. (1963) as a *bayanihan* society because of the people's stress on personal, face-to-face, and neighborly relationships. The obligation and commitment to others was also expressed in *utang na loob*, which describes the bond between the receiver and the provider of help. Within the obligation network, one is morally bound to repay the person who extends help (Kaut, 1961). Lynch (1964) coined the phrase *pakikisama* to describe the Filipinos' high regard for getting along and maintaining harmony. Enriquez (1986) later suggested that the term *pakikipagkapwa* is the superordinate Philippine value because it strikes at the heart of the Philippine core value, which is attention to others. *Kapwa* (in English, the closest equivalent is "others") recognizes the shared identity between self and others. According to Enriquez, this concept emphasizes the similarity of others' dignity and being to one's own, and thus exemplifies the Filipinos' strong awareness of others. Respect is another fundamental value that is inculcated from a very early age. Filipino children are taught to respect others, especially the elderly and persons in authority.

Respect is manifested in manners and behaviors, in the tone of voice, and in the use of respectful terms such as *po* when talking with elders or authority figures, or the use of *ati* or *kuya* to address an older sister or brother respectively (Landa-Jocano, 1972).

ANGLO-AMERICAN AND PHILIPPINE AMERICAN NURSING CARE VALUES

The nursing care values and caregiving practices of the Anglo-American and Philippine American nurses are described here in terms of the four themes I found most representative of each group. Identification (Code ID) and data on informants are in Tables 3–1 through 3–4.

Anglo-American Nursing Care Values: Themes

Promotion of Autonomous Care or Self-Care. The Anglo-American nurses demonstrated a strong value for patients' independence. They encouraged patients to do as much for themselves as possible, and self-care was often mentioned as a desirable patient outcome. The following statements from the Anglo-American nurses exemplify this care value:

KAA04: The first thing patients must do is participate in their own care. You know, they have to take care of themselves.

KAA07: We practice self-care here. We encourage our patients to do things for themselves. We encourage them to wash themselves. It is good for patients to stretch their muscles and do things for themselves. . . . Of all the nursing theories, I like Orem best. I like her theory because one of the ways you get better is by helping yourself.

The Anglo-American nurses' promotion of patient independence is congruent with the value Americans place on self-reliance. The Anglo-American nurses exhibited a strong belief in helping patients gain independence and achieve the ability to care for themselves.

Value for Patient Education. Nineteen of twenty-two (86 percent) of the Anglo-American nurses mentioned patient education as an important nursing care practice. In contrast, only 30 percent of the Philippine nurses mentioned patient education as a nursing care value and practice. These examples of statements made by the Anglo-American nurses provide support for the value placed on patient education:

KAA01: In my nursing school, patient teaching was emphasized. We all had to prepare a teaching plan for certain disease conditions.

KAA04: We had a man who had bilateral amputation of the legs. His circulation was very poor. He was supposed to stop smoking but he continued to smoke. We constantly told him about the effects of smoking on his circulation. We realized that he will not stop immediately, but we kept reinforcing our teaching.

GAA13: Patient teaching—that is not done enough.

The Anglo-American value for patient education was also reflected in the requirements of the Joint Commission on Accreditation of Hospitals Organizations (JCAHO). To satisfy the patient education requirements of JCAHO, the hospital nursing educators added patient education in the revised nurses' daily flow sheet, to underscore the importance of providing patient and family education. Patient education is a nursing care activity that Anglo-American nurses acquired and learned cognitively in their professional nursing education. However, patient education is also consistent with the value of self-reliance because acquiring knowledge and skills is necessary for optimal self-care.

Expectation That Patients Will Comply. The Anglo-American nurses' value for autonomous care and patient education was accompanied by an expectation that patients would comply with the prescribed health regimen. Some statements made by the Anglo-American nurses illustrated this point:

KAA01: Nothing bothers me more than having a few patients come back to the hospital because they are not taking their medicines. We have a patient here who is actually a doctor. He just won't take his cardiac meds. Of course, he came in all the time in worse and worse condition.

GAA02: Patients must get as much information as possible. They must comply, they must do what the health care professionals tell them.

GAA03: Patients must comply—cooperate. If they do not, they will not get better.

The statements above showed the frustration of Anglo-American nurses when they perceived their patients as noncompliant. Although they wanted patients to take care of themselves, they wanted the patients' decisions and choices to be consistent with the scientifically established knowledge of the health professionals.

Control of Situations and Conditions.   The last theme that characterizes the Anglo-American nurses is control. This theme was expressed in the Anglo-American nurses' desire to be "on top of things" or to have control over situations and events. The nurses anticipated changes and prepared for them through careful assessment, regular monitoring of vital signs, and recognition of abnormal laboratory values. These statements from Anglo-American nurses exemplify this care value and practice:

> KAA01: Patients' stable status is the most important thing to me. That comes above anything else. For my priority? I check vital signs and I monitor their SMAs [laboratory values].

> GAA08: Nursing care is more than baths, it is also assessment. I come from a [nursing] program where assessment is a big thing. When I was a new nurse, I was very pompous. When I discussed a case with a nurse who was a diploma grad, I asked, "How does the lung sound?" If she said, "I do not know," that was like a blasphemy. I said, "How could you not know?" I am not that way anymore, but I still think that assessment is very important because that is the best way we can plan and handle patients' problems.

The Anglo-American nurses' acts of assessment, monitoring, and interpretation of laboratory values are professional acts learned during their professional education; however, the basic value for control is consistent and is embedded in the American value for "mastery of nature."

The Philippine American Nurses' Care Values: Themes

Expressed Seriousness and Dedication to Work.   The Philippine American nurses expressed a sense of "duty," "conscience," and a "vocationlike" commitment to work.

KPA06: Filipinos put their hearts in their work. There is satisfaction when you give.

KPA09: Because of conscience, we make an effort to do our best even if the task is menial.

GPA15: I have worked with real caring Americans, but I think that they are less sensitive and more easygoing than us. I think we take our jobs and patients more seriously.

The Philippine nurses' dedication and commitment to service were consistent with the Philippine cultural tradition, which emphasizes respect for authority, social acceptance, group orientation, and sacrifice of individual interests in favor of group or communal interests. The Philippine nurses' recent arrival and precarious status in the United States (H-1 visa) may have added to their emphasis on obligation or duty. Many stated that they had fewer rights to make demands.

Attentiveness to Patients' Physical Comfort.   The majority of the Philippine nurses emphasized the importance of promoting physical comfort. Examples of Philippine nurses' statements are:

KPA02: To us, the comfort of the patients is number one. Filipinos are very clean with patients.

KPA05: Filipino nurses have conscience. They cannot simply let patients drown in their own secretions, or soak in their own urine, or keep flat in bed.

KPA06: Culture influences care. I think that is true because we see to it that patients are comfortable. Patients here say that Filipino nurses are attentive to their needs. We are more conscientious about leaving patients and bedside clean and orderly. We see to it that patients are comfortable.

The stress on physical comfort comes from the Filipinos' high value for cleanliness. Filipinos are meticulous about their bodies and they take pride in keeping clean, tidy, and organized surroundings. A Filipino folk song, which all Filipino children learn in school, expresses pride in keeping a tiny bamboo home so clean that people can eat off its floor.

Care as Respect.   The Philippine nurses cited respect as a value they learned early in life; they said it prevailed in their care of patients. These selected statements from the Philippine nurses illustrate the significance of respect in their culture and in their practice of nursing:

> KPA09:   Even if the patient is comatose, you show your respect for them. You give them the same respect you would give an awake and alert patient.

> KPA05:   When I care for elderly patients here [in the United States], I do what I know I would do for my grandparents. Maybe this is the area where Chinese and Filipinos are different from Americans. Chinese and Filipinos show more respect for the elderly patients.

The Philippine nurses explained that respect is an integral part of their culture and that their families inculcated the value of respect when they were growing up. Even the two Philippine nurses who described their upbringing as "not typical Philippine upbringing" stated that respect was highly emphasized. The Philippine nurses reported that respect was taught as an important dimension of caring: respect was to be accorded to all human beings, especially older persons and persons in position of authority. Respect was therefore a generic care, and the Philippine nurses integrated it in their care of patients in a professional hospital context.

Care as Patience.   The Philippine nurses claimed that they were patient by nature and that this characteristic influenced their relationship with patients. Here are some of their comments:

> KPA03:   I think we are more patient than Americans. They tell us this too. For example, we are slower to complain about work, we take our time, we do not rush people. Oh, I do not know; maybe it means that we take abuses more easily [laughter].

> KPA09:   When I encounter demanding patients, I do not answer back. I just let them talk. I find that after their catharsis, they feel better and are less demanding. American nurses tell me to put those patients in their places. I find that, when you answer back, they just get agitated and angry; nothing is accomplished. Of course, I also get mad when patients scream or say insulting things, but I remind myself not to take their remarks personally. Often, they are upset about their illness.

The Philippine nurses indicated that patience was inherent in their nature (generic) and was manifested in their professional care of patients.

CONCLUSION

The study demonstrated the potency of Leininger's theory of culture care for discovering and making explicit the meaning and interpretation of care values and caregiving practices from the perspectives of culturally different nurses. It also provided some support for the interlinking of professional and generic care in nursing. Leininger suggested that generic care may be the epistemic base of professional caring. This idea found support in the influence of culture and social structure on the professed values of the nurses. The Anglo-American and Philippine nurses cited professional education as well as cultural and childhood upbringing as the sources of their care values. The professional or the cognitively learned care values of the nurses were consistent with the values of the culture in which the nurses were nurtured. The linkage between generic and professional care has also been suggested by Brown, Kitson, and McKnight (1992):

The natural capacity of the individual to care and their ethical response to the caring relationship are the foundations upon which professional care is built (p. 37).

REFERENCES

Aamodt, A. (1979). Social-cultural dimensions of caring in the world of the Papago child and adolescent. In M. Leininger (Ed.), *Transcultural nursing* (pp. 47–56). New York: Masson International Nursing Publications.

Benner, P., & Wrubel, J. (1989). *The primacy of caring.* Menlo Park, CA: Addison-Wesley.

Brown, J. M., Kitson, A. L., & McKnight, T. J. (1992). *Challenges in caring: Explorations in nursing and ethics.* Melbourne: Chapman & Hall.

Buber, M. (1970). *I and thou* (Walter Kaufmann, Trans.). New York: Scribner's.

Du Bois, C. (1955). The dominant value profile of American culture. *American Anthropologist, 57,* 1232–1239.

Enriquez, V. G. (1986). *Kapwa:* A core concept in Filipino social psychology. In V. G. Enriquez (Ed.), *Philippine world view* (pp. 6–19). Singapore: Institute of Southeast Asian Study.

Frankena, W. K. (1983). Moral-point-of-view theories. In N. Bowie (Ed.), *Ethical theory in the last quarter of the twentieth century* (pp. 39–79). Indianapolis: Hackett.

Fry, S. (1990). The philosophical foundations of caring. In M. M. Leininger (Ed.), *Ethical and moral dimensions of care* (pp. 13–24). Detroit: Wayne State University Press.

Gadow, S. (1988). Covenant without cure: Letting go and holding on in chronic illness. In J. Watson & M. A. Ray (Eds.), *The ethics of care and the ethics of cure: Synthesis in chronicity* (pp. 5–14). New York: National League for Nursing.

Gaut, D. A. (1981). Conceptual analysis of caring: Research method. In M. Leininger (Ed.), *Caring: An essential human need* (pp. 17–24). Detroit: Wayne State University Press.

Gaut, D. A. (1984). A theoretic description of caring as action. In M. Leininger (Ed.), *Care: The essence of nursing and health* (pp. 27–44). Thorofare, NJ: Slack.

Gaylin, W. (1979). *Caring.* New York: Knopf.

Heidegger, M. (1962). *Being and time* (M. J. Robinson, Ed.). New York: Harper & Row.

Hunt, C., Pal, A., Collier, R., Espiritu, S., de Young, J. E., & Corpuz, S. F. (1963). *Sociology in Philippine setting.* Quezon City, Philippines: Phoenix.

Hsu, F. L. K. (1983). *Rugged individualism reconsidered.* Knoxville: The University of Tennessee Press.

Kaut, C. (1961). *Utang na loob:* A system of contractual obligation among the Tagalogs. *Southwestern Journal of Anthropology, 17,* 256–272.

Kelly, B. (1990). Respect and caring: Ethics and essence of nursing. In M. M. Leininger (Ed.), *Ethical and moral dimensions of care* (pp. 13–24). Detroit: Wayne State University Press.

Kluckhohn, C. (1949). *Mirror for man.* New York: McGraw-Hill.

Landa-Jocano, F. L. (1972). Filipino social structure and value system. *Silliman Journal, 19*(1), 59–70.

Leininger, M. (1978). *Transcultural nursing: Concepts, theories, and practices.* New York: Wiley.

Leininger, M. (1985). *Qualitative research methods in nursing.* New York: Grune & Stratton.

Leininger, M. (1988). Leininger's theory of nursing: Cultural care diversity and universality. *Nursing Science Quarterly, 1,* 152–160.

Leininger, M. (1990). Ethnomethods: The philosophic and epistemic bases to explicate transcultural nursing knowledge. *Journal of Transcultural Nursing, 1*, 40–51.

Leininger, M. (1991). The theory of culture care diversity and universality. In M. Leininger (Ed.), *Culture care diversity and universality: A theory of nursing* (pp. 5–68). New York: National League for Nursing.

Lynch, F. (1964). *Social acceptance. Four readings on Philippine values* (IPC Papers No. 2). Manila: Ateneo de Manila University Press.

Mayeroff, M. (1971). *On caring.* New York: Harper & Row.

Noddings, N. (1984). *Caring: A feminine approach to ethics and moral education.* Berkeley: University of California Press.

Ray, M. (1991). Caring inquiry: The esthetic process in the way of compassion. In D. Gaut & M. Leininger (Eds.), *Caring: The compassionate healer* (pp. 181–189). New York: National League for Nursing.

Spangler, Z. (1991). Culture care of Philippine and Anglo-American nurses. In M. Leininger (Ed.), *Culture care diversity and universality: A theory of nursing* (pp. 119–146). New York: National League for Nursing.

Watson, J. (1985). *Nursing: Human science and human care: A theory of nursing.* Norwalk, CT: Appleton-Century-Crofts.

Vezeau, T., & Schroeder, C. (1991). Caring approaches: A critical examination of origin, balance of power, embodiment, time and space, and intended outcome. In P. L. Chinn (Ed.), *Anthology of caring* (pp. 1–16). New York: National League for Nursing.

4

Caring in Birthing: Experiences of Professional Nurse and Generic Care

Julianna Finn

Childbirth is, at the same time, a commonplace biological process and a unique sociocultural event for women everywhere. Every society and culture provides ways of handling and organizing the life event of birth for the mother and the infant. Childbirth beliefs and practices that usually vary by culture include: the content of prenatal and postnatal care; who is an appropriate caregiver; diet; clothing; the management of labor; use of medicines and herbs; behavioral restrictions; support mechanisms; and birth attendants. Cosminsky (1978) contended that, in addition to the cultural proscriptions associated with childbirth, the birthing woman and her family, and the attendant(s) chosen, should have similar, compatible beliefs associated with this process (p. 116). The cultural practices associated with birth are of major interest to nurses and nurse midwives.

A typical childbirth in the United States is greatly influenced by American beliefs and cultural values, which have generally integrated the Western biomedical model and related practices. Within this biomedical model, pregnancy and birth are often viewed as an illness requiring careful observation and management by intervention and the use of technology. Most births in the United States occur in hospitals, and the women choosing this setting, and their physicians, usually subscribe to the biomedical interventionist model of birth.

Because most women choosing to birth in hospitals in the United States have adopted the biomedical view of the body as a series of separate parts, requiring medical surveillance and quality-controlled observations and maneuvers, the women tend to expect the application of high-technology instruments routinely, even for normal, healthy childbirth. Women who select a hospital birthing setting generally rely on the use of the latest technology and instrumentation, in the hope that this will ensure the health and safety of both the mother and baby. The major questions of interest are: What can nurses do to make the high-technology hospital birth experience more humanistic and more caring? In spite of the prevailing interventionist perspective, can the care given by professional nurses ameliorate the technological environment that predominates in hospital births in the United States? Can the caregiving by professional nurses convey a new vision to parents who deliver in hospitals? This new perspective would envision each childbirthing woman (and her family) as a valued, unique, holistic human being in need of family-centered care, rather than as a composite of separate body parts, including a uterus that requires treatment, interventions, and "deliverance" in order to birth a healthy baby. Can nurses selectively employ appropriate caring expressions that convey a holistic attitude toward women and birthing? Can nurses provide a model of competent care and caring that meets the care expectations of the childbirthing woman and her family in a high-technology hospital birthing environment?

Historically, women birthed in their homes or villages, in the company of supportive family, friends, and other women who had successfully birthed (Anderson, 1986). In hospital settings in the United States, female nurses are often the only women present to assist and support the childbirthing woman. Additional support comes from the woman's spouse or significant other and the physician, both usually male. Can a nurse form an alliance with the childbirthing woman and establish a caring relationship based on meeting her care expectations? Can the care provided by the professional nurse meet the woman's caring needs in a way reminiscent of and yet surpassing the care provided by the network of women from home who guided and supported their childbirthing comrade in other times and in other cultures?

It is my belief that the professional nursing care provided by the nurse during childbirth can create a nurturing, supportive, helping environment in the high-technology context of hospital labor and delivery settings. Nurses employing scientific knowledge about the care expectations and needs of the childbirthing woman can cognitively and creatively choose among caring modes and practices in order to select the most meaningful care expressions and activities for a particular childbirthing client. How will nurses know which caring modalities to select? One of the primary questions for this study was to discover and explicate professional nurse care and caring modalities as they are experienced by the recipient of that care, the childbirthing woman. Professional nurse caregiving must be appropriate to the care and caring expectations of the client. Leininger (1988a) held that each client's care expectations are largely culturally learned and determined and that culturally based care by professional nurse caregivers will make a difference to the client.

While working with a variety of women in different urban hospital obstetrical units, I have frequently noticed and contrasted the various caregivers offering different types of care to women during labor and childbirth. These women experience care from both the professional nurse and the woman's lay caregiver from home (usually her spouse and/or the father of the baby). The nurse's contact with the client is usually episodic, and involves assessment, alert surveillance, teaching, facilitating, empowering, coaching, volitional touching, and performing other selected activities or tasks. The lay caregiver, on the other hand, usually provides continual care for the woman during eight to twelve hours of labor, by coaching, encouraging, protecting, helping the woman make decisions, comforting, witnessing, supporting, and often relating these care modalities to the woman's home and natural living context. How does the woman understand and interpret these two types of care? Is the care from the professional nurse recognizably different from the care provided by the woman's spouse or caregiver from home?

Leininger (1991) stated that generic care has existed since the beginning of humankind and that humans could not have survived without care. Generic care is learned as part of growing up, in all cultures throughout our global environment, and is particularly evident in woman-to-woman care during childbirth. In the majority of the world, birth continues to be an event handled by women in home or village settings. However, in the United States, as women moved from home birthing to hospital delivery, some lay care practices that had been provided by family and friends acting as caring birth attendants were lost when physicians and nurses "took over" and focused on professional caregiving practices.

Leininger (1991) defined these two types of care in her Theory of Culture Care Diversity and Universality. Generic care she defined as:

Those culturally learned and transmitted lay, indigenous (traditional) or folk (home care) knowledge and skills used to provide assistive, supportive, enabling, facilitative acts (or phenomena) toward or for another individual, group or institution with evident or anticipated needs to ameliorate or improve a human health condition (or well-being), disability, lifeway, or to face death. (p. 38)

Professional nursing care was defined (Leininger, 1991) as:

Formal and cognitively learned professional care knowledge and practice skills obtained through educational institutions that are used to provide assistive, supportive, enabling, or facilitative acts (or phenomena) to or for another individual or group in order to improve a human health condition (or well-being), disability, lifeway or to work with dying clients. (p. 38)

PURPOSES OF THE STUDY

The primary purpose of this study was to discover childbirthing women's lived experiences of professional nurse care and noncare, and generic care and noncare, using Leininger's Theory of Culture Care Diversity and Universality, so that nurses can learn ways to provide culturally congruent care. Another purpose of this research was to look for congruence between the finalized descriptions of the structure of professional nurse care and generic care and Leininger's definitions of these two concepts within her culture care theory.

RESEARCH QUESTIONS

Some of the research questions that guided this study were:

1. What are the childbirthing woman's lived experiences of care received from the professional nurse and from the generic caregiver from home?
2. What are the childbirthing woman's lived experiences of noncare received from the nurse and from the generic caregiver from home?
3. What are the essential features, whether similarities or differences, of professional nurse care and generic care as identified by childbirthing women, and how are they possibly congruent with the definitions of these concepts within Leininger's culture care theory?

4. What are the implications, for nursing and for the recipient, of these different modes of care?

LITERATURE PERSPECTIVES ON CARE

Komorita, Doehring, and Herchert (1991) found that few studies focus on the client's perceptions of caring, and that a lack of agreement exists between nurses and clients regarding what are caring behaviors. Riemen (1986b) and Larson (1984) found a discrepancy in care expressions and values between nurses and clients. Brown (1986) discovered that nurses identify expressive behaviors (touching, listening) as indicators of care, whereas clients identify instrumental nursing behaviors (administering medications accurately, managing equipment efficiently) as more important care indicators. Leininger (1981) found that some Anglo-American professional nurses in the United States tend to emphasize the following caring constructs in their caregiving: concern, compassion, alleviation of stress, nurturance, comfort, and protection.

CONCEPTUALIZATION WITHIN LEININGER'S THEORY

This study was conceptualized within Leininger's Theory of Culture Care Diversity and Universality. This theory is based on a distinct concept of care that can describe, explain, and predict nursing practice. Leininger's (1988b) firmly held position has been that "care is the essence of nursing and the central, dominant, and unifying feature of nursing" (p. 152).

Leininger's (1991) Sunrise Model (see Figure 1–1) depicts the elements and concepts of the theory. According to the model, generic and professional nurse care are revealed through the worldview, cultural values, and social structures that influence these care patterns and expressions. The social structures consist of seven types of factors: technological, religious and philosophical, kinship and social, cultural values and lifeways, political and legal, economic, and educational factors.

Because of the uniqueness of each culture and the manifestations of care and caring, nurses cannot assume that all clients will view the nurse's intended caring actions positively. Leininger (1988b) contended that it is a myth that whatever is perceived by the nurse as a caring action or attitude will necessarily be viewed as care by the client. In fact, this myth may be viewed as a limiting factor that interferes with the nurse's therapeutic effectiveness and, as a consequence, can impede client satisfaction.

Care and caring are generally manifested in different care constructs among various cultures. To minimize the impact of culturally diverse care constructs on the outcomes of this research, I limited the informants, spouses, and nurses in my study to persons of European-American culture.

METHODS

In order to learn about professional and generic care (and noncare), I interviewed three women, after childbirthing, on the postpartum unit of a large urban hospital in the United States. A hospital childbirthing setting was selected because women usually experience the two relevant types of care during labor and childbirth in this setting. The registered nurse is expected to provide professional nurse care and caring during childbirth. The woman's significant other, usually her spouse, provides generic (or lay) care and caring during childbirth. The birthing unit of the hospital provided a special opportunity to explore and discover these two types of care as experienced concurrently by the childbirthing women.

Informants

The criteria for selection of informants were:

1. English-speaking, European-American, married women.
2. Ages twenty to thirty-five years old.
3. Multiparas and primiparas.
4. European-American spouses and nurse caregivers.
5. Attendees at childbirth classes with spouses.
6. Minimum of two hours in labor/delivery/recovery.
7. Normal vaginal births and normal newborns.
8. Agreeable to talking and to signing informed consents.
9. Consenting to follow-up interviews in their homes.

The three informants, their spouses, and the nurses providing care during childbirth were all of European-American culture and met the criteria for this study. The ages of the informants ranged from twenty to twenty-eight. Two informants were multiparas and one was a primipara. The length of time for labor and birthing for these three women in the hospital's labor/delivery/recovery rooms ranged from six to nine hours. Each informant (and her infant) met normal criteria and was cared for during childbirth by the woman's spouse and a registered nurse.

Phenomenological Method of Data Analysis

The phenomenological method delineated by Colaizzi (1978) was used to analyze the data. This method was chosen because it is a qualitative method that utilizes a humanistic, people-centered approach to focus on the clients' experience rather than the nurses' perspective. It is important when using phenomenological analysis that the researcher deliberately bracket or set aside any preconceived ideas about the meanings of professional nurse care and noncare and of generic care and noncare.

The Colaizzi steps (1978, p. 59) used for analysis were as follows:

1. Read through the descriptions.
2. Extract significant statements.
3. Formulate meanings from the significant statements.
4. Organize the meanings into themes.
5. Organize the themes into an exhaustive description of the phenomena.
6. Formulate a statement of the structure of the phenomena.
7. Validate the analysis by interviewing each informant at home and ascertaining whether this analysis describes her experiences accurately.

The informants confirmed the accuracy of the descriptions.

Sample Steps of Analysis

Table 4–1 is an example of some of the steps used in the process of analysis: sample quotations from the informants, extraction of significant statements,

Table 4–1
Sample Steps Used in Analysis of Birthing Process

Quotes	Significant Statements	Themes
	Professional Nurse Care	
1. Explained everything she was doing and why. Knowledgeable about what affected contractions. Considerate of what I was going through.	Conveyed own knowledge about anticipated events and feelings associated with childbirth.	Drew on a reservoir (base) of knowledge and experience of events and feelings associated with childbirth. Prepared woman in early labor and helped her anticipate and cope with childbirth.
2. Could tell she was in the profession because she wanted to be, not because it was a job.	It was evident the nurse viewed her profession as a calling rather than a job.	There because of a conscious choice to invest herself in caring for others.
	Generic Care (Spouse)	
1. His biggest help was being there for me, holding my hand. He helped me breathe and push, and held my leg. He used touch and eye contact to coach and encourage me during labor.	Used hand and eye contact and words to coach and encourage me during labor. Remained with me throughout labor and birth, gently caring, encouraging, offering moral support. Coached and held me during pushing.	Offered self by constant presence and moral support, verbal encouragement, touch an eye contact, and gentle caring. Physically held and coached mate during birth.
2. Said he wished he could take the pain for me. He was scared for me. Let me squeeze his hand hard. Got upset to see me hurting. Felt helpless, not knowing how to help.	Felt helpless, worried, distressed, and scared for me. Endured actual discomfort himself to help me and even wished he could take on my pain of labor and birth.	Communicated his empathy, distress, helplessness, and fear at seeing his mate in pain. Willingly endured actual discomfort himself and conveyed wish to take on all the pain of childbirth in place of his mate.

Table 4–1 *(Continued)*

Quotes	Significant Statements	Themes
	Nurse Noncare	
1. Attitude was cold and uncaring, not wanting to be bothered. She did her job, like that's all she was there for, not to see that I was comfortable, which I thought was wrong.	Attitude was cold and uncaring, not wanting to be bothered. Rather than seeing me as a person needing comforting, I was treated like just one more set of tasks that needed doing, part of the job, which I thought was wrong.	The nurse did not see the laboring woman as a person, as an individual in distress needing assistance and comforting. Rather, the nurse's attitude conveyed to the woman that she was an object, stripped of personhood, that required time and attention, a series of necessary tasks to be done, the demands of the job. The nurse communicated an attitude of remoteness and routine objectivity, putting forth the minimum required effort. This attitude by the nurse was viewed by the woman as not in accordance with the care expected by the laboring woman.
2. I wasn't very happy with the nurse. She wasn't very nice. I was looking for comfort and she didn't give it to me. She left me alone for long periods of time during labor.	Short and curt in communications; avoided; minimally present; only available when absolutely necessary. It wasn't what she said that wasn't nice, it was her attitude. I was looking for comfort and she didn't give it to me. Left me alone for long periods of time during labor.	The nurse withheld involvement, avoided contact physically and verbally, and was minimally present for the laboring woman so that the woman felt isolated and abandoned for long periods of time. The nurse chose to remain apart and presented herself only when absolutely necessary. The laboring woman communicated an urgent need for the nurse's presence, comfort, and caring.

Table 4–1 (*Continued*)

Quotes	Significant Statements	Themes
	Generic Noncare (Spouse)	
1. At home, he wasn't very good when I woke him because labor had begun. He was crabby and upset at first because he didn't think it was the real thing. He said, "Better be sure it's the real thing. I don't want to sit at the hospital and then go home." I cried and then he changed right away.	Acted noncaring initially at home; reluctant to undertake a possibly unnecessary trip to the hospital if there was a possibility of being sent home.	During early labor at home, the woman's spouse communicated an unwillingness to accompany her on a possibly fruitless trip to the hospital. Initially, her spouse was motivated more by a fear of possible rejection by the hospital than by his mate's need for his presence and support. The woman felt pressured to make a decision alone about whether this was "the real thing" and necessitated a trip to the hospital.

and development of themes. This process is depicted in the table for each phenomenon of the study: professional nurse care, generic (spouse) care, nurse noncare, and generic (spouse) noncare. A full description of the structure of each phenomenon was developed.

Structure of the Phenomena

Professional Nurse Care. The essence of the nurse—her presence, knowledge, and even her own body—became intimately involved with and functioned in harmony with the childbirthing woman. The nurse's entire reservoir of knowledge and experience was selectively drawn on and willingly presented to the laboring woman and her mate for the sole purpose of aiding and facilitating safe passage through labor and the birth of a healthy baby. The nurse made a deliberate choice to invest herself in caring for others, both through her own ministrations and by forming an enabling partnership with family members. Using efficacy, sensitivity, and comforting compassion, the nurse functioned with and in behalf of the woman, her mate, and the newborn.

Generic (Spouse) Care. The caring spouse was a sensitive and comforting companion, quietly protecting, present with the woman, and accepting her pain as his own. He offered her his total being, including his love and his intimate knowledge of her. He grasped any possible means of assisting her, including relieving her of responsibilities at home, collaborating with and imitating the actions of the nurse, embracing her body during birthing, and beholding their baby with awe and reverence.

Nurse Noncare. The nurse did not respond to the laboring woman as a person, as an individual in distress who needed assistance and comforting. Rather, the nurse's attitude conveyed to the woman that she was an object requiring time and attention. The laboring woman felt transformed into a thing, a burdensome obligation to be minimally dealt with. Her yearnings for authentic human presence, compassion, and tenderness were ignored by the nurse. The nurse distanced herself, not giving of herself either physically or emotionally, and seemed to deliberately withhold that which the laboring woman most craved. The attitudes and actions of the nurse resulted in the woman's feeling devalued and abandoned.

Generic (Spouse) Noncare. As her body signaled the beginnings of labor, her spouse minimized her requests for his caring support and instead focused on his own physical and emotional needs. She felt alone and unimportant.

Qualitative Evaluation Criteria

Evaluation of the data was done according to Leininger's (1985) criteria for evaluation of qualitative research. The criteria chosen were: credibility, meaning-in-context, recurrent patterning, saturation, transferability, and confirmability.

An example of the use of one of these criteria, saturation, follows. Saturation is the criterion especially pertinent to evaluation of phenomenological analysis. Saturation is achieved when words, actions, and patterns repeat, when there is no more to know. The researcher may begin to hear duplication in the informants' comments; however, additional research with a larger group of informants is necessary to provide evidence that saturation has been achieved.

DISCUSSION OF RESULTS

The nonverbal expressions and attitude of the nurse were discovered to be a crucial factor in whether the professional nurse care was interpreted by these informants as care or noncare. The caring nurses' attitudes were described as: "wonderful, pleasant, real good, considerate." Additional positive comments were: "You could tell she [the nurse] was in the profession because she wanted to be, not because it was a job." It was evident from these comments that caring expressions referred to the nonverbal attitudes of the person as well as to the overt actions. This finding is supported by Graham (cited in Stevenson and Tripp-Reimer, 1990), who declared that caring touches simultaneously on who you are and what you do.

One informant's experience of noncare from her nurse provided even stronger evidence that the attitude of the nurse was more important than the actions. The experience of noncare was described as:

> *The nurse not seeing me as a person needing comforting. . . . I was treated like just one more set of tasks that needed doing, part of the job. . . . Her attitude was cold and uncaring, not wanting to be bothered. . . . It wasn't what she said that wasn't nice, it was her attitude. . . . I was looking for comfort and she didn't give it to me.*

Watson and Ray (1988) specifically addressed the treatment of the person as an object and stated that "caring is a moral ideal that entails commitment. . . . Caring is attending and relating to a person in such a way that the person is protected from being reduced to the moral status of object" (p. 2). Riemen (1986a) also described noncaring as treating clients as objects. The findings from this study about noncare are consistent with these other researchers' results.

The failure by one nurse to maintain the dignity and personhood of one of the informants was given the assigned meaning of noncare by that informant. This finding was supported by Kitson (1987), and Swanson-Kauffman (1990). Kitson who stressed the importance of maintaining the integrity of the recipient of care. Swanson-Kauffman validated that caring preserves a person's integrity during dignity-stripping, painful, and embarrassing situations.

The informant's experience of noncare was also consistent with Forrest's (1989) research on objectification and "doing to" a client. Forrest correlated the relationship of caring and "doing to" a client with the belief system and practice of nurses. She discovered that caring involvement and interaction incorporates, on the part of the nurse, a preference for "being with" rather than "doing to" a client. Additionally, Forrest's research led her to conclude that sometimes even these caring nurses resorted to an approach that involved a focus on tasks, routines, and "doing to," as a protection when the demands of caring seemed too great. An important discovery of Forrest's research was:

> More than being physically present to a patient, a particular quality of interacting denotes caring; interaction that often develops from anticipating needs and responding to subtle cues of which the patient may not even be aware. Woven into the fabric of the essential structure of caring are the threads that affect a nurse's involvement and interaction with a patient or patient's family (p. 822).

The experience of noncare in the present research included objectification and "doing to" the woman. This treatment of the client as an object was described in the following words by the informant:

> She [the nurse] did her job, like that's all she was there for, not to see that I was comfortable, which I thought was wrong. . . . She was short and curt in her communications. . . . She only came in when absolutely necessary.

These comments are consistent with, and supported by, Forrest's (1989) findings.

The nurse whose actions and attitudes were interpreted as noncare by one informant had actually performed competently (according to the researcher's interpretation of the informant's descriptions of this nurse's actions). However, competence in practice is necessary but not sufficient to be a caring nurse. Van Hooft (1987) insisted that it is not sufficient for professional activities to be competently carried out. More important than the expertise are the motivations or attitudes underlying nursing actions:

> We can accept that the mere exercise of caring behaviors without regard to the spirit in which these activities are engaged is not adequate. . . . The manner in which nurses exercise the activities of their profession does seem to be of ethical importance and the attitudes of the nurse will be partially constitutive of the manner in which nursing is exercised. (Van Hooft, 1987, p. 34)

Roach (1987) also discussed the necessity of an attitude of compassion along with competence in professional nursing care. Roach considered compassion indispensable to caring, and stated that compassion operates from human care:

> While competence without compassion can be brutal and inhumane, compassion without competence may be no more than a meaningless, if not harmful, intrusion into the life of a person or persons needing help. (p. 61)

Griffin (1983) focused on the relationship of activities and attitudes, especially cognitive and emotional attitudes, to the concept of care:

> Before the nurse can provide care, he/she must have developed a particular way of thinking about and perceiving the situation and circumstances of the patient. Such cognitive and moral considerations—attitudes—affect the way the nurse views and responds to the patient's situation. Indeed, it is only when the cognitive and moral ideas are clearly established that the nurse can begin to understand his/her emotional involvement in the provision of care. (p. 292)

Griffin specifically linked the formation of caring attitudes to cognition, which is a key descriptor in Leininger's definition of professional nurse care and differentiates professional from generic care.

The findings from this research study are supported by the body of research cited above. The attitude of the nurse providing care and caring is critical to the client's interpretation of the meaning of the caring interventions. This finding contrasts with the conclusions of other nurse researchers. In particular, Larson (1984) discovered that clients valued technological knowledge and competence as indicators of professional nursing care in preference to psychosocial skills such as talking and listening. Brown (1986) documented that clients identify instrumental nursing behaviors as care indicators more frequently than do nurses. These discrepancies in research findings indicate a need for further study using appropriate methods. Nurses must not assume that their intended care and caring expressions will necessarily be recognized and interpreted as such by the recipient.

CONCLUSION

The nonverbal expressions and attitudes of the nurse were discovered to be a crucial factor in whether the nursing care was interpreted by these informants as care or noncare. The client assigns meanings and interprets care expressions and patterns, and nurses must examine the process of caring from the perspective of the client, not from the viewpoint of the nurse. The interpretation of this one nurse's attitude as "noncaring" validated Leininger's (1990) prediction that "if there is a discrepancy between the care provided by the nurse and care expectations of the client, stress and conflicts will result and the client will not value professional nursing care and not feel cared for" (p. 29).

This study discovered evidence indicating recognizable differences between professional nurse care and generic care and supporting Leininger's definitions of these two concepts within the Theory of Culture Care Diversity and Universality. This support can be viewed as providing an important direction for clinical practice so that nurses throughout the world can use scientific care knowledge as a firm base on which to build their practice decisions. Implementation of research-based care knowledge in clinical practice will help nurses confirm the effect their planned care has on clients.

The future of nursing everywhere depends on nurses' promoting the unique role of the nurse as the provider of exemplary care. By applying knowledge gained from this research, nurses can focus their energy and take pride in their ability to provide outstanding care. As nursing care knowledge and practice become increasingly grounded in research, the care provided by nurses to clients everywhere in our global village will result in enhanced support and prestige for the nursing profession.

Drew (1986) stated that the essence of care is still something that happens between people. A relationship of care nourishes the humanness of both the caregiver and care receiver, wherever this encounter occurs in our global environment.

REFERENCES

Anderson, S. (1986). Traditional maternity care within a biosocial framework. *International Nursing Review, 33*(4), 102–109.

Brown, L. (1986). The experience of care: Patient perspectives. *Topics in Clinical Nursing, 8,* 56–62.

Colaizzi, P. (1978). Psychological research as the phenomenologist views it. In R. Valle & M. King (Eds.), *Existential-phenomenological alternatives for psychology* (pp. 48–71). New York: Oxford University Press.

Cosminsky, S. (1978). Midwifery and medical anthropology. In B. Velimerovic (Ed.), *Modern medicine and medical anthropology in the U.S.–Mexico border population* (Scientific Publication No. 359, pp. 116–125). Washington, DC: Pan American Health Organization.

Drew, N. (1986). Exclusion and confirmation: A phenomenology of patients' experiences with caregivers. *Image: The Journal of Nursing Scholarship, 18,* 39–43.

Forrest, D. (1989). The experience of caring. *Journal of Advanced Nursing, 14,* 815–823.

Griffin, A. (1983). A philosophical analysis of caring in nursing. *Journal of Advances in Nursing, 8,* 289–295.

Kitson, A. (1987). A comparative analysis of lay-caring and professional (nursing) caring relationships. *International Journal of Nursing Studies, 24,* 155–165.

Komorita, N., Doehring, K., & Herchert, P. (1991). Perceptions of caring by nurse educators. *Journal of Nursing Education, 30,* 23–29.

Larson, P. (1984). Important nurse caring behaviors perceived by patients with cancer. *Oncology Nursing Forum, 11,* 46–50.

Leininger, M. (1981). Some philosophical, historical, and taxonomic aspects of nursing and caring in American culture. In M. Leininger (Ed.), *Caring: An essential human need* (pp. 133–143). Thorofare, NJ: Slack.

Leininger, M. (Ed.). (1985). *Qualitative research methods in nursing.* New York: Grune & Stratton.

Leininger, M. (1988a). Caring: A central focus of nursing and health care services. *Nursing and Health Care, 10,* 135–176.

Leininger, M. (Ed.). (1988b). *Care: Discovery and uses in clinical and community nursing.* Detroit: Wayne State University Press.

Leininger, M. (1990). Historic and epistemologic dimensions of care and caring with future directions. In J. Stevenson & T. Tripp-Reimer (Eds.), *Knowledge about care and caring* (pp. 19–31). New York: American Academy of Nursing.

Leininger, M. (Ed.). (1991). *Culture care diversity and universality: A theory of nursing.* New York: National League for Nursing.

Riemen, D. (1986a). Noncaring and caring in the clinical setting: Patients' descriptions. *Topics in Clinical Nursing, 8,* 30–36.

Riemen, D. (1986b). The essential structure of a caring interaction: Doing phenomenology. In P. Munhall & C. Oiler (Eds.), *Nursing Research* (pp. 85–108). Norwalk, CT: Appleton-Century-Crofts.

Roach, Sister M. (1987). *The human act of caring: A blueprint for the health professions.* Ottawa, Ontario: Canadian Hospital Association.

Stevenson, J., & Tripp-Reimer, T. (1990). *Knowledge about care and caring: State of the art and future developments.* Kansas City, MO: American Academy of Nursing.

Swanson, K. M. (1990). Providing care in the NICU: Sometimes an act of love. *Advances in Nursing Science, 13*(1), 60–73.

Swanson-Kauffman, K. M., Roberts, J., Aamodt, A., et al. (1990). *Knowledge about care and caring: State of the art and future development.* Kansas City, MO: American Nurses Association, American Academy of Nursing.

Van Hooft, S. (1987). Caring and professional commitment. *Journal of Advanced Nursing, 4,* 29–38.

Watson, J., & Ray, M. (Eds.). (1988). *The ethics of care and the ethics of cure: Synthesis in chronicity.* New York: National League for Nursing.

5

Education: One Means for Caring for Clients and Nurses in Isolated Northern Settings

Elizabeth H. Thomlinson

*C*aring, as the essence of nursing, integrates the need for the protection, strengthening, and preservation of client and family within the context of their environment. When caring for clients, nurses must be cognizant of the commonalities among all human beings while respecting the uniqueness that sets each person apart. When the client in question is the indigenous community, transcultural education becomes an essential part of any program. The prevalent medically based health care system does not foster or facilitate a transcultural approach to client care.

In many isolated areas of the Canadian north, nurses serve as primary health care providers. However, all but one of the nursing education programs in Manitoba, as in most of Canada, are urban-based and prepare nurses to function within technologically advanced health care facilities. Many of the health care interventions performed in outposts, nursing stations, and health centers are beyond the curriculum objectives of these programs. When nurses practice in remote settings, both clients and nurses become discouraged because neither group's needs are met if nurses lack required clinical skills and knowledge of their clientele. Often, a result of this frustration is high nurse turnover and discontinuous provision of health care. One tribal council translated caring into the need for an education program that would provide clinical skills and cultural education for nurses who provide primary health care in remote settlements in northern Canada.

This chapter reviews the historical context and health care issues of the aboriginal peoples of Canada, which resulted in the lobby for a nursing baccalaureate program in northern Manitoba. The program, adapted from the undergraduate program on the main campus of the University of Manitoba, provides additional clinical courses in conjunction with enhanced cultural content. This description of the first offering of the program examines course content as it relates to facilitating student success in the northern settings.

THE CONCEPT OF CARE

The focus of nursing care has been the amelioration of illness-oriented needs. Several nursing theorists have identified caring as an essential human need covering the life span (Benner & Wrubel, 1989; Leininger, 1988). Caring is considered the necessary component, the essence, of professional nursing. Leininger (1988) noted that caring behaviors and needs are culture-specific. To provide appropriate care, nurses would then require "culturally based knowledge and skills for efficaciousness" (Leininger, 1988, p. 6). Culturally sensitive and responsive care necessitates that the caregiver be aware that each response to a situation or illness is affected by the culture of the individual receiving the care. However, this awareness alone is not sufficient to prepare health care workers to care for their clients. There remains a need to delve more deeply into the effect of the cultural beliefs and practices, beyond the cognizance that culture has an impact on persons and families.

According to Leininger (1988), professional nursing care is a learned process to help or enable individuals, families, and communities, through culturally specific means, to improve or maintain as favorable a life or death as possible (p. 9). Key components of the definition are: *learned, culturally specific*, and *means* or "processes, techniques, and patterns" (p. 9). To effect this definition, nurses would require education incorporating not only clinical skills but knowledge about how culture affects care.

The multicultural nature of Canada is well-recognized. In nursing education, all too often, vague concepts of multiculturalism are taught and it is assumed that these principles are sufficient to be applied across cultures. Leininger (1990) noted that "cultural factors of ethical care are conspicuously missing in most nurses' curricula and clinical decisions" (p. 51). The differences in values and beliefs as they govern behavior within each culture often are addressed only in limited fashion in nursing education (Toumishey, 1991). Practice issues that result from the lack of awareness and consideration of these differences may create barriers between nurses and the clients with whom they are working.

Nurses practice from their own cultural perspective—a major factor of which they are often unaware (Leininger, 1988). The inherent beliefs and values that nurses develop, not only from their ethnic background but also from within the culture of "nursing," must be understood and shared with clients.

An issue important to nursing practice within aboriginal communities is the nurses' lack of awareness of traditional healing methods. Leininger (1988) noted that there is a need to link traditional and professional caregiving practices (p. 52). To prepare nurses to collaborate with aboriginal community members in the development of health care programs, it is imperative that the nurses develop an appreciation for elders and healers and a willingness to incorporate them into the system.

The cultural component of care is one factor within the broad concept of care, which includes commitment, knowledge and skill, the need to preserve the honor of those for whom care is provided (Clarke & Wheeler, 1992), and responsibility and regard for the patient (Gaut, 1983). Although a greater emphasis in nursing education has been placed on the psychosocial aspects of care, to the detriment of biological/medical care (Drew, 1988), patients continue to emphasize the importance of the latter content (von Essen & Sjoden, 1991). Before nurses can feel confident in their caring, they must acquire the knowledge and skills to encompass both realities, the physical and the psychosocial.

HISTORICAL CONTEXT

The approximately one million aboriginal peoples who comprise 4 percent of the population of Canada encompass (1) status Indians who are registered with an Indian band; (2) nonstatus Indians who have lost registered status; (3) Metis, who are descendants of mixed marriages between aboriginal women and French fur traders; and (4) Inuit of the Arctic. In 1986, of the 403,000 status Indians in Canada, about two-thirds lived on reserves. The remainder lived off reserves, mainly in urban centers. The aboriginal peoples of Canada are actively pursuing a course to change the physical and cultural devastation that misguided governmental policies of the past three centuries have inflicted on them through a recurring pattern of disintegration and dislocation of entire communities.

Paternalistic and ethnocentric policies and administrations governed interactions with aboriginal peoples for over 200 years. The nonaboriginal population has pursued greater wealth through mining, flooding for hydroelectric power, and logging, all of which led to the demise of the traditional way of life, hunting and fishing. The national and provincial governments denied that problems existed and delayed compensation while the economy in aboriginal communities floundered. Forced relocations resulted in social disorganization, a loss of culture, and a high incidence of substance abuse (Siggner, 1988). A paternalistic attitude has resulted in the imposition of programs on aboriginal communities without consultation or consideration of cultural relevance (Clayton, 1991).

In the late nineteenth and early twentieth centuries, Canadian Indian Affairs encouraged aboriginal people to become full Canadian citizens by giving up their ties to the aboriginal community (Gibbins & Ponting, 1988). Although the policy of assimilation into mainstream society persisted over a number of decades, the aboriginal peoples faced discrimination that rejected their integration into the dominant society. Of greater importance is the fact the aboriginal peoples resisted the total annihilation of their culture and way of life.

A major loss of language and traditional life skills, which further separated children from their families, occurred when the Canadian Indian Act of 1920 made school attendance compulsory. Because small isolated communities did not have schools, many children were sent to residential schools where they were prevented from speaking their native language. Those who survived the education system, however, were not allowed to attend school past the age of sixteen. This policy controlled access to higher education, and, as a result, the children fit in neither arena; they could not survive by using traditional skills and they were not allowed to obtain higher education. Child sexual and physical abuse, perpetrated in many residential schools (York, 1989), resulted in long-term social consequences that are only now beginning to be addressed.

The aboriginal peoples have had no control of education, justice, health care, and child welfare systems in their communities. Day-to-day management decisions on reserves required approval from Canadian Indian Affairs. The pursuit of aboriginal self-government, as yet not fully defined, is favored by many Canadians (Gibbins & Ponting, 1988). Negotiations continue toward this end.

Loss of self-esteem, poverty, denigration, and destruction of their cultures are common to aboriginal peoples around the world. The common goal of self-determination is shared by native Hawaiians, native Americans, and the aboriginal peoples of Canada, Australia, New Zealand, and South America. Aboriginal controlled schools, in which native languages are taught, produce increasing numbers of secondary school graduates. Education is viewed as the primary means for any peoples to become self-reliant.

In this entire process, it must be noted that the reserve lands set aside for aboriginal peoples have been too small to support the traditional way of life of hunting and fishing and too infertile for farming. Several recent large land-claim settlements are slowly reversing this situation. However, infrastructure deficiencies regarding roads, water supplies, sewage, housing, and garbage disposal have contributed to health care problems in the populations and have not yet been adequately addressed.

HEALTH ISSUES

Despite increased spending for health care, at a level that may exceed the Canadian population at large (Young, 1988, p. 126), socioeconomic conditions contribute to health care problems in aboriginal peoples (York, 1989). A comparison of selected causes of death among registered Indians and the total Canadian population showed that aboriginal peoples have three times the death rate due to accidents, poisoning, and violence, and twice the death rate due to infections and parasitic diseases. Substance abuse contributes to a murder rate four times as high as in the general population and a suicide rate that may be six times higher (York, 1989, p. 97). These rates are comparable to Native American peoples, among whom accidental deaths related to substance abuse are four to thirteen times the national rate (Ivey & Duyan, 1991; Larson, 1991).

Many small isolated communities are microcosms of the process of dislocation and self-destruction common to indigenous peoples around the world. Gasoline sniffing, which is one of the most dangerous addictions in the world, is an endemic problem in the Canadian north and is prevalent even in young children (York, 1989, p. 9). Gasoline sniffing is associated with permanent damage to the nervous system, the brain, the kidneys, and the liver. It has been suggested that 70 percent of children in northern Manitoba have sniffed gasoline. These problems are not unique to Canada: studies have found that 40 percent of American Indian youths and 20 percent of Australian northern territory aboriginal children have tried inhalants

(York, 1989, p. 17). In these regions, between 60 and 70 percent of juvenile crime is associated with sniffing. In addition, the escalation of substance abuse of drugs ranging from alcohol to "crack" and cocaine is occurring at a phenomenal rate. In an attempt to combat these problems, aboriginal people are demanding the control of their health care.

Despite major problems, the Canadian model of health care delivery to remote and isolated communities is recognized as one of the most comprehensive in the world (Young, 1988, p. 135). Health care facilities, communication systems, and transportation are technically superior to those of other nations. The shift to community participation and self-reliance is a necessary step to promote community development. Young (1988) noted that, despite the ineffectiveness of the medical system in reducing morbidity and mortality, the "'caring' role—in providing relief for pain and anxiety, reassurance, comfort and sympathy" remains important (p. 135). McLean (1991) suggested there is little evidence that the health of a community is improved by more frequent physician visits or technologically advanced facilities. A change in health status begins when members have input into the development and implementation of health care programs, as will transpire under devolution of health care by health transfer to local Indian band control (Connell, Flett, & Stewart, 1991). This shift from professional control of health care services to community control creates a focus on local strengths and builds programs based on local needs (Eng, Salmon, & Mullan, 1992). Health care professionals must be educated to assist individuals and communities to take control of their own needs and to seek solutions concurrently. This process requires the acknowledgment by health care professionals that they are not omnipotent decision makers but partners in change.

According to Flynn (1988), nurses working with community members to solve problems identified by the community members will be better able to promote health and community self-reliance. Education in the health transfer process, in political systems, and in community assessment enables nurses to participate in the empowerment of community members long accustomed to the imposition of programs. The integration and involvement of local persons and resources enhance community acceptance and ownership.

PROGRAM BACKGROUND

As early as 1982, The Pas Indian Band and the Swampy Cree Tribal Council (SCTC), in Manitoba, recognized that, for the health transfer process to succeed, aboriginal persons educated in the health care professions were needed (Stewart, 1986; Thomlinson, Gregory, & Larsen, 1991). At that time, there were approximately 200 aboriginal health care professionals throughout the entire country. A positive change is demonstrated by current statistics: among the 200,000 nurses in Canada, it is estimated there are now 350 aboriginal nurses. Nurses practicing in the north often experience cultural shock and physical and psychological isolation from family, friends, and colleagues. They may lack the clinical skills required for primary health care delivery, and supervision and assistance may be hundreds of miles away by telephone. Canitz (1991) found that because of work pressures and limited social contacts, nurses are frequently unable to build social support systems in local communities.

These problems have resulted in high nurse turnover with a resultant lack of opportunity to build long-term health promotion and prevention programs. The SCTC postulated that aboriginal nurses educated at the baccalaureate level would not experience the same culture shock and would remain in communities to provide health care over a longer term. This health care provision would include the active participation of community members in a comprehensive process.

THE PROGRAM

The Northern Bachelor of Nursing Program (NBNP) was instituted to meet the following objectives:

1. To provide aboriginal nurses, who are to comprise at a minimum one-half the student body, with a baccalaureate education;
2. To integrate traditional healing and culture-specific education in the program;
3. To include advanced assessment and clinical skills within the curriculum.

The conceptual framework on which the NBNP was based focused on providing to individuals and families, within their communities, care by nurses possessing the skills and knowledge that strengthened their abilities to develop long-term community commitments. This conceptual framework included content that specifically addressed isolated, northern, and cultural aspects of care within a baccalaureate program that integrated theory, research, and practice and was commensurate with programs throughout Canada.

Viewed in its broadest context, caring may be considered to include not only the client population but the nurses themselves. The baccalaureate program as it meets the educational and cultural care and knowledge needs of nurses will benefit both clients and nurses. Nurses who have additional clinical skills and culture-specific knowledge are better able to care for clients and, in turn, are better equipped to cope with the exigencies of their tasks. According to Nyberg (1989), the concept of caring requires that caring persons develop strong self-esteem, feel cared for within their personal and professional lives, and recognize that they are able to offer something to others through the caring process. An interest in others develops, through knowledge, into a commitment to work with, and to assist, the others toward growth. Employers carry a responsibility to support and provide additional educational opportunities for nursing staff. Nurses must be confident that they are able to bring a unique perspective to the overall development of health in a community.

Curriculum

Patients, community members, nurses, and educators have recognized that nurses need expanded clinical skills if they are to perform as front-line workers. To address this area, courses in primary health care skills and applied therapeutics, based on a thorough foundation of health assessment, were developed. Nurses must assess not only the health of individuals but also of the communities in which they practice. This assessment provides them with the background necessary for assisting the community in program development.

Within the courses in the NBNP are imbedded the aboriginal holistic perspective of health that includes the mind, the body, and the spirit. The community and the individuals are inextricably linked; one does not function without the other. Community assessments and practice recognize that hospital-based care—the curing model—is not adequate to address needs. Acute care provides "stopgap" measures until the sources of the problem— environmental issues (sewage/water/housing), poverty, and the lack of educational and employment opportunities—are addressed. Students' completed assessments of local communities are returned to leaders in the community for use in health care planning. This process is beginning to develop a connection between students and the community leaders, who see a practical benefit from what has often been merely an academic exercise for students.

Because demands on nurses' time are so great at stations, there is little opportunity to meet the nurses' own needs (Canitz, 1991). A result is that nurses often withdraw and insulate themselves from the community. Caring for the self is primary to building internal resources to care for others. The issue of recognizing and allowing for a need for personal time is important because many of the nurses carry multiple roles and responsibilities. Affirmation of this principle is integrated in several courses in the program.

The knowledge and skills to effect change through the enhancement of others' potential is integrated in several courses. This component is based on the premise (in opposition to paternalism) that the "other"—the community and its members—is a partner capable of growth and change, not a child requiring care and protection. Information on political processes, leadership theory, and empowerment is emphasized to aid nurses in challenging the status quo of the health care system and in interacting and collaborating with community members and political leaders in the health care system at large.

Aboriginal history in relation to Western dominance and influence forms the basis for native studies. Traditional medicine, rituals (including songs and dance), and art are taught at a primary level and offer a beginning cognizance of the breadth and depth of aboriginal culture. The opportunity to participate in sweetgrass and sweat lodge ceremonies occurs during the cultural camp held each fall and in the term of Introductory Native Studies.

The curriculum, however, would be remiss if content were limited to geographic and culture-specific content. Issues affecting nursing globally, nationally, and provincially form one course. A professor in this course has incorporated content that challenges students to analyze how their own history and culture influence their view of issues and health, and then to share their perspectives with their colleagues.

Student Body

Students within the program bring diverse backgrounds and skills developed during one to twenty-two years in nursing practice. Some have worked in nursing stations in northern Manitoba as well as the Arctic; others have practiced in rural and urban settings. Most are attending a university while balancing family and work obligations.

The students share a number of common goals:

1. They all intend to remain in the north.
2. They are seeking further education because they have identified:
    a. a lack of requisite clinical skills,
    b. a desire to increase their knowledge of aboriginal culture,
    c. a need for increased community assessment capability,

d. a wish to become participants in change by increasing their
skills and abilities.

The students are cognizant that learning is a lifelong process. Within the
context of the nursing program, they will only begin their learning of traditional health practices and of aboriginal political processes. As one of the
healers noted, the students must remain open to continued learning and
growth. Interaction with aboriginal healers and elders provides the opportunity for a variety of experiences. As guest lecturers, local political and administrative personnel share their knowledge and perceptions of health care
delivery and community management with students.

Collegial networks are being established within the student body. In the
future, these networks may provide professional and social support when
the graduates spread throughout the north. Jennings (1987) noted that people who experience support are better able to withstand stresses. Knowing
that one can seek assistance from others who share a common educational
and occupational background will be invaluable.

CONCLUSION

It is anticipated that the graduates of the Northern Bachelor of Nursing
Program (NBNP) will be more than providers of care and educators in
health promotion and disease prevention. They will be expected to collaborate in the holistic planning and integration of community health care with
community members and political leaders.

Morse (1992) proposed that the concept of nursing practice is the provision of comfort to clients. The concept of comfort is not broad enough to
include the tasks the nurses graduating from the NBNP will be called on
to perform, particularly with the challenge of change in the current health
care delivery system. Morse, Bottorff, Neander, and Solberg (1991) suggested that caring should be divided into separate and disparate behavioral
outcomes. Caring demonstrated in the indigenous communities must include the total person, the family, and the community. Therefore, caring as
envisioned in the NBNP is a more pervasive whole that embraces strategic
planning, political action, and community leadership, as well as individual
supportive behaviors. The interconnectedness of these behaviors may pre-
clude analysis or description of discrete behavioral outcomes.

As nurses learn culture-specific care, there is an obligation on employers,
community members, and coworkers to educate and assist the nurses in this

process. If communities expect nurses to "know" or to learn through their own means the culture of a specific group/region/community, the responsibility rests on one side. A mutual teaching/learning would benefit both sides. The opportunity to teach health care professionals about one's culture is empowering to the community while at the same time valuable in providing the professionals with new insights into the skills and abilities of the teachers.

If nurses are not taught in curricula culture-specific values/beliefs/models, there must rest on all of us an onus to seek information but also an obligation to share. One cannot expect culturally appropriate care without the obligation to teach. This obligation rests not only with the dominant society but also with the culture being served. Members of the communities served by SCTC have accepted this obligation. They not only participated in the education of health care professionals but were the proactive thinkers and lobbyists who promoted the need for such a program. It is hoped that, as self-determination becomes entrenched, other communities throughout the world will participate in this education.

REFERENCES

Benner, P., & Wrubel, J. (1989). *The primacy of caring: Stress and coping in health and illness.* Menlo Park, CA: Addison-Wesley.

Canitz, B. (1991). Health care in crisis: Understanding nursing turnover in northern Canada. In B. D. Postl, P. Gilbert, J. Goodwill, N. E. K. Moffatt, J. D. O'Neil, P. A. Sarsfield, & T. K. Young (Eds.), *Circumpolar Health 90, Proceedings of the 8th International Congress on Circumpolar Health* (pp. 177–80). Winnipeg: University of Manitoba Press.

Clarke, J. B., & Wheeler, S. J. (1992). A view of the phenomenon of caring in nursing practice. *Journal of Advanced Nursing, 17,* 1283–1290.

Clayton, H. J. (1991). Indian health and community development: Notes for an address. In B. D. Postl, P. Gilbert, J. Goodwill, N. E. K. Moffatt, J. D. O'Neil, P. A. Sarsfield, & T. K. Young (Eds.), *Circumpolar Health 90, Proceedings of the 8th International Congress on Circumpolar Health* (pp. 42–43). Winnipeg: University of Manitoba Press.

Connell, G., Flett, R., & Stewart, P. (1991). Implementing primary health care through community control: The experience of the Swampy Cree Tribal Council. In B. D. Postl, P. Gilbert, J. Goodwill, N. E. K. Moffatt, J. D. O'Neil, P. A. Sarsfield, & T. K. Young (Eds.), *Circumpolar Health*

90, *Proceedings of the 8th International Congress on Circumpolar Health* (pp. 44–46). Winnipeg: University of Manitoba Press.

Drew, B. J. (1988). Devaluation of biological knowledge. *Image: The Journal of Nursing Scholarship, 20,* 25–27.

Eng, E., Salmon, M. E., & Mullan, F. (1992). Community empowerment: The critical base for primary health care. *Family Community Health, 15*(1), 1–12.

Flynn, B. C. (1988). The caring community: Primary health care and nursing in England and the United States. In M. Leininger (Ed.), *Care: Discovery and uses in clinical and community nursing* (pp. 29–38). Detroit: Wayne State University Press.

Gaut, D. (1983). Development of a theoretically adequate description of caring. *Western Journal of Nursing Research, 5,* 313–324.

Gibbins, R., & Ponting, J. R. (1988). Historical overview and background. In J. R. Ponting (Ed.), *Arduous journey: Canadian Indians and decolonization* (pp. 18–56) Toronto: McLelland & Stewart.

Ivey, G. H., & Duyan, K. R. (1991). The Alaska area native health service: Improving the health status of the native people of Alaska. In B. D. Postl, P. Gilbert, J. Goodwill, N. E. K. Moffatt, J. D. O'Neil, P. A. Sarsfield, & T. K. Young (Eds.), *Circumpolar Health 90, Proceedings of the 8th International Congress on Circumpolar Health* (pp. 66–69). Winnipeg: University of Manitoba Press.

Jennings, B. M. (1987). Climate of caring. *Nursing Administration Quarterly, 11*(4), 63–71.

Larson, K. (1991). The evolution of a village-based health education project. In B. D. Postl, P. Gilbert, J. Goodwill, N. E. K. Moffatt, J. D. O'Neil, P. A. Sarsfield, & T. K. Young (Eds.), *Circumpolar Health 90, Proceedings of the 8th International Congress on Circumpolar Health* (pp. 153–158). Winnipeg: University of Manitoba Press.

Leininger, M. M. (1988). Care: The essence of nursing and health. In M. Leininger (Ed.), *Care: The essence of nursing and health* (pp. 3–16). Detroit: Wayne State University Press.

Leininger, M. M. (1988). Caring: A central focus of nursing and health care services. In M. Leininger (Ed.), *Care: The essence of nursing and health* (pp. 45–59). Detroit: Wayne State University Press.

Leininger, M. (1990). Culture: The conspicuous missing link to understand ethical and moral dimensions of care. In M. Leininger (Ed.), *Ethical and moral dimensions of care* (pp. 49–66). Detroit: Wayne State University Press.

McLean, C. L. (1991). The health status of communities employing paraprofessional indigenous community health workers as the primary health care providers. In B. D. Postl, P. Gilbert, J. Goodwill, N. E. K. Moffatt, J. D. O'Neil, P. A. Sarsfield, & T. K. Young (Eds.), *Circumpolar Health 90, Proceedings of the 8th International Congress on Circumpolar Health* (pp. 170–172). Winnipeg: University of Manitoba Press.

Morse, J. (1992). Comfort: The refocusing of nurse care. *Clinical Nursing Research, 1*(1), 91–106.

Morse, J., Bottorff, J., Neander, N., & Solberg, S. (1991). Comparative analysis of conceptualizations and theories of caring. *Image: The Journal of Nursing Scholarship, 23*(2), 119–126.

Nyberg, J. (1989). The element of caring in nursing administration. *Nursing Administration Quarterly, 13*(3), 9–16.

Siggner, A. J. (1988). The socio-demographic conditions of registered Indians. In J. R. Ponting (Ed.), *Arduous journey: Canadian Indians and decolonization* (pp. 57–83). Toronto: McLelland & Stewart.

Stewart, P. (1986). *Swampy Cree Tribal Council, Bachelor of Nursing Feasibility Study Report.* Unpublished report.

Thomlinson, E., Gregory, D., & Larsen, J. (1991). The Northern Bachelor of Nursing Program: One solution to problems in health care provision. In B. D. Postl, P. Gilbert, J. Goodwill, N. E. K. Moffatt, J. D. O'Neil, P. A. Sarsfield, & T. K. Young (Eds.), *Circumpolar Health 90, Proceedings of the 8th International Congress on Circumpolar Health* (pp. 145–148). Winnipeg: University of Manitoba Press.

Toumishey, H. (1991). *Report of the multicultural health curriculum project committee,* Downsview, Ontario: Canadian Council on Multicultural Health.

von Essen, L., & Sjoden, P. (1991). Patient and staff perceptions of caring: Review and replication. *Journal of Advanced Nursing, 16,* 1363–1374.

York, G. (1989). *The dispossessed: Life and death in Native Canada.* Toronto: Lester, Orpen and Dennys.

Young, T. K. (1988). *Health and cultural change: The Indian experience in the central subarctic.* Toronto: University of Toronto Press.

6

Care: What It Means to Lithuanian Americans

Rauda Gelazis

This study focused on caring within a distinct cultural group in the United States: Lithuanian Americans. In 1990, Lithuania came into prominence when the nation declared its independence for the second time in this century. Lithuania and the other Baltic countries, Estonia and Latvia, came to the attention of the world in their dramatic struggle for freedom from Soviet oppression. Nurses have become aware of the country but few may have an understanding of the Lithuanian culture and people. Caring has been studied in various cultural groups, but no one to date has considered caring in this particular group.

LITHUANIAN AMERICANS: HISTORICAL BACKGROUND

The Lithuanian American people studied came to the United States between 1949 and 1951. Lithuania had been an independent nation from

1918 to 1940. During World War II, Lithuania was taken over by Russia and was forcibly annexed to the Union of Soviet Socialist Republics (U.S.S.R.). When the communist regime took over, all private ownership was eliminated. Hundreds of thousands of Lithuanians, along with Estonians and Latvians, were killed. Still others were deported to U.S.S.R. prison camps in Siberia. Under communist rule, most people were suspect, especially if they had positions of authority, were educated, or owned any property. Those who could, escaped to the West. As a result, approximately 800,000 Lithuanians are in exile in various free countries throughout the world. There are about 650,000 Lithuanians in the United States, living mostly in industrial and metropolitan centers in the East and Midwest. Lithuanians also live in Brazil, Argentina, Uruguay, Canada, Great Britain, and Australia (Alilunas, 1978).

In 1990, Lithuania regained its freedom. When the Soviet Union began its policy of openness (*glasnost*) during 1988, Lithuania began to work for its freedom. On March 11, 1990, the official Act of the Restoration of the Lithuanian State was signed, declaring independence from the Soviet Union. When the Soviet Union was finally dissolved in late 1991, the United States, the United Kingdom, and other countries officially recognized Lithuania as a sovereign nation. Russia, however, continues to try to maintain its hold on Lithuania. Even today, 300,000 Russian troops are stationed in Lithuania and the other Baltic countries (Sliesoriunas, 1991). Russia, reluctant to pull these troops out, continues to send new replacements for those whose tour of duty has ended. Lithuania is working toward a market economy under a democratic form of government. The various changes occurring in Lithuania were closely followed by the Lithuanian American subjects of this study.

PURPOSE OF STUDY

I studied Lithuanian Americans in a field study and doctoral dissertation for the purposes of (1) describing, analyzing, and interpreting the experiences, expressions, and meanings of care from their worldview, social structure, language, and environmental contexts; and (2) determining whether a relationship exists among care, well-being, and humor, from the emic perspective of the Lithuanian American.

RESEARCH QUESTIONS

The research questions related to care were:

1. What are the experiences, expressions, meanings, and patterns of care to Lithuanian Americans, as influenced by their particular environmental contexts?
2. Are there, for Lithuanian Americans, any interrelationships among care, well-being, and humor?

THEORETICAL FRAMEWORK

The theoretical framework for this study is Leininger's Theory of Cultural Care Diversity and Universality (1988b). Leininger's theory, model, and ethnonursing research method were developed and used within a qualitative, naturalistic perspective to study culture care. Leininger's theory of culture care holds that care is central to nursing. The theory's goal is "to provide cultural congruent nursing care" or care that fits with the client's culture and lifeway (Leininger, 1988b, p. 155). In order to achieve this goal, Leininger (1991) predicted three dominant modes to guide nursing:

1. Cultural care maintenance or preservation (care that helps to preserve clients' values and health care beliefs).
2. Cultural care accommodation (care that attempts to adapt to clients' values and health care beliefs).
3. Cultural care restructuring and repatterning (care in which some change in clients' beliefs and actions is needed).

Leininger (1991) identified care as essential to the growth, well-being, and survival of human beings. Ideas about care and well-being are embedded in the worldview and social structures of particular cultural groups (Leininger, 1978). Leininger developed the Sunrise Model (see Figure 1–1) to depict the various aspects of worldview, culture, and social structure dimensions that influence care and health through the cultural contexts identified. Cultural and social structure dimensions include technological factors, religious and philosophical factors, kinship and social factors, cultural values and lifeways, political and legal factors, economic factors, and educational factors

(Leininger, 1991). These factors influence and, in turn, are influenced by care expressions, patterns, and practices, and by health or well-being, as can be seen by the two-way arrows in the model. In this study, the Sunrise Model was used as the basis for assessing important elements of the social structure and worldview of Lithuanian Americans.

ASSUMPTIONS

The assumptions underlying this investigation were as follows:

1. Care is defined, experienced, and expressed according to the Lithuanian American culture.
2. Care is embedded in and is an integral part of the worldview and environmental context.
3. Culturally congruent nursing care can be achieved by a thorough knowledge of the lifeways and culture of a people.

These assumptions relate directly to the theoretical framework for this study and are based on Leininger's conceptualization of person within a culturally diverse environment.

ORIENTATIONAL DEFINITIONS

This research was done under the qualitative research paradigm, therefore orientational definitions (Leininger, 1988c) are appropriate rather than the operational definitions used in the quantitative research paradigm. Orientational definitions give an orientation or direction that indicates the starting point of the inquiry, but they may change as the research progresses and new information is discovered. The orientational definitions for this study were:

Care (noun) refers to phenomena related to assisting, supportive, or enabling behavior toward or for another individual (or group) with evident or anticipated needs, to ameliorate or improve a human condition or lifeway (Leininger, 1988b, p. 156).

Cultural care refers to the cognitively known values, beliefs, and patterned expressions that assist, support, or enable another individual or group to maintain well-being, improve a human condition or lifeway, or face death or disabilities (Leininger, 1988b, p. 156).

Culturally congruent care refers to a meaningful fit of creatively designed nursing decisions and actions with the lifeways of individuals, families, or groups, thereby providing meaningful, satisfying, and beneficial care to clients (Leininger, 1988b, p. 155; 1988c, p. 27).

Emic refers to the "inside view," using language and actions of the people of a particular group or culture (Leininger, 1988b).

Etic refers to the external, more universal, and generalized view (Leininger, 1988b).

Lithuanian American refers to a person who was born in Lithuania and now lives in the United States; one whose parent or parents are Lithuanian; or one who identifies himself or herself as a Lithuanian American.

SIGNIFICANCE OF THE STUDY

This investigation is important to nursing because it helped to discover and describe the dimensions of care for Lithuanian Americans. To date, very little has been written about this culture. As more is known about it, appropriate culturally congruent nursing care for Lithuanian Americans can be planned and given in light of the values and social structure contexts held by this group of people.

REVIEW OF LITERATURE

Nurses have been interested in care and caring since the beginning of nursing itself (Valentine, 1988). Care is a basic part of being human; it is viewed by nurse theorists such as Watson, Leininger, and others, as central to nursing, but care has not been researched in nursing until recent decades.

Nurse scholars have studied care from various perspectives. Philosophical consideration and investigation of care and caring have focused on the identification of the nature of care and caring. Gaut, for example, developed the philosophical analysis of caring by starting with a conceptual analysis of caring (1981) and later proposing a philosophical method for studying caring (1984) in order that nurses might achieve a comprehensive, penetrating, and flexible understanding of the concept of caring. Ray (1981) also did a concept analysis of caring from a more metaphysical perspective. Other scholars who have identified the attributes of care are Mayeroff (1971), Carper (1979), Gaylin (1976), Riemen (1983, 1986), and Noddings (1984). More recently, nurse scholars have expanded the philosophical foundations of the knowledge of care by developing an ethics of caring (Fry, 1989, 1990; Gadow, 1987; Pellegrino, 1985; Yarling & McElmurry, 1986).

Nurse researchers have also studied care, formally and informally, from the vantage point of care in nursing practice (Benner & Wrubel, 1989). Nursing literature contains examples of nurses' differentiations of care in nursing from care in other professions. For example, Weiss (1986, 1988) differentiated nurses' from physicians' perceptions of caring. Morrison (1989) described a British study of nurses' perceptions of themselves as professional carers. Research has also been done in a continuing attempt to better assess care in nursing practice. Larson (1981, 1987), for example, studied cancer patients' and nurses' perceptions of caring and developed a tool, the CARE-Q, for the assessment of caring. Wolf (1986) developed the CBI (Caring Behavior Inventory) to identify nurses' caring behaviors.

Fry (1990) pointed out that the nursing literature on the study of care and caring can be grouped into three models that illustrate how thought about care and caring phenomena has developed from different perspectives. The three models of caring are the humanistic, feminist, and cultural models. The humanistic model of caring includes Watson's (1985, 1988) humanistic nursing theory, in which she emphasizes the caring occasion as central in the nurse–patient encounter. Watson's carative factors (1979) are given as guidelines for nursing interventions. Another example of the humanistic model of caring is that of Patterson and Zderad (1988).

The feminist model of caring is theoretically based on ethics and social psychology and stresses the ethics and morality of gender-related caring. Noddings' (1984) work is an example of the feminist model of care. In recent years, more interest in this model has become evident. Fry (1989) saw the need for developing a model of caring as a nursing ethic that is broader and is free of the limitations of the biomedical model of ethics, which is still common today.

The cultural model of caring was developed from anthropological and sociological studies of care. Leininger (1991) and others have developed the transcultural nursing approach to care knowledge. In this model, humanistic and scientific caring behaviors, values, and expressions are seen as present in all cultures but expressed differently according to each culture. Numerous scientific studies have been done to systematically discover the caring phenomenon in various cultures. Leininger (1991) has studied over forty-five cultures and has discovered care meanings and expressions in her research. Other studies of care include: Horn's study of the Muckleshoot people (1978), Boyle's study of caring practices in a Guatemalan population (1984), Aamodt's study of care in children and adolescents in the Papago Indian culture in Arizona (1978), Wenger's identification of care in an Old Order Amish group (1988), and Luna's study of care in three contexts among Lebanese Arab-American Muslims (1989). This study of care in a Lithuanian American population follows in this tradition and fills a knowledge gap about Lithuanian Americans.

RESEARCH METHODS

The ethnonursing research method under a qualitative research paradigm was the primary method used in this study. Leininger (1985a, 1985b, 1991) developed this method to systematically document, describe, explain, and interpret transcultural nursing phenomena such as cultural care. Ethnonursing is defined as "the study and analysis of the local or indigenous peoples' viewpoints, beliefs, and practices about nursing care behavior and processes of designated cultures" (Leininger, 1985b, p. 38).

SETTING

The setting for this study was a metropolitan area in the Midwest that has a Lithuanian American population of approximately 12,000. The setting was selected because the numbers of Lithuanian Americans are large enough to help them maintain their cultural identity. The natural setting of informants' homes was used when possible. A full cultural context can be appreciated in natural settings and a truer picture can be obtained of informants' lifeways (Spradley, 1980).

Because I speak, read, and write the Lithuanian language, elderly Lithuanian Americans who did not have a good command of the English language found it easy to talk with me. My knowledge of the language and culture also helped to gain the trust of informants. My Lithuanian background had the above advantages, but also had some disadvantages, such as bias; these were kept under check via the use of a mentor and field notes.

INFORMANTS

As Werner and Schoepfle (1987), Spradley (1980), and Lincoln and Guba (1985) have indicated, informants should be persons involved and well-versed in their culture and able to communicate their knowledge to a researcher. Lincoln and Guba (1985) pointed out that informants are sought until there is redundancy, that is, until no new information is obtained and previously learned material is repeated. Leininger (1988a) advised that because informants represent a broad part of the culture to be studied, persons of various ages, sexes, and professions need to be selected.

Key informants are those who are most knowledgeable about the phenomenon and culture to be studied; general informants, who are also well-informed about the culture, help to verify general information given by key informants (Leininger, 1988a). Usually, about twelve to fifteen key informants (Leininger, 1991) are considered to be a desired number, while twice that number of general informants is used. In this study, there were twelve key informants and sixteen general informants, for a total of twenty-eight informants. The key informants selected were known to be knowledgeable about their culture and able to verbalize their knowledge. The general informants also had a good knowledge of and familiarity with the culture, but were interviewed only once. Both key and general informants represented a variety of ages, sexes, and generations, identified themselves as Lithuanian or Lithuanian American, and lived in the selected Lithuanian American community. The key informants provided in-depth knowledge of the culture; the general informants helped to substantiate the data through their broad, general knowledge of the culture. A general interview guideline was followed, but interviews were open-ended in order to gather as much informant information as possible. Informed written consent was obtained from all informants.

OBSERVATION PARTICIPATION

Spradley (1980) and Leininger (1985a), among others, have suggested that in-depth informant interviewing is best for research when it is closely integrated with participant observation. Leininger's (1985b) suggested moving from primarily observation (when first entering the field) to observation with some participation and finally to primarily participation with some observation. Leininger's (1985b) and Spradley's (1980) suggestions and guidelines for participant observation in research were initially considered, and Leininger's (1985b, p. 52) four phases of observation were finally followed:

1. Primarily observation.
2. Primarily observation with some participation.
3. Primarily participation with some observation.
4. Reflective observation as the researcher prepares to withdraw from the field.

Activities that proved useful to observe included church religious and social functions, meetings of some of the organizations in the Lithuanian American community, social events related to special events, Lithuanian holiday observations, and similar occasions.

DATA ANALYSIS

Data were analyzed in this ethnonursing study by means of the Leininger four-phase method of analysis (Leininger, 1988a). Themes and patterns related to care expression in daily life, and patterns of care in the Lithuanian American community were identified. The suggested sequential format and steps for thematic and pattern analysis of nursing and ethnonursing data given by Leininger (1991) were used. This four-step process (see Figure 6–1) begins with the identification and listing of cognitive data, combines related data and patterns into meaningful units, moves to formatting themes or pattern statements to test or reaffirm, and ends with the use of confirmed themes in decision making and intervening.

The computer software that is now available (the Leininger–Templin–Thompson program for coding and classifying data) was used throughout this study. The use of a computer program facilitated the long and tedious process of dealing with a large amount of data. (In qualitative research, the data analysis process is an ongoing process throughout the study.)

The following evaluation criteria for qualitative studies were used in this study: credibility or the "truth value" of findings; confirmability or auditability; meaning-in-context or the avoidance of context stripping; recurrent patterning or repetition of themes and patterns; saturation (when all data are taken in about a phenomenon); redundancy or repetition of ideas; and transferability or relevancy to similar contexts (Leininger, 1988; Lincoln & Guba, 1985; Sandelowski, 1986).

FOURTH PHASE

Themes, Major Research Findings, and Theoretical Formulations

This is the highest phase of analysis and synthesis of data. It requires synthesis of thinking, configuration modeling and creative analysis of data from previous phases. The researcher abstracts major themes research findings, and may offer theoretical formulations and recommendations.

THIRD PHASE

Pattern and Contextual Analysis

The data is scrutinized to discover patterns of behavior, structural meanings and contextual analysis. Interpretations, components or categories of data are examined to show recurrent patterning. Research looks for *saturation,* consistencies and credibility of data.

SECOND PHASE

Identification of Descriptors and Components

Data are studied to find similar or dissimilar statements or behavior that can be coded or classified to understand the domain(s) or inquire, or the questions under study. Data may be classified (*emic* or *etic* data) or in a special way that retains the *meaning-in-context.* Confirming information and establishing the *credibility* and *preserving accuracy* of data and are of major importance.

FIRST PHASE

Collecting and Documenting Raw Data (Use of Field Journal and Computer)

The researcher collects, records and begins to analyze data related to the purposes, area of inquiry, or questions being studied. This phase includes recording data from *key* and *general* informants including interviews, observations with participant experiences; noting analyzing contextual meanings; making interpretations; identifying symbols; and recording daily (and nightly) lifeways related to the phenomenon under study mainly from an *emic* focus. The data from the condensed of full field record directly into the computer.

Figure 6–1
Leininger's Phases of Analysis for Qualitative Data (1987)

FINDINGS

Regarding the first research question, the findings of this study indicated that care had specific meanings, experiences, and expressions for Lithuanian Americans. These care meanings were experienced and expressed according to the cultural values and lifeways of the Lithuanian American informants. The following cultural and social structure dimensions were viewed as highly important by the informants: first, the dimension of kinship and social factors; second, the dimension of religious and philosophical factors; third, cultural values and lifeways. Educational factors, political and legal factors, and technological factors were frequently mentioned. Economic factors were also seen as important, but in ways that related to other values such as family and hard work.

The following were highly valued by the Lithuanian American informants and were important in their lives: family; religion and faith; Lithuanian culture and language; hospitality; hard work and industriousness; education; a sense of community (a caring community); endurance and persistence; suffering economic and other hardships; and charity to others. Care meanings related to these values—for example, to many Lithuanian Americans, care meant presence. In describing how this was experienced and evidenced, informants would give examples of what a caring presence meant. Most used family examples. For instance, one man said that he took off from work when there was illness in his family. When his wife was ill with the flu, he stayed home to take care of her and their three children until his wife was better. Also, when his father was ill, he took time off from his job to take him to the doctor and to the hospital. Many times, informants mentioned that care was demonstrated "in the little things that you can do for each other" in the family. Family may be a universal value among people, but it was highly emphasized by the informants and was evident in participant observations.

Other meanings of care to Lithuanian Americans included: listening attentively; being responsible for; looking after (*priežiūra*); concern for (*rūpestis*); sharing with others; hospitality to others; and helping in times of need. Hospitality was very frequently noted to be a characteristic trait of Lithuanians. Both young and old informants gave many examples of the hospitality experienced in Lithuania and in Lithuanian American homes. Some jokingly said that Lithuanians were "too hospitable," referring to the custom of the host or hostess frequently pressing guests to eat or drink. Some of the older informants noted that hospitality customs were different in America. When they first came to the United States, they would refuse the first offer of food or drink only to discover that further offers were not forthcoming. In the Lithuanian custom, the host offers something to eat, the guest politely refuses one or two times, and the host continues to offer. Eventually, the guest takes the offered food or drink. After a few experiences with American hosts who took them at their word when they first refused and did not continue to offer, the informants learned that American customs were different. Younger informants noted that they had assimilated some American viewpoints and did not press their guests to eat and drink as much as their parents' generation did. Those who had visited Lithuania noted that their relatives would save for months, borrow money, and share foods with their friends and relatives in order to receive their "American" guests as lavishly as possible, even if it meant deprivation for themselves. All Lithuanian American informants who had visited Lithuania noticed and commented about the warmth and hospitality of the Lithuanian people.

In the process of data analysis, the following care theme emerged: care for Lithuanian Americans is a basic orientation and attitude of concern for others. These patterns related to care were noted in this study:

1. Care is expressed and intertwined with daily lifeways as expressed in interactions with family and friends.

2. Care is sometimes expressed in an organized caring community effort through Lithuanian organizations.

Lithuanian Americans have a strong network of organizations that help to maintain the community. The Roman Catholic parishes are centers for meetings and for various concerts and social activities. The Lithuanian Community is a worldwide organization through which Lithuanian Americans are linked to one another throughout the world. Folk festivals are held at regular intervals at various places. For example, in July 1992, a Lithuanian Folk Dance Festival was held in Chicago in the United States. Two years earlier, a Lithuanian Folk Dance Festival had been held in Vilnius, Lithuania. On these occasions, Lithuanians of all ages gather to put on dance and song programs or scouting jamborees, and other organizations gather from various cities or countries. Thus, the values, customs, and language of this culture are preserved.

The second research question was answered affirmatively: the findings indicated that Lithuanian Americans saw a relationship among care, well-being, and humor. Lithuanian Americans viewed well-being in a broad fashion that included physical, emotional, and spiritual health as well as an approach to life. Many included contextual or environmental influences on their well-being, such as community support and family support. When

Lithuanian American informants gave examples of how these dimensions added to their sense of well-being, male informants tended to cite economic security and being able to provide for the needs of their families as important to the well-being of the entire family.

Informants noted that the care they received from family and friends was vital to their well-being. Older informants seemed to emphasize the importance of caring experiences and persons in their lives. Many informants valued the sense of caring that they had noted or experienced through the Lithuanian American community and its activities. Younger informants said that participation in the Lithuanian American community enriched their lives and, although participation in their cultural activities along with participation in the broader American culture was demanding, they highly valued the experiences within their own cultural group. Some informants expressed a desire to see more caring in the way that organizations functioned, indicating that disagreement among their own cultural group members was distressing to them.

Humor was seen as desirable because it adds to health and well-being, as well as to caring, by helping to give new perspectives on the situations or issues under discussion. Some informants expressed a wish to have more humor in their lives. They admitted that Lithuanian Americans are viewed as serious, but all could think of friends or family members who had highly developed humor and made it an integral part of their lives. Humor was also viewed by some as a way of demonstrating caring to others, especially in stressful situations. Some older informants described how humor had helped them through the many hardships they had experienced in life—leaving their homeland to avoid death, adjusting to a new country, and changing their lifeways. Even informants who had been imprisoned in concentration camps said that humor had been used as a way of helping to survive inhuman conditions. Lithuanian Americans characterized Lithuanian humor as subtle and wry in nature, sometimes to a point where persons from other cultures, such as Germans or Americans, did not get the humor until an explanation was given. Because humor was used to help deal with conflict, oppression, and other difficult situations, humor was linked to the preservation of well-being and, sometimes, to life itself.

IMPLICATIONS

The above findings have various implications for the nursing profession. Nurses who take care of the needs of Lithuanian American clients need to be aware of the values as well as the meaning and expressions of care held by this cultural group. In qualitative research, findings are not generalized to other groups, but the above findings may hold true for Lithuanians living in various countries, as well as for clients from Estonia and Latvia. Further investigation needs to be done in order to determine what holds true in a more universal way for all Lithuanians—or possibly, for people from other Baltic countries.

Because Leininger's theory and model were used, the nursing implications are reported in terms of the three modes in giving cultural care: cultural care accommodation, cultural care repatterning, and cultural care preservation.

Presence means caring to Lithuanian Americans, so it is important for the professional nurse to make her presence felt by both the client and the family. The nurse needs to spend time with the family during visiting hours. The nurse should not wait until the Lithuanian American client asks for help, because this client may be reluctant to ring the call bell. Hard work, industriousness, and endurance of pain and hardships may be so ingrained in the clients, especially the elderly, that they may not want to "bother" the nurse with valid requests and complaints.

Because education is highly valued and doctors and nurses are seen as highly educated, professionals tend to be highly respected. Any instructions that the nurse gives will probably be closely followed. Nurses should, therefore, be sure that all instructions, such as medication teaching, are correctly understood. Getting feedback from the client and family, to be sure instructions have been correctly interpreted and understood, is advisable.

Lithuanian American clients may be reticent to complain about or call attention to any problems they may be having with the health care system. Frequently, the nurse is in a position to help clients express themselves. Subtle humor may sometimes be used with these clients to help them communicate. Negative comments and feelings may not be directly expressed by these clients, and indirect communication through humor may be very helpful.

The family and kinship system is highly valued by Lithuanian Americans. This means that nurses need to make every attempt to include family members whenever nursing care is needed, whether in acute care settings or home settings. Nurses may need to accommodate to the presence of family members by extending visiting hours and giving family members a role in the care of Lithuanian American clients. Many Lithuanian American clients will choose to care for chronically ill family members in their own homes rather than place them in nursing homes or extended care facilities. Such care is given even if deprivation of the caregiver, such as an elderly spouse, must be endured. Nurses need to be sure that professional follow-up is provided to the client and that the family is aware of and takes advantage of all government and other health programs that are available. For example, respite care may be something that the family can use as needed, or day care programs for Alzheimer's clients may help family members to maintain their jobs.

Lithuanian Americans value education and technology. They tend to be aware of current medical practices and will usually cooperate with prescribed medical and nursing care regimes. Health and well-being are valued. Should any changes be needed, these clients are likely to cooperate, provided that the nurse carefully explains the reason for the changes and includes the entire family in such instructions. For example, many traditional Lithuanian foods are high in fat and cholesterol and may need be eliminated from diets for cardiac clients. Nurses need to plan with the client and family how substitutions can be made, such as using skim milk instead of whole milk and cream for making farmer's cheese. Careful discussion of how a food can be baked instead of fried is another example of changes in food and eating patterns that may be needed.

CONCLUSION

Culturally congruent care is possible for people from different cultures. Little-known cultures need to be studied further in the future so that their care can be better understood and carried out. Future studies of related cultures, such as those of Latvia and Estonia, would be beneficial. Contrasts and comparisons are needed to reveal possible universal care features. Lithuanian Americans are better understood as a result of this study of care and care meanings and expressions in this culture.

REFERENCES

Aamodt, A. (1978). Social-cultural dimensions of caring in the world of the Papago child and adolescent. In M. M. Leininger (Ed.), *Transcultural nursing: Concepts, theories, and practices* (pp. 34–39). New York: Wiley.

Alilunas, L. J. (1978). *Lithuanians in the United States: Selected studies*. San Francisco: R. & E. Research Associates, Inc.

Benner, P., & Wrubel, J. (1989). *The primacy of caring: Stress and coping in health and illness*. Menlo Park, CA: Addison-Wesley.

Boyle, J. (1984). Indigenous caring practices in a Guatemalan Colonia. In M. M. Leininger (Ed.), *Care: The essence of nursing and health* (pp. 123–132). Thorofare, NJ: Slack.

Carper, B. A. (1979). The ethics of caring. *Advances in Nursing Science, 1*, 11–19.

Fry, S. T. (1989). Toward a theory of nursing ethics. *Advances in Nursing Science, 11*(4), 9–22.

Fry, S. T. (1990). The philosophical foundations of caring. In M. M. Leininger (Ed.), *Ethical and moral dimensions of care*. Detroit: Wayne State University Press.

Gadow, S. (1987). Nurse and patient. In A. H. Bishop & E. Scudder (Eds.), *Caring, curing, coping: Nurse, physician, patient relationships* (pp. 31–43). Birmingham: University of Alabama Press.

Gaut, D. A. (1981). Conceptual analysis of caring: Research methods. In M. M. Leininger (Ed.), *Caring: An essential human need* (pp. 17–24). Thorofare, NJ: Slack.

Gaut, D. A. (1984). A philosophic orientation to caring research. In M. M. Leininger (Ed.), *Caring: The essence of nursing and health* (pp. 17–25). Thorofare, NJ: Slack.

Gaylin, W. (1976). *Caring*. New York: Knopf.

Horn, B. M. (1978). Transcultural nursing and child-rearing of the Muckleshoot people. In M. M. Leininger (Ed.), *Transcultural nursing: Concepts, theories, and practices* (pp. 223–237). New York: Wiley.

Larson, P. J. (1981). *Perceptions of important nurse caring behaviors*. Doctoral dissertation, University of California, San Francisco.

Larson, P. (1987). Comparison of cancer patients' and professional nurses' perceptions of important nurse caring behaviors. *Heart and Lung, 16*, 187–193.

Leininger, M. M. (1978). *Transcultural Nursing: Concepts, theories, and practices*. New York: Wiley.

Leininger, M. M. (1985a). Transcultural care diversity and universality: A theory of nursing. *Nursing and Health Care, 4*, 209–212.

Leininger, M. M. (1985b). *Qualitative research methods in nursing*. New York: Grune & Stratton.

Leininger, M. M. (1988a). Class presentation. Wayne State University, Detroit.

Leininger, M. M. (1988b). Leininger's theory of nursing: Cultural care diversity and universality. *Nursing Science Quarterly, 1*(4), 152–160.

Leininger, M. M. (1988c). *Care: Discovery and uses in clinical and community nursing*. Detroit: Wayne State University Press.

Leininger, M. M. (1991). *Culture care diversity and universality: A theory of nursing.* New York: National League for Nursing.

Lincoln, Y. S., & Guba, E. G. (1985). *Naturalistic inquiring.* Beverly Hills, CA: Sage.

Luna, L. J. (1989). *Care and cultural context of Lebanese Muslims in an urban U.S. community: An ethnographic/ethnonursing study conceptualized within Leininger's theory.* Doctoral dissertation, Wayne State University, Detroit.

Mayeroff, M. (1971). *On caring.* New York: Harper & Row.

Morrison, P. (1989). Nursing and caring: A personal construct theory study of some nurses' self-perceptions. *Journal of Advanced Nursing, 14,* 421–426.

Noddings, N. (1984). *Caring: A feminine approach to ethics and moral education.* Berkeley: University of California Press.

Patterson, J. G., & Zderad, L. T. (1988). *Humanistic nursing.* New York: National League for Nursing.

Pellegrino, E. D. (1985). The caring ethic: The relation of physician to patient. In A. H. Bishop & E. Scudder (Eds.), *Caring, curing, coping: Nurse, physician, patient relationships* (pp. 8–30). Birmingham: University of Alabama Press.

Ray, M. (1981). A philosophical analysis of caring within nursing. In M. M. Leininger (Ed.), *Caring: An essential human need* (pp. 25–36). Thorofare, NJ: Slack.

Riemen, D. (1983). *The essential structure of a caring interaction: Phenomenological study.* Unpublished doctoral dissertation, Texas Woman's University, Denton.

Riemen, D. (1986). The essential structure of a caring interaction: Doing phenomenology. In P. Munhall & C. Oiler (Eds.), *Nursing research: A qualitative perspective* (pp. 85–108). Norwalk, CT: Appleton-Century-Crofts.

Sandelowski, M. (1986). The problem of rigor in qualitative research. *Advances in Nursing Science, 8*(3), 27–37.

Sliesoriunas, G. (1991). Lithuania's steps to independence. *Lietuva* (Lithuania), 1, 17–24.

Spradley, J. (1980). *Participant-observation.* New York: Holt, Rinehart and Winston.

Valentine, K. L. (1988). History, analysis, and application of the carative tradition in health and nursing. *Journal of the New York State Nurses Association, 19*(4), 4–9.

Watson, J. M. (1979). *Nursing: The philosophy and science of caring.* Boston: Little, Brown.

Watson, J. M. (1985). *Nursing: Human science and human care, a theory of nursing.* Norwalk, CT: Appleton-Century-Crofts.

Watson, J. M. (1988). New dimensions of human caring theory. *Nursing Science Quarterly, 1*(4), 175–181.

Weiss, C. J. (1986). *Perceptions of nurse caring.* Unpublished doctoral dissertation, Texas Woman's University, Denton.

Weiss, C. J. (1988). Model to discover, validate, and use care in nursing. In M. M. Leininger (Ed.), *Care: Discovery and uses in clinical and community nursing.* Detroit: Wayne State University Press.

Wenger, A. F. (1988). *The phenomenon of care in a high context culture: The Old Order Amish.* Doctoral dissertation, Wayne State University, Detroit.

Werner, O., & Schoepfle, G. M. (1987). *Systemic fieldwork: Foundation of ethnography and interviewing.* Beverly Hills, CA: Sage.

Wolf, Z. R. (1986). The caring concept and nurse identified caring behaviors. *Topics in Clinical Nursing, 8*(2), 84–93.

Yarling, R. R., & McElmurry, B. J. (1986). The moral foundation of nursing. *Advances in Nursing Science, 8*(2), 63–73.

PART II

WOMEN, CARING, NURSING

7

In the War Years: Women, Caring, and Economic Rationalism

Margaret Dunlop

*T*he title of this chapter is adapted from Cherie Moraga's book of poetry and prose, *Loving in the War Years,* in which she explores the tensions inherent in loving in a context of war, a war that is metaphorical of her experience as a woman, a Hispanic, a feminist, and a lesbian. In an earlier article (Dunlop, 1986), I argued that, in considering caring, we should not lose sight of the structures in which people, predominantly although not exclusively women, are expected to care. If we lose sight of the broader picture, caring failures can too easily be seen by the carer, the one cared for, and significant others as personal defects for which guilt and blame should be individually assigned. Individual faults are then seen as requiring individual remedies, in line with a radical form of the individualism that has shaped modern Western societies.

A *reductio ad absurdum* of that radical individualism is apparent in the development of a powerful ideology of economic rationalism—an almost global phenomenon that insists that the state has interfered too much in our lives and that the answer to our problems lies in privatization of much of the responsibility that governments have increasingly accepted over the past two centuries for our well-being. While not without its critics, it provides a context for considering the ways in which nurses and others have begun very self-consciously to focus on caring—one of the central concepts that might be threatened by re-privatization, at least caring as it exists in the public world. Economic rationalism threatens to annihilate nursing as a public occupation, at least to the extent that it focuses on caring, and it remains to be seen whether the simplistic worldview of economic rationalism will prevail or be interred in the graveyard of other dead economic theories. Unless it does or until it is, it seems perfectly appropriate to analogize from Moraga's title and speak of caring in the war years.

Although I have written about caring, I do not consider myself a caring theorist and I remain deeply committed to the caring practices on which we and our world depend for our very being—invisible though they often are in the smokescreen that passes for the economy. But such practices are difficult—even embarrassing—to talk about.

Why should this be? One answer may lie in the background nature of these caring practices. Like women, they are just there, excluded from what Frye (1989) called "phallocratic reality," which takes place in the foreground, as if in a dramatic production. As Frye argued:

> Foreground figures are perceptible, are defined, have identity, only in virtue of their movement against a background. . . . The background is unseen by the eye which is focused on foreground figures, and if anything somehow draws the eye to the background, the foreground dissolves. What would draw the eye to the background would be any sudden or well-defined motion in the background. Hence, there must be either no motion in the background, or an unchanging buzz of small, regular and repetitive motions. The background must be utterly uneventful if the foreground is to continue to hang together. (p. 88)

When we wish to focus on caring practices, as at this conference, we have to turn our gaze away from the center stage, where predominantly male actors "strut their stuff," and concentrate on what the world sees as inconsequential, even if, in a subliminal way, necessary. To the extent that we have been incorporated in the drama of phallocratic reality (female professors of nursing are to some extent incorporated in the play), our attention is stranded between background and foreground, drawn by the background from which we emerged but drawn also into the play.

Neither feminism nor nursing has any neat answers to this dilemma. To the extent we draw some of the caring practices into the foreground, which is hard to do, we leave most of them behind, because we in turn need a background. Thus, one way of understanding nursing's current preoccupation with caring is to see it, rather unkindly, as a marketing strategy aimed at upping the visibility and price of certain caring practices in the public world. However, it is clear from this conference that there are those who are attempting the even more difficult task of making visible the background connections with the wider range of unremunerated, use-value, caring practices.

Backgrounds should not be embarrassing. Perhaps an embarrassment results from the all-pervasive sentimentality that hangs around a notion of caring as some sort of idealized affect and often conceals even from its practitioners the knowledge, skills, and understanding embedded and embodied in caring. Fisher and Tronto (1990) recalled a class of women discussing caring. The middle-class White women discussed caring in strongly affective terms—"communicating with your child," "showing love and affection," "facilitating their development as people"—until it got too much for one African American woman, who burst forth into a description of the very physical things her mother did, as a sole parent, that meant care for herself and her siblings. Care is easily etherealized, particularly in Western middle-class rhetoric. The term caring practices, although also subject to etherealization, provides more sense of embodiment: caring practices flow from the live bodies and are practiced with live bodies. As nurses, we understand this; it has been the strength of our practice in comparison with other, more disembodied forms of caring, but, as Lawler (1990) illustrated, it has also been a source of embarrassment and loss of caste. Clean caring is a higher status activity than dirty caring—hence its popularity in White middle-class discourse, even among women.

Another problem for those of us who would foreground caring is its sheer complexity, the way it defies Occam's razor, so beloved of empirical science. Attempts to treat caring as a science have run into difficulties because of the tight relationship between caring and context. Decontextualized or universalistic accounts of caring do seem to be contradictions in terms, as Noddings (1984) pointed out. What is caring in one context may be quite uncaring in another, as most of us recognize readily. Most of what we can say about caring, rich as it often is, gestures toward rather than defines a range of activities that resist being impaled by academic, phallocratic discourse. Caring practices are as diverse as the corporeal practices of the body itself and, similarly, have a history—a genealogy, as Foucault would put it. This genealogy still lacks exploration.

Fisher and Tronto (1990) attempted to provide some form in which to analyze the meanings of caring. I find their work helpful in understanding the modern Western cluster of concepts covered by the term, particularly in elucidating its hierarchical nature in our own societies. They put forward four phases of caring:

1. Caring about.
2. Caring for/taking care of.
3. Caregiving.
4. Care receiving.

Caring about, the most general phase, denotes a disposition of concern toward. It is closest to the purely affective meaning of care and is the sense we pick up when we are challenged to do something and respond, "Of course I care." We can care about situations that are quite outside our ability to ameliorate—for example, the war in what was Yugoslavia—and we can also care about things we have no intention of doing anything about. Generally, caring about denotes some disposition toward doing something.

Caring for or taking care of involves taking up the burden of responsibility, making sure the work of care is done. More often than not, particularly for women and nurses, this slips into "plugging the gaps" in provision by personal caregiving, as in the third category.

Caregiving is the actual, physical, hands-on work of care. Care receiving is the onerous work of being suitably grateful to those who provide one's care—an obligation from which only unconsciousness (or, sometimes, being of the male gender) frees one!

At the family level (and I deliberately stereotype), a husband may care about his sick mother, his wife may take responsibility for seeing that his mother is cared for, which may involve some personal caregiving and some delegated caregiving. The mother feels grateful to her son and rows with her daughter-in-law/caregiver or with other caregivers employed by her!

At the level of the state, concern about different problems and groups of problem people filters through the political process to give rise to policies whereby the government takes some responsibility for those problems and problem people. The government "takes care of," thereby lifting the burden of the general feeling of public concern. Something is now being done. But manifestly, the government now has to delegate the actual care down the line. Typically, conflicts arising from differing expectations are played out at the interface of caregiver and care recipient.

We often talk about caring as if it were a harmonious process, despite our experiences to the contrary. The persons who care about the original situation may believe their intentions have been distorted by those "taking care of" or those giving care. Those who delegate caregiving may be dissatisfied with the level and quality of care provided, as may the care recipients.

Caregivers may be blamed by care recipients for deficiencies of care for which they are not responsible. Care receivers may expect more than is physically available or financially possible within the constraints of a system that is organized above them. Caregivers may strive, at great personal cost, to make up the deficiencies, yet still feel guilty that their care is less than optimal. Care recipients who are sensitive to this response may themselves feel guilty about their level of need for care. Indeed, one could say that caring systems work most efficiently on the potent fuel of guilt and blame, whether we are talking about mothers raising their children, nurses caring for patients, or caregivers, predominantly but not inevitably female, who care at home for the disabled, chronically ill, or frail aged.

Waring (1988) attacked the systematic way in which women's traditional work and the environment (both, not coincidentally, seen as natural) are omitted from public accounts and measures of economic activity. Both are part of the background against which activity is seen as taking place. The environment only enters in its destruction (for example, when a hill becomes an open-cut mine, or an oil-spill has to be cleaned up) and women only enter when their work moves into the market economy. Thus, the nurse working in a nursing home counts, but a women caring for her very disabled child or elderly parent does not. The situation is even worse than this brief outline suggests because, in economies that rely mainly on subsistence, the major contribution that women make to that subsistence does not count in the reckoning of the gross domestic product. Besides seriously understating the available resources of such countries, this approach means that international aid agencies direct their attention to the work of men and then wonder why their aid has so little effect! Waring pointed to the paradox that making weapons of war is productive activity, but bearing and raising children is not. While it could be argued that the world has too many children, the same *a fortiori* could be said about weapons of war.

Our economy, according to its describers, remains largely care-free (in the most literal sense) and this is seen as rational accounting! Imputed worth, particularly in subsistence economies, is given to men's activities, and under that heading are subsumed some female activities now attributed to the male. Aid agencies bring men in to talk to them about improved agricultural methods, overlooking that, in subsistence economies, women are the core primary producers.

Perhaps there is some rationality in refusing to even impute value to women's unpaid work. Governments can pass the buck on caring back to "the community" (largely a code for women as unpaid carers) in a predominantly "cost-free" fashion. After all, if women are outside the economy proper, what cost can there be? Even if governments provide a few rudimentary support services, the cost will still be "cheaper" than institutional care, particularly in a climate of concern about the quality of institutional care. The real costs are hidden: the cost to the carers of providing care will disappear from the ledger into that great sea of work that "counts for nothing."

In a book edited by Finch and Groves (1983), some feminist sociologists started working out what the costs to the carers were. Families who provided the most care had the smallest incomes on which to do so. Moreover, the carers, predominantly women, not only forewent current income by leaving work or dropping back to part-time work, but they also lost future superannuation entitlements, going a long way toward ensuring that they themselves would, in turn, be in need of care. In addition, their health suffered through the burden that care placed on them, again helping to ensure that, in time, they too would require care. Caring can thus become "the tender trap" in all senses of that phrase (Dunlop, 1988).

Should this concern us as nurses? Nurses are part of the market economy, at least in our employment as nurses, although many of us have second, unpaid jobs. Yet the closeness of what we do to what counts for nothing often means that our work is seriously or even severely undervalued. What this might mean in salary is one thing. It has been possible to raise nursing remuneration considerably because of the way in which we have become necessary in the increasingly more acute, more short-stay end of health care provision. It is primarily there that our contribution is valued (because of its importance to modern medicine) and that value, at least in the Australian centralized wage structure, then flows through to other areas of registered nursing work, including much of our not-specifically-medical caring. But in other settings, the development of a range of undertrained, underqualified personal carers is now proliferating—a product, I believe, of the general belief that caring is unskilled work. Where women cannot be coerced into doing it for nothing as kin of the cared-for, they are paid to do it for a pittance, with a scattering of registered nurses to oversee the work. In this way, the cost to the public purse is reduced, but the costs to the private purses of both women and nurses are increased. We are witnessing just such an economic rationalization of caring work. The next steps in that process of rationalization are deregulation of the wage structure and privatization of public utilities. As these processes take effect, nursing comes under threat of being restructured economically according to a hierarchy of high-technology skills rather than in terms of its caring practices and the needs they meet.

Pusey (1991) argued that the discourse of economic rationalism seems to have arisen with the evolution of a complex set of problems that exceed the problem-solving resources of the planners, the policy makers, and the service deliverers. Stumped for answers, the system has retreated to the mysticism of the market and market forces. They will be the *deus ex machina* that sorts the whole thing out and puts the world to rights. Along with this naive faith has developed an unreflecting empiricism that reduces politics to economics and economics to econometrics. In this context, Waring's book, important as it is, can be seen as symptomatic of the global political scene where what counts must count economically to be worthy of our concern, and what counts economically is what involves dollars and cents.

In his study of the Australian bureaucracy, Pusey (1991) found top bureaucrats to have a predominantly scientist attitude with no coherent concept of society, a mind-set in which values are seen as being a matter of subjective choice. This mind-set was most marked in areas that dealt with economic policy, but was still frighteningly strong in relation to government services and programs. In this context, social policy, discussion about social ends, and any form of social consensus or agreement are lost in overriding demands for system rationality in economic terms.

As Pusey pointed out, this accords with what Habermas called "mediation of the life-world," "the process by which cultural meanings and social action are uncoupled and converted into system structures" (Pusey, 1991, p. 175). The process leads to social and psychic "colonization" as the values of the economic system are imported back into the life-world. The economy takes on a facticity of its own. Apparently impersonal market forces are set over culture and civil society.

In the period following the chaos of the industrial revolution in the West, societies gradually built up structures to ameliorate the most destructive elements of the industrial system. There was some dawning recognition that the welfare of the poor and the working classes affected the welfare of all. From *noblesse oblige,* privatized forms of charity developed some notion of the rights of the citizen to a certain level of care and sustenance in time of need. What had previously been privatized charity work developed into the health, education, and welfare systems; new professions and occupations developed—among them, modern nursing. (I will leave aside, although it is compelling, Foucault's argument that this represented an increasingly internalized form of surveillance of the citizenry. It is possible to recognize the truth of such a reading and yet see the major benefits of such amelioration of the market economy. If we doubt this, some rereading of Dickens might well be in order.)

Today, there has arisen a new faith that the market economy will do what it manifestly did not do before. The market has, however, moved from a predominant emphasis on production to a predominant emphasis on consumption. Automation has reduced the need for citizens as industrial fodder, but the abundance of goods produced has increased the need for consumers of those goods. Services become increasingly constructed as goods. The citizen is thus constructed less as a worker and more as a consumer.

The marketplace, which is to solve all our woes, is now geared toward consumption. Caring will be increasingly marketed as a commodity, a consumer "good." Our exploration of caring is now situated within this rather bleak context.

Despite the front-stage antics of technological medicine as it presents ever new miracle cures, it is slowly dawning on more and more of us that the front stage is not really where the action is at. When we are watching a play that starts to pall, our attention begins to wander and we focus on some aspect of the background—in this case, the caring practices that we recognize as nursing.

As we draw them out of the background, describe and label them, we are in fact packaging them as commodities for the consumer culture in which we now all live.

Like the air-hostesses in Hochschild's study (1983), nurses are now finding their emotional labor—their caring in its emotional labor sense—being packaged as a commodity. As the competition between private hospitals has heated up, they have begun marketing along the lines of "our nurses are the most caring." The ongoing privatization of our public health services seems likely to strengthen this trend.

As Ehrenreich and English (1978) pointed out, the rise of modern medicine broke up the web of human healing by packaging cure as a marketplace commodity. The concern of the practitioner for the patient became packaged as "bedside manner," importing a high level of alienation into the practice of modern medicine. To some extent, nursing was caught up in this process but was somewhat sheltered by its salaried status. Within this shelter, we developed our theories of nursing, which were highly idealistic and ran counter to the trends evident in medicine.

However, our practice, influenced by dominant trends in the health marketplace, developed differently. It is no coincidence that the ideas that have gained most purchase in nursing practice—nursing process and nursing diagnosis—are those that fit most comfortably with ongoing commodification of nursing. This conference can be usefully regarded as a site of resistance of such commodification.

We do not live in a monolithic culture, either as people or as nurses. Cultures, even apparently simple cultures, are not internally consistent. Our own cultures are incredibly complex; indeed, Western countries like our own have become experiments in multiculturalism. The richer the cultural mix, the more possible lines of resistance are opened up, and there has been ample evidence in this conference that some of these are being actively explored. Sometimes, these resistances will arise almost spontaneously and subliminally from the sense that something is wrong, or from weariness with the old and desire for the new. We are not always rational calculators, as Habermas sometimes seems to suggest. In other words, it is not always or perhaps not even commonly the case the emancipatory actions issue from reflective practice. Furthermore, actions intended at the time to be emancipatory can become captive to forces tending in other directions. A simple example is the use of women's liberation to sell cigarettes and other consumer goods.

Yet it is important to get as good a handle as we can on the context within which we as nurses are now exploring the concept of caring. It is not sufficient to simply explore and amplify caring itself—to create a body of caring knowledge. Human beings do create and continually recreate the world they inhabit, but they do not create it just as they like. In the complex world we inhabit, our best intentions can have unforeseen results. To have some chance of avoiding such a fate, we need to take in as much of the picture as we can.

If we wish, as nurses, to continue to develop our knowledge and understanding of our caring practices in the hope of improving them, we need also to recognize the environmental threats to our caring in the structures in which our caring is embedded. Perhaps destruction is the least of our worries; new phoenixes rise from the ashes and, if human beings continue to exist, caring will be needed and new modes of care will arise. Perhaps the greatest danger is the colonization of our practices by the values of the technological, rationalizing imperative that colonizes ourselves as nurses.

In the past, we have been colonized by biopower—the biomedical model, a colonial yoke from which we are not yet free. As I have tried to suggest, other modes of colonization may now pose a greater threat to our integrity and the integrity of the care we provide.

REFERENCES

Dunlop, M. J. (1986). Is a science of caring possible? *Journal of Advanced Nursing, 11*, 661–670.

Dunlop, M. J. (1988). Science and caring: Are they compatible? In *Shaping nursing theory and practice: The Australian context*. Monograph, School of Nursing, Latrobe University.

Ehrenreich, B., & English, E. (1978). *For her own good—150 years of the experts' advice to women*. Garden City, NY: Doubleday.

Finch, J., & Groves, D. (1983). *A labour of love: Women, work and caring*. London: Routledge & Kegan Paul.

Fisher, B., & Tronto, J. (1990). Toward a feminist theory of caring. In E. Abel & M. Nelson (Eds.), *Circles of care—work and identity in women's lives* (pp. 35–62), New York: SUNY Press.

Frye, M. (1989). To see and be seen: The politics of reality. In A. Gary & M. Pearsall (Eds.), *Women, knowledge and reality* (chap. 5). Winchester, MA: Unwin Hyman, Inc.

Hochschild, A. R. (1983). *The managed heart—commercialization of human feeling.* Berkeley: University of California Press.

Lawler, J. (1990). *Behind the screens.* Melbourne: Churchill Livingstone.

Noddings, N. (1984). *Caring—a feminine approach to ethics and moral education.* Berkeley: University of California Press.

Pusey, M. (1991). *Economic rationalism in Canberra—a nation-building state changes its mind.* Cambridge, England: Cambridge University Press.

Waring, M. (1988). *Counting for nothing—what men value and what women are worth.* Wellington, NZ: Allen & Unwin.

8

Healthworld Theory: A Universal Language of Caring

Jill Hill

WHO CARES?

"Nurses don't care anymore!" This cry, heard widely in recent years, reflects an accusation that nursing is an occupation that has somehow fallen from grace during the course of the dramatic shifts that have recently overwhelmed nursing's professional, educational, and clinical world. The implication is that nurses normatively *should* care, even if the world around their occupational roles is becoming technologized, distant, impersonal, alienated, and *system*atized.

The vested interests of the accusers are usually not far from the surface of their expression of "concern":

- Politicians have used the maxim as an argument against admitting nursing students to higher education; a U.S. senator was reported to have uttered the phrase in this context ("Walsh . . . ," 1990).
- Led by doctors, professional peers of nursing have used the expression to argue against the continuing professionalization of nursing

since the beginning of the century; doctors particularly have expressed a fear that they would lose their hegemony within medical practice because of "nurses being taught too much" (Anon., 1926).

• The lamentation that nurses don't care has been heard from those responsible for the organizational and managerial state of the health care system; it serves to obscure the structural flaws that increasingly make it impossible for nurses to carry out caring nursing activities (Valentine, 1989). This observation was developed by the Director of the Nursing Division of the International Council of Nurses (Broe, 1959).

More insidiously, however, caring is under threat within the profession itself. Some, at least, have had their own assumptions colonized by the attributed status that accrues in contemporary society from scientific rationalism and "technique," and disavow caring as the core of nursing purpose. As Godden, Curry, and Delacour (1990) suggested, this is an action of "defensive compensation" against the "poor status and hidden undervalued work" that has traditionally confronted the occupation.

What we find in the accusation, therefore, is a *hidden language of interest, of power, and of co-optation.* Behind the lamentations that reach the surface of discourse have been deep and societywide *processes* of change in the "grammar" of nursing action. Within a wider political discourse of economic rationalism, "care" is expensive, subjective, and inefficient. It is therefore subject to continuous cost-cutting as the health system is financially pruned. Within a wider professionalization discourse, nursing interests have sought to acquire status and legitimized power through adopting the empiricist values of science and technique. In the name of assumed objectivity, nurses' detachment from their client-subjects follows, a trend in direct opposition to the subject–subject relations that are intrinsically implied in caring. Behind the professionalization discourse stands its philosophical grammar in the empiricist perspective, which holds that truth about the world can only be discovered through cognition—a position that by definition excludes nonrational thought, intuition, emotion, or, in short, the "art" of caring. In other words, the hidden languages of power that lie behind discourses of caring are deeply set in the macro level of contemporary society's philosophic, institutional, and political assumptions. The result is confusion—between nurse professionalism and patient care—both for nurse practitioners and for those who gain advantage from holding them in thrall to their own interests.

The confusion is real. However, when seen as a confusion that arises from not understanding the language that is embedded in discourses of power that underlie nursing practice, it can be resolved. The purpose of this chapter is to provide a theoretical framework by which the language of nurse–client interaction can be used to explain the process of caring and increase our understanding of the nurse's function to care.

Habermas's theoretical perspective on communicative action is a very useful starting point (Habermas, 1984, 1987). Within Habermas's observation of the increasing *system*atization of the world—where activities of the everyday world are institutionalized into "systems" of food production, education, health care, and so on—the systems that arise and surround everyday life *stand outside the language of everyday life*. In other words, the individual's "lifeworld," or domain of everyday action, is subject to a system discourse that the individual can have no part in. System discourses are dominated by the language and logic of the marketplace, of administrative power, and of technique—all largely independent of individual intentions. In Habermas's terms, systems "drop out" of language at the same time as they increasingly take over those parts of the lifeworld that have yet to be colonized. This has been a continuous process that directly parallels the global historic discovery and implementation of the power of technique and scientific understanding.

Caring involves subject–subject hearing, listening, and response, which Habermas describes as the main characteristics of communicative action. With the *system*atization of health care, the assumptions of communicative action that are intrinsic to caring are therefore "colonized" by systems assumptions that, although dressed in clothes of professionalism and scientific validity, intrinsically attack the language of caring. With the encroachment of specialist technique, for example, a *whole* human subject is "heard" and dealt with within a grammar of *fragmented* "expert" knowledge assumptions. A psychologist will concentrate on the objectification of subjective elements of client interaction. The dietician, physician, and physiotherapist will concentrate on the physical-objective elements of client interaction, and so on. They may, to a greater or lesser degree, hold concern for the whole of the patient, but their top priority must be to achieve the professional objective of applying the disciplined technique that they are employed to provide, whether this objective is control of disease, realignment of bones, counting of calories, or relief of aberrant mental symptoms. The language of technical specialization is the language of intervention and power. In Habermas's terms, this is the language of "strategic action," not of communicative action, and thus involves intentions that are not open to scrutiny on the part of the patient. The client is disempowered from entering the linguistic domain as an equal; the language of the system stands outside his or her lifeworld.

The nurse, of all health professionals, is left to *care*. Caring, intrinsically, has to do with the whole of the patient, not only an appendix or a trapezoid muscle. The actions (and interactions) of caring therefore lie firmly within the lifeworld, where the person captures understanding of the world, constructs meanings, communicates, feels, and *chooses* how to live. Many within nursing are aware of a loss of caring that pervades the occupation in the interest of technical performance efficiency and scientific ways. For example, the National League for Nursing passed a unanimous resolution, in June 1989, encouraging the development of nursing curricula that enhanced caring practices and asserted social values, participation with patients, and critique of the system (National League for Nursing, 1989; Tanner, 1990). The danger the nurse confronts today is very real; in exercising her professional expertise, the language of caring may itself be dropping out of discourse and being co-opted into system language. It would then control the assumptions of the lifeworld rather than engage with lifeworld assumptions as equal partners. Under these conditions, nurses will indeed "not care anymore," for they will have lost the language by which they can care.

Much has been written on the definitions of caring, which are basically dichotomized between affective feelings (Watson, 1979) and behaviorist action. However, the universal nature of caring and how it works remains highly problematic, and the language of human caring remains little understood. Leininger has said that, although nurses are "the professional group who repeatedly use the expressions, 'nursing care,' 'care' and 'caring' in everyday parlance, the linguistic, semantic and professional usages of these terms are still limitedly understood and studied" (Leininger, 1988b, p. 48). Derbyshire (1991, p. 16) stated that the problem of (1) the public image of nursing and of nurses themselves and (2) the reclaiming of the realm of humanistic caring is the lack of a "vocabulary for excellence": "How can we value ourselves and our work when we don't even have a language that speaks of how good it is and how we do well?" Nurses in clinical praxis, like Parker (1990), search for a universal, relational language and still find themselves "fumbling for the right words."

TOWARD A NEW LANGUAGE OF HUMAN CARING

The nursing profession must be able to theorize these tensions and conflicts in order to know how to prevent the language of caring from dropping out of nurse–patient discourse, which would mean the dismemberment of the core purpose of nursing. At the heart of this theorization is a need to recognize the boundary assumptions that are put into practice *within* interactions. At these horizons to real linguistic discourse, colonization by system is occurring and the language of caring is being disempowered and appropriated into the system.

Toward such a theory, it is helpful to conceptualize caring as being the activity not of a health system, but of a *healthworld*. The distinction is absolutely critical. System is the domain in which communicative interaction has been lost in the face of assumptions of technique. Healthworld is the domain where lifeworld is lived; however, for the sake of theory as well as a guide in nursing practice, lifeworld is focused within domain assumptions that impinge on *living* health. The assumptions of Habermas about lifeworld and its associated communicative action discourses can be mirrored in the development of the healthworld theoretical framework. As this chapter will demonstrate shortly, with attention on healthworld rather than health system, the "grammar" of disempowerment can be demonstrated *within* the linguistic activities of responsive caring. For example, "strategic action" (implying hidden control) can be demonstrated in the "perlinguistic" shadows that lie behind the immediate nurse–patient and other health professional interactions. Healthworld is able to provide a guide to caring nurse *praxis*—the enjoining of action, consciousness, and theory in professional action. Healthworld is a theory that can be applied immediately in the practical world of being a nurse professional.

Some definitions are useful in laying down the introductory groundwork for such a healthworld theory.

Central to a *healthworld theory of caring* is Habermas's assertion that people relate to three domains of reference *simultaneously* in each and every act and utterance:

1. The objective domain, referring to objects and facts.
2. The social domain, referring to normative rightness.
3. The subjective domain, referring to authenticity of inner experience.

These domains can be differentiated by formal linguistic structures.

The healthworld theory of caring asserts that caring involves breaking down barriers to the person's understanding of his or her own healthworld assumptions and to autonomous action in conscious recognition of these assumptions. Because it asserts that health implies empowerment, the healthworld theory requires *holistic* analysis of the integrated set of assumptions the person applies within his or her own healthworld. The theory does not stop with analysis, however. The healthworld theory is intrinsically a theory of *praxis,* for assumptions can only be identified by testing them in action. Consciousness of both the person and the health practitioner with whom the person interacts is joined with *communicative action* in both understanding and applying healthworld principles. Within the healthworld theory, the nurse is a conscious actor involved in communicative action with the client. Fundamentally, the nurse's role is more than that of a dispenser of professional technical skill. The nurse is a person who has a professional "response ability" for the holistic caring of a person, group, or community. She has as her focus the *sustainable potential* of her client, with whom she enters a client-centered interaction bound by the social/legal "being careful," the physical "giving care," and the subjective "caring" obligations to potentiate the ideal health situation for each client. ("She" is used in the generic sense for the nurse throughout the chapter.)

Health is defined as the inbuilt thrust of an individual, group, or community to realize a sustainable potential—physically, socially, mentally, and spiritually—throughout the passage of life. It can be seen, therefore, as an inbuilt thrust for the ideal health situation. The health of an individual, group, or community can be compromised by environmental structures such as public policy, unrestrained air, water and earth pollution, unsafe work practices, or inefficient infrastructure (poor drainage in overcrowded areas, and so on). The *health situation* of an individual, group, or community can be measured at any one time by established indicators such as epidemiological studies, documentations and reports, statistics, clinical investigations, and self-reports and descriptions.

Healthworld is the domain of everyday experience. Each person *lives* his or her health based on meanings constructed within taken-for-granted domain assumptions that the person makes about physical, mental, social, cultural, environmental, cosmological, and "unknowable" worlds, or interconnected "spheres of reference."

The person *lives* health within frameworks of meaning and assumptions of which he or she is rarely conscious. The lived experience—and the consciousness of its meaning—forms the boundary beyond which the person cannot go in assembling information and constructing meaning about a health situation and sustainable potential. The person may master all the elements or concepts within each of the healthworld's spheres of reference to a greater or lesser degree, depending on their exposure and relevance to the person's lived experience. (See Figure 8–1.)

A person's construction of meaning within the healthworld is continuous. Health is lived, through the manner in which the person responds to life environment: smoking or not smoking, choosing stressful or nonstressful work activities, adopting high-fat or low-fat diet, and so on. In equal mea-

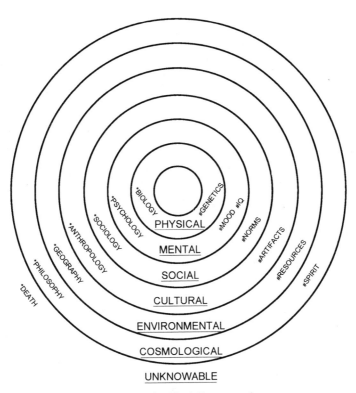

* Traditional epistemological categories/discipline examples
# Common element examples

Figure 8–1
Healthworld Context of Relevance

sure, the person is constrained by factors that impinge on health but are imposed by the environment: pollution, noise, access to healthy foods, and education, among others. In *any* environment, the individual has healthworld choices; however, in some environments (for example, a poverty-stricken family in a developing country), health choices are more limited and are likely to be *assumed* as low priorities.

Apart from involvement in more general public awareness campaigns, the nurse–client interaction does not occur as the person goes about normal everyday life. Instead, it is part of a situation that is *problematized* by a *theme*. The theme acts like a spotlight on the field of general assumptions the person has tended to take for granted; it lights up those that are most directly evoked by the problem situation they confront. A *segment* of the healthworld contexts of relevance therefore colors the person's way of viewing and dealing with the situation theme.

A brief story will illustrate this point.

Case Study: Dealing with Cancer

One Friday, a sixty-five-year-old man talked to a nurse after having just been informed by his doctor that he must return the following Tuesday to have a malignant kidney removed. He had wanted to know about the effects of possible subsequent chemotherapy on his quality of life and the possibility of alternative medicines. In response, he had been told that he would live for one to two years with the operation and three months without it, and he had better get on with it. He was upset. He and his wife were about to fulfill a long-term plan to travel around Australia. He was resigned to the issue of dying; he said he had been luckier than most and would rather enjoy the time he had left. He had been made to feel that he had let the doctor down. He felt he *should* follow medical instructions but he did not want to have the operation. He was asymptomatic, and the diagnosis of cancer of the kidney had been incidentally derived. After being enabled by the nurse to verbalize and discuss all of his concerns in-depth, he was able to weigh up all facets (theme and elements of context of relevance) of his health situation. He made the decision not to have the operation and now, twelve months on, after consulting with his family and making appropriate life-style changes (particularly in regard to alternative medicine and diet), he is happily traveling around Australia with his beloved wife. Ultrasound and CAT scan demonstrate that his tumor has shrunk significantly.

On analysis of the interactions, the *meaning* of the theme malignant kidney was quite different for the patient, doctor, and nurse. These differences were leading the participants in the health situation in entirely different directions for plans, actions, and goals.

For the physician, meaning was derived from a purely bio-techno-efficient background of lived experience and a healthworld of tacit assumptions. The assumptions from which the physician had drawn meaning regarding the tumor (the health situation theme) were based in the traditions of the Western medical model: preservation of life regardless of choice or quality. (See Figure 8–2, segment A.) The doctor's goal was to destroy the tumor with surgery, and his action was to stand on his medical "expert" authority and demand that the client "get on with it." He geared his communication to the objective

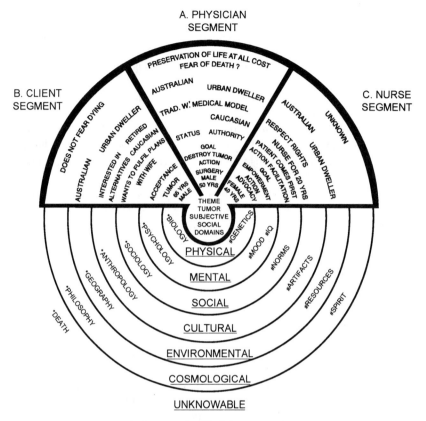

* Traditional epistemological categories/discipline examples
# Common element examples

Figure 8–2
Healthworld Context of Relevance—Communication Boundaries

domain: "The fact is that you must come back next Tuesday. You have a malignant tumor on your left kidney and it must be removed." His action denied the holistic nature of the meaning the theme held for the client's healthworld and sought to foreclose any discussion or recognition of other possibilities. His action was disempowering to the client, making him feel that he had "let the doctor down."

The theme in this health situation for the client was not only the tumor, but also the effect the tumor had on his mutual commitments with his wife (referring to the social domain) and his concern about quality of life, not quantity and fulfillment of plans and desires (referring to the subjective domain). His goal was to make a decision that would maximize satisfaction in *all* areas of his life. To do this, he needed to re-evaluate his healthworld and re-examine his assumptions about his *sustainable potential* and how it was to be sustained. His action was to weigh up the impact of the health situation theme in all areas of his life. (See Figure 8–2, segment B.)

Analysis of the nurse–client interaction revealed that this physical manifestation (the malignancy) would have important consequences in the social and subjective domains as well as the physical domain of the patient's life, and the patient had some important self-determining and autonomous decisions to make. The nurse acknowledged and validated his social and subjective domains of reference by accepting his concerns as legitimate *for him*; she also acknowledged the seriousness of the physical problem and what could be done about it. Her interaction reflected her lived experience and revealed values of client-centered holistic caring and respect for the patient. In healthworld terms, the subjective, objective, and social domains of reference are embedded in every speech utterance and every action. Because a health situation theme simultaneously refers to objective, subjective, and social domains of reference, they must be addressed simultaneously to maintain *holistic* care. (See Figure 8–2, segment C.)

Holistic caring does not stop with the validation of the patient's representational meanings of experience. It also involves a linguistic evolutionary thrust of empowerment, a challenge to the assumptions from which the client derives the meaning that guides his or her action. Empowerment is brought about by linguistic analysis (verbal and nonverbal), the swapping and challenging of validity claims associated with each domain of meaning in language. The next section explains how it works.

A UNIVERSAL LANGUAGE

Language has a *cognitive function* (related to objects and facts), an *expressive function* (related to inner experiences of the sender), and an *appeal function* (communication from the sender to the receiver). Language constitutes an action that describes something and refers to the user's doing something: I warn, I promise, and so on. These acts have *locutionary* aspects (the statement of a proposition with a certain sense) and *illocutionary* aspects (what is done in saying things: making a promise, issuing a warning). Illocutionary aspects indicate the reference world to which the speech act specifically refers (objective, social-normative, or subjective (inner) world). Locutionary and illocutionary elements of action can be revealed from the speech act itself.

The *perlocutionary* element, on the other hand, represents the hidden intention of the speaker and requires knowledge outside the speech situation if it is to be understood. The speaker does not reveal or declare his or her aims as such. The perlocutionary element is therefore associated not with communicative action, where "discourse" between equals is possible, but with "strategic" action, where the speaker is seeking to have a certain effect on the listener, a *control of outcomes* that indicates covert strategic action. The speaker wants to frighten or embarrass or coerce, an intent to which he or she cannot admit.

Language geared to shared understanding and empowerment, whereby power differentials are neutralized and each speaker can participate freely, requires criticizable validity claims that encompass more than one world. Claims to *truth* refer to the objective world, claims to *rightness* refer to the social world of legitimately regulated interpersonal relations, and claims to *sincerity* or *authenticity* refer to the individual's own subjective world of experiences. The listener reacts to a claim by understanding the meaning, taking a yes or a no position, and following up with action, usually affirmative. If not affirmative, then the interaction can stop or be converted into discourse whereby both can modify their positions (Habermas, 1987).

In many "crossed" communications, the world to which speech action is referred is confused. In the case study given above, one person attempted to persuade another of the rightness (within the social world of norms) of a course of action: have an operation. The appeal to "fact" (objective world), "You have cancer," was supported entirely by the appeal of the voice of authority rather than by rational exchange of validity claims. The medical professional sought to retain power, in the interest of technical efficiency, rather than allow the patient to make a choice about his own life. In fostering this power, the doctor had employed perlocutionary "threat" and had sought to invoke "guilt" within what otherwise appeared a communicative action.

In the healthworld empowerment model, the nurse breaks down the communication boundary of the client's healthworld by exposing perlocutionary effects—elements that lie outside of the client's awareness and tacit assumptions. Perlocutionary effects lie in technical jargon, social structures, the behavior of others, the grammar that is used, and the client's internal representational system. When we superimpose the earlier example on the model, we see how the nurse's interaction has drawn the full meaning (subjective and social, as well as objective) into the grasp of the client. (See Figure 8–3.) In the nurse–client interaction, the nurse exposed the perlocutionary effect that the doctor–client interaction had had on the client. In response to the nurse's asking the client why he felt he *should* have the operation, the client said, "Well, the doctor knows all about it and what should be done and he told me to have the operation."

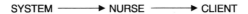

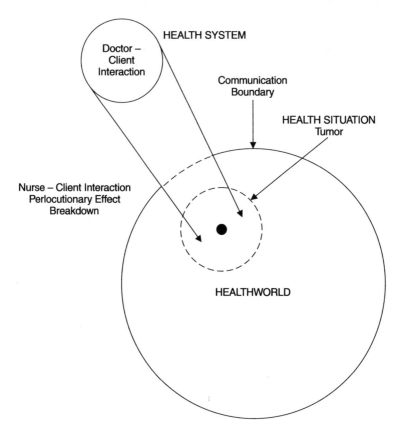

Figure 8–3
Empowerment Model

The following dialogue is extracted from the exchange:

NURSE: An oncologist is a medical practitioner with extra training in the medical intervention of cancer. Nobody knows all about cancer; for instance, we still don't know what causes it. He is a physician; he may not know all about it.

CLIENT: But he is a doctor and he knows what is best.

NURSE: And you are upset with his decision?

CLIENT: [nods and looks down]

NURSE: He is a medical practitioner who has acquired knowledge about the workings of the systems of the body, and skills in medical and surgical procedures. Does he know what is best for your life?

CLIENT: Uhh, well, he doesn't know me. Now that reminds me of a workmate. I wasn't close to him but I do remember him telling us that he had cancer. . . somewhere. . . and he was told that he would die within the year if he didn't have an operation and he would live for years if he did. He was very confident. . . had the operation. . . was in agony for three weeks and died. I owed him a pack of cigarettes. I was going to pay him back when he came back to work.

NURSE: Each situation is different. That may not happen to you. Do you feel badly that you did not have the opportunity to pay him back?

CLIENT: No. Everybody lends cigarettes; you usually don't get them back. You know, I heard of someone who was supposed to die years ago but they're still going strong on herbs or something.

NURSE: There are different approaches called alternative medicines, and they are not held in high esteem by medical professionals. I don't know much about them, but you may wish to discuss your options with someone.

The nurse consciously and subconsciously cued in on nonverbal messages that also relayed meaning and, through the interaction, sometimes used these keys to clarify or challenge. For purposes of this chapter, I do not need to go into details.

The medical professional had sought to retain power. His action was therefore disempowering. The nurse, holding a *holistic* client-centered approach, *analyzed the language structure of interaction*, elsewhere labeled as "uncharted wisdom" (Benner, 1988), and revealed the embedded perlocutionary effects.

These, in turn, empowered the client to take a self-determining role in his own health care.

Case Study: Elderly Need

A more simplistic case involves a nurse who was caring for an elderly man who had fractured his hip. He did not want to do anything. His continuous cries of "I can't!" in response to every suggestion that he physically could (and, implied, *should*) do things, were getting his primary nurse down to such a point that she had requested reassignment to someone else. On her last day with him, she looked at him more closely. He was sitting in bed with a full breakfast tray in front of him. "I can't eat this," he responded to inquiry as to how he was feeling. "Do you feel overwhelmed looking at so much food on this breakfast tray?" she asked. He nodded. "Does eating three bites seem overwhelming?" she asked. "No, I can do that," he answered (Holt, 1992, p. 53). This simple interaction changed both nurse and client: the nurse went on to break down all of his daily activities into manageable steps.

The real problem about achieving activities lay in the subjective and social/normative domains of the activities. When the nurse moved from her technical focus—trying to coerce the client to complete set objectives relating to the objective/physical world—and acknowledged and addressed the other domains, she was able to understand the impasse. She used language that acknowledged and referred to the subjective domain: "Do you *feel* overwhelmed . . . ?" The client affirmed her inquiry and they reached a shared understanding related to the situation theme. She then was able to break down the perlocutionary effect that the situation held for both herself and the client. The social/normative expectations that were too demanding and disempowering in the client's subjective world were then broken down, and successful action coordination between nurse and client was achieved.

The core *language problem* for the "caring" health practitioner follows from not recognizing that embedded in each situation theme are *three* domains of reference. Together, they make up the *integrated meaning* the client holds for that situation theme. The tendency of health professionals to deal with the client's healthworld through the disciplined technical interpretation of the situation theme, rather than in communicative action with the client (defining the theme together), is the heart of the problem.

CONCLUSION

The healthworld theory of caring ensures holistic care by focusing on the integrated meaning held by the principals in a health situation theme. Holistic caring acknowledges and addresses three domains of reference that are simultaneously embedded in each and every act and utterance. Because the healthworld theory looks behind cultural diversity to the universal dynamics of language, it adds explanatory strength to Leininger's idea of the universality of nursing (Leininger, 1988a), and it explains how the exemplars of Benner's and Watson's carative factors (Benner, 1988; Watson, 1979) operate in the nurse–client interaction. For the first time, the power relations embedded in the social/normative domain of reference for meaning are *directly* addressed, theoretically and operationally. Operational tools for dealing with the hidden normative rules embedded in the interactions of a health client will ensure that the distortive potential of both the practitioner's and the client's definition of a health situation are dealt with. Empowerment gained by the exposure of perlocutionary effects embedded in language ensures that the client's interests are always placed first, thus demonstrating that true *holistic* caring and empowerment are inextricably linked. The role of language analyst needs to be added to the nurse's function in order to legitimize what nurses have done all along: care.

REFERENCES

Anon. (1926). Theory and practice. *Nursing Times, 22,* 224.

Benner, P. (1988). *From novice to expert.* Menlo Park, CA: Addison-Wesley.

Broe, E. (1959). Nursing education. *Australasian Nurses Journal* (10), 250–257.

Derbyshire, P. (1991). In H. Gaze (Ed.), RCN Congress: Changing images. *Nursing Times, 15,* 16–17.

Godden, J., Curry, G., & Delacour, S. (1990). The decline of myths and myopia? Recent trends in nursing historiography. *Proceedings, The Discipline of Nursing: New Horizons in Nursing Theory, Education, Practice and Research.* University of Sydney Faculty of Nursing, National Conference, Sydney, Australia.

Habermas, J. (1984). *The theory of communicative action. Volume 1: Reason and the rationalization of society* (Thomas McCarthy, Trans.). Boston:

Beacon. Habermas, J. (1987). *The theory of communicative action. Volume 2: Lifeworld and system: A critique of functionalist reason.* Boston: Beacon.

Holt, J. (1992, April). Mr. McLean had two words for us: "I Can't." *Nursing 92, 52–53.*

Leininger, M. (1988a). *Caring: An essential human need.* Detroit: Wayne State University Press.

Leininger, M. (1988b). Caring: A central focus of nursing and health care services. In Leininger, M. (Ed.), *Care: The essence of nursing and health.* Detroit: Wayne State University Press.

National League for Nursing. (1989). Resolution No. 12: Support for innovative curricula for nursing education (news). *Nursing Health Care, 10,* 386.

Parker, R. S. (1990). Nurses' stories: The search for a relational ethics of care. *Advances in Nursing Science, 13*(1), 31–40.

Tanner, C. A. (1990). Caring as a value in nursing education. *Nursing Outlook, 38*(2), 72.

Valentine, K. (1989). Caring is more than kindness: Modeling its complexities. *Journal of Nursing Administration, 19,* 28–34.

Walsh hits nurse-training move. (1990, September 1). *The Age.*

Watson, J. (1979). *Nursing: The philosophy and science of caring* (pp. 9–10). Boston: Little, Brown.

9

Caring: Beyond the Dyad

Robin Watts

I invite you to accompany me on a voyage around this global village in which we live. Given the pressure of time, there will be only four brief stops. All you will need to take with you on this voyage is an openness to new perspectives and insights. On our return, we will reflect on what questions are raised and what can be learned from this experience as it relates to the concept of caring.

The Voyage

For our first stopover, we have gone back in time. It is the year 1988 and we are in Burma, or Myanmar as the country is now called. Just down the street from where we are standing is the General Hospital, the major health care center in the capital of Rangoon. The pro-democracy movement, inspired by Aung San Suu Kyi, has swept the country but the army refuses to give up its power and is in the process of crushing the democratic movement.

There is a group of people on the front steps of the hospital. Let us draw as close as we can, to observe what is happening. There is a small group of staff, some of whom are obviously nurses, arguing vehemently with a larger

group of heavily armed soldiers. Our translator tells us that the staff are
refusing to allow the soldiers to enter the hospital to arrest injured civilian
protesters who were admitted after a street clash with the army earlier that
morning. The argument becomes more and more heated with the staff
steadfastly refusing to give way. Suddenly, several soldiers raise their guns
and mow down the hospital staff. All die instantly.

Our next stop is a little more cheering in terms of outcome. We are now
in Santiago, Chile, with its backdrop of mountains. It is April 24, 1991, a
sunny but blustery Wednesday morning. We are standing outside the main
gates of the women's section of the city's prison. As we gaze at the forbid-
ding walls, a pale, thin woman emerges through a side door. Two women
cross the street and embrace her, then hurry her to a waiting taxi. We follow them to a nearby café and listen in on their conversation.

From the excited exchange, we learn that the former prisoner is Patricia
Herrero Mediavilla. She had been incarcerated for four years, four months,
and six days. Following her arrest in December 1986, she was subjected to
interrogation and torture. Her "crime" was to provide nursing care for sick
and injured individuals who opposed the Pinochet junta. She was charged
under the antiterrorist act and sentenced by a military tribunal to 39 years
of imprisonment. Her cause, and that of two other nurses imprisoned under similar circumstances, was taken up by groups of nurses throughout the
world. In a letter-writing campaign to the President of Chile, they de-
manded her release. Other nurses contributed to the support network in a
variety of ways. That support and solidarity over these long years had finally paid off.

Now let us travel back into the present and northward to the United
States. It is 6 o'clock in the evening in one of the country's northeast cities.
We are in the staff room of a health center in one of the less salubrious
areas of the city. A group of nurses are sitting around the table animatedly
discussing a document. You peer over one of the nurses' shoulders and note
that it is a draft position paper on health care financing.

Equity in access to health care for all members of this country's population has become a problem of increasing concern to many different groups
of stakeholders in the health care system. To date, the political response to
what is fast becoming a problem of massive proportions could best be described as constipated.

One positive reaction to the political inaction and rhetoric has been the
stimulation of groups of health care providers to seek possible solutions.
Nurses have been in the forefront of this action. A number are working on
a vision of what would constitute a just and caring health care system,
identifying barriers to achieving that system, and discussing ways of opera-
tionalizing the vision.

Our last stop is Australia. It is a Saturday and we are traveling through some of the farming areas of the country. Those of us who are city folk are totally dismayed at the extent and severity of the salinity problem that is spreading rapidly from the marginal wheat growing areas into more established farming districts. Even to those of us with no farming background, the surrounding paddocks in many of these latter areas look undernourished and degraded.

We stop for afternoon tea. Working their way toward us along the fenceline are a small group of people in working clothes. Half are armed with shovels. Others are planting young trees in prepared holes. When they reach our group, they call a halt to their labors and we start chatting. We discover that the workers are a group of city nurses who are members of HEAL, an acronym that stands for Hospital Environmental Awareness Link.

To date, their activities have been confined to addressing environmental concerns within the boundaries of their own hospitals. However, a felt need to widen their contributions, based on a broadened definition of health and factors that will affect the population's health in the future, stimulated them to volunteer to spend a weekend in the bush on a regeneration project. They all commented on how regenerated they themselves felt, albeit with varying degrees of stiffness and soreness, as a spinoff of this exercise.

REFLECTION

Storytelling can serve a number of purposes at different levels (Boykin & Schoenhofer, 1991; Parker, 1990; Sandelowski, 1991). In this case, the narrative provides a vehicle for the reflective process.

What do these stories tell us about caring? Do they illustrate potential problems and limitations with the description of caring as it is currently being explicated? What pointers do they give us in terms of new directions for the development of caring in practice, theory, and research? What do these stories confirm about current knowledge and the practice of caring?

CARING BY NURSES

Before we move to attempting to provide some answers to these questions, we must ask whether these stories even constitute caring by nurses. To answer this fundamental question, let us examine how the postulated examples of caring at the group or macro level fit with essential elements or characteristics of caring identified by theorists. Although a number of frameworks could be employed for this purpose, only those of Roach (1987) and Gaut (1986) will be used to illustrate this point.

Roach (1987) identified the *five Cs*—compassion, conscience, commitment, competence, and confidence—as the attributes of caring. The first three attributes—compassion, conscience, and commitment—are obvious in all four stories. Illustrations of the remaining two characteristics, however, are not universal. For the core members of the Free Herrero movement, for example, given the reputation of the dictatorship they were dealing with, faith or supreme optimism would be a more appropriate attribute than confidence. Mayeroff's (1972) ingredient of hope is probably more meaningful in this context.

Confidence is defined as "the quality which fosters trusting relationships" (Roach, 1987, p. 63), and reference is made to an environment and conditions of mutual trust and respect. The element of relationships will be explored later. Suffice it to say for now that, in the Chilean situation, the development of mutual trust and respect was not possible. The one being cared for, Patricia Herrero, was, in all likelihood, totally unaware of the efforts being made on her behalf.

The attribute of competence is described by Roach as "having the knowledge, judgment, skills, energy, experience and motivation required to respond adequately to the demands of one's professional responsibilities" (1987, p. 61). For the purpose of analysis, let us examine "experience." If we take the Burmese vignette, attempting to protect patients from the army is hardly something one could expect or would even want nurses to have experience in. Unfortunately, this experience is probably far more common than we would want to imagine. For political reasons, information of this kind is suppressed by those in power. Does this type of action even constitute one of the "demands of one's professional responsibilities"? The prospect of injury or even death is hardly an outcome we can expect professionals to face in a caring situation. As the study by Bäck-Pettersson and Pryds Jensen (Chapter 17) illustrates, another C could be added to Roach's five: courage.

The same point can be made in relation to the first of Gaut's (1986) essential elements: knowledge. The remaining elements are choice and implementation of action(s), and intention to produce positive change. These are governed by the criterion of welfare of the recipient. This criterion is obviously met, although in the plural, in three of the stories. The initial choice in all four situations was between acting and doing nothing. The intention to produce positive change for those in need is clear in three of the stories. It could be suggested that, indirectly in the Burmese and Chilean situations, the long-term positive change being contributed to was the replacement of repressive regimes with a just and democratic system of government. Each individual was making a small contribution to that goal.

Can we argue that fighting for democracy is related to caring in health? If it is intended to implement a democratic system in the health care system, then I believe we can answer that question in the affirmative. I have addressed the issue of democracy in health care in another forum (Watts, 1990), so suffice it to say that, in Australia at least, we still have a long way to go before we can say we have achieved a truly democratic system where paternalism no longer dominates the health care provided to individuals and communities.

Does the lack of a neat fit between what the stories demonstrate and what two theorists have identified as the characteristics of caring negate these as examples of caring by nurses, or does it indicate the need for further development of the concept? I would argue for the latter.

CARING AND NURSING

The nomination of these activities as caring raises a further question. The nurse side of the equation is not in question but is the other side—the nursed—a justifiable label for these disparate groups? In other words, do these actions fall within the definition of nursing?

The first two examples were actions taken by nurses, if not to save lives, to attempt to protect individuals from injury through torture. Given the history of the repressive and murderous regimes in those two countries, there would have been no question in the minds of the nurses who acted that that was the fate these individuals were facing or already experiencing. In the Burmese situation, the protected individuals were clearly a responsibility of the staff: they had been admitted to their hospital. In the Chilean example, the moral imperative to care arose out of the responsibility that nurses have to fellow nurses and to fellow human beings.

The other two examples of caring in nursing can also be defended on the grounds that nurses have a responsibility to protect and promote the health of fellow human beings through both direct and indirect means. In the past few years, many nurses have become more comfortable with the notion that professional nursing practice encompasses involvement in the formulation and analysis of health care policy (Courtney, 1987; McPherson, 1987; Milio, 1984; Schultz & Schultz, 1987). However, we still often hear the characterization, in Australia at least, of a "real nurse" as one who gives "hands-on" care to clients.

THE NATURE OF RELATIONSHIPS IN CARING

As indicated earlier, these stories raise the issue of relationships in the context of caring. To date, with a few notable exceptions (Leininger, 1988; Ray, 1989), the dyadic relationship, with its direct, personal involvement, has dominated the literature on caring in nursing. Many nurses, at least in Western countries, well may assume that the direct, dyadic relationship is essential for caring to occur. This perception of caring as being of an individualistic nature may reflect, as Dunlop (1986) suggested, the historico-cultural emphasis in both nursing and our society. These four stories illustrate that caring can and does occur outside those boundaries.

Direct, Personal Knowledge

Let us re-examine the four stories from the perspective of direct, personal knowledge of those being cared for. The Burmese nurses may or may not have known or taken care of the injured civilians. We have no way of knowing that information. I would suggest that previous personal contact was not a factor in the decisions they took in their attempts to protect the sick assigned to their collective care. In the case of the imprisoned Chilean nurse, the individual was clearly identifiable, although personally unknown, to the many nurses who directed their energies to obtaining her release. In most cases, their paths will never cross.

The action being taken by nurses in the United States to influence health policy is political. Nurses from all over the country are being stimulated to act for the disadvantaged and the at-risk members of the nation's population. The motivation to do so could well be born out of their personal experience with individuals requiring health care, but their actions are being taken on behalf of the entire nation. The outcome sought is at the collective, community level, not at the level of a specific, known individual.

Those taking environmental action are caring on an even more general level. Those persons at whom the actions of these nurses are directed are, in a sense, faceless, unknown members of the world's future population. The "Act locally, think globally" environmental slogan does, however, indicate a more immediate, identifiable focus to their activities. The actions of these nurses in respect to people are also indirect (via the environment). This story illustrates very clearly that caring "about" and caring "for" are inextricably linked.

In relation to the environment, Schuster (1990) raised the issue of anthropocentricity, given that the current exploration of the concept of caring in nursing has been restricted to human-to-human relationships. In contrast to the means-to-an-end argument that caring for the environment constitutes true caring in that it is a means, albeit indirect, of caring for the health of human beings, a number of environmental groups would adopt the position that, as an end in itself, caring for the environment is a valid form of caring for nurses.

Some have specifically rejected an extension of the concept of caring to all constituents of the environment. Noddings (1984), for example, maintained that plants are not, as humans are, potentially ones-caring. However, she did point out that it is entirely another matter "if one's behaviour toward the plant world or the natural world in general affects human beings deleteriously" (1984, p. 160). In other words, the human–human connection is the essential element. We need to remember that nursing's raison d'être is people.

Interpersonal Interaction

Tschudin (1992) stated that caring is only possible in a relationship, and this in turn is defined by the sharing of feelings. Parker (1990) questioned whether a relational ethic of care can be effective beyond the dyad of the nurse–patient relationship. Morse, Bottorff, Neander, and Solberg (1991), in their analysis of the current conceptualizations of caring, identified one of the 5 categories as being interpersonal interaction.

Do these stories of caring in action challenge this position, answer the question, fit into the category? The definition of "interpersonal," pertaining to relations between persons, does not exclude them. However, the implications of "interaction," defined as action on the other or reciprocal action, are not so clear. Strictly speaking, the action of the Burmese nurses did not fit the criterion of interaction. There was no opportunity for those they were attempting to protect to reciprocate or interact with those nurses. However, in all probability, the sacrifice of those nurses has acted on others in the sense that their action has contributed to keeping the flame of democracy alive in the country while the rest of the world turned a blind eye, until very recently, to that nation's suffering. Whether this constitutes action on the other is the question.

The effect of the experience of fighting for Patricia Herrero's release from prison is identifiable in respect to those who orchestrated the battle and who met up with her after her release. But what about those who were only marginally involved—those, like me, who only wrote a letter from thousands of miles away? What, if any, effect has the experience had on me? I certainly felt good when I read that she had been released. The news re-energized my belief that these sorts of actions can have results. Does this constitute action on the other, reciprocity, mutual exchange?

The same question can just as validly be applied to the remaining two situations. Again, in none of these cases were feelings shared with the other. Does this mean that caring did not occur? Although Marek (1990), in her discussion on therapeutic reciprocity, argued that the sharing of positive meanings between the nurse and client in the dyadic relationship is required for genuine caring to occur, she concluded with a quote that opens up the possibility of extending the meaning of reciprocity to include these examples. The quote comes from a short story by Goyen in which he described reciprocity as "the way human beings work upon each other" (1975, as cited in Marek, 1990, p. 58). These stories provide illustrations of how people work on others in positive ways.

Noddings stated that the caring relation requires a form of "responsiveness or reciprocity" (1984, p. 150) on the part of the person cared-for. She emphasised, however, that this reciprocity is not characterised by mutuality, that is, it is not contractual in nature—it does not dictate or require a direct response to the one-caring. The response or receptivity to caring may be demonstrated in some other indirect way.

Campbell encouraged a view of helping relationships as covenants rather than contracts. In this context, he described the nature of reciprocity in the following terms: ". . . parties to a covenant are recipients of gifts: neither is just a selfless giver" (1984, p. 105). Campbell identified some of the gifts or rewards that the professional receives from such a relationship as support, enlightenment, and personal development. These gifts can arise from caring in a nondirect, nondyadic situation. This discussion also raises a question as to whether reciprocity is even an essential element of caring in these types of situations. The philosopher Frankener's position that caring includes duty to care but not reciprocity may well be applicable here. (See Chapter 11.)

Caring and Comfort

Analysis of these stories highlights the unavoidable reality that caring in these contexts is political. That conclusion leads to another insight contained in these stories: caring is not necessarily comfortable.

One of the common, often implicit images of caring these stories bring into question is that caring results in "warm fuzzies" for those concerned. This image is encouraged by the use of such phrases as "the beauty of the caring moment" (Boykin & Schoenhofer, 1990, p. 21), or the use of the metaphor of instrumental friendship defined as "a relationship in which the other is loved primarily for incidental features that permit the actualisation of mutual expectations or goals" (Badhwar, 1987, as cited in Rawnsley, 1990, p. 46), to connect the theory and practice worlds of nursing as caring. The use of these two examples is not to deny that caring moments can be beautiful or that those involved are left with warm feelings in many situations. What is being questioned is whether this image of caring translates into a definitional requirement.

Obviously influenced by the assumption that any action that does not result in immediate warm feelings does not meet the acid test of caring, Morse, Solberg, Neander, Bottorff, and Johnson (1990) argued that a paradox can arise in relation to caring and safe practice. They maintained that, to inflict pain, nurses must become divorced or disembodied from the patient's experience while the patient is totally immersed in the experience. That is, nurses must become detached from caring to perform pain-inflicting nursing procedures.

Many nurses may well divorce themselves from the patient's experience in situations like this, but it does not mean that this approach is taken all the time by all nurses or that it should be. Parker's (1990) account of her personal experience in caring for a patient during his long and painful sojourn in ICU is a prime example that this is not necessarily so. Gaut drew the conclusion that caring "is best discussed in terms of actions to achieve goals rather than in terms of specific caring behaviors" (1986, p. 78). Does the longer-term outcome sometimes demand caring actions that do not generate warm feelings?

It is argued that these types of feelings are not an ever present, inherent, and essential characteristic of caring. Caring is not, as Street (1992) clearly illustrated, synonymous with niceness or feeling good. Caring can in fact be very discomforting.

The loss of one's life as an outcome of caring is thankfully not a sacrifice that many nurses are called on to make. The other stories, however, also hint at varying degrees of discomfort. For example, a colleague who had left Chile some years before struggled within herself as to whether she should become involved with Patricia Herrero's case. To petition the Chilean president could well result in her immediate family members, still in Chile, being placed under surveillance. On the other hand, she felt very committed to assisting this fellow nurse and citizen. Finally, she decided that her contribution would have to be confined to translating letters her colleagues had written into Spanish, in the hope that this would facilitate the contents being read by the authorities in Chile.

In respect to political issues, involvement in lobbying for a change in health policy may well generate varying amounts of discomfort for individual participants. For a number of nurses, any form of political involvement requires a change in behavior. Politics means public activity. Some find the move into the public arena, however limited in scope, difficult and sometimes painful.

There are other possible sources of discomfort in seeking policies that provide a means of achieving a just and effective outcome. We may well be required to examine and discard beliefs and positions to which we have held firmly up to this point. For example, the history, dominant culture, and experience of the United States have resulted in a deeply entrenched suspicion, if not outright rejection by many citizens, of any policy that might be construed as contributing to the development of "socialized medicine." The problem is that the most effective solutions to the current lack of equity in access to health care for large segments of the U.S. population—for example, the adoption of a form of national health insurance—are perceived by many as leading to that very outcome. One could question the definition of socialized medicine that is operative; however, that type of approach does not alter the fact that many health care professionals are, in all likelihood, going through a very personal and uncomfortable process in the course of demonstrating their caring for the disadvantaged and the at-risk.

In a recently published book (Hobson, 1992) is a Persian poem that is pertinent to this discussion. The book is the autobiography of a woman who for 20 years headed the first school for social workers in Iran. She was one of the first arrested after Khomeini came to power and only chance saved her from execution. For 20 years, she had studiously avoided political involvement of any kind. With the benefits of hindsight and exile, she came to the self-knowledge that she, like all the others from the educated middle class in that country, had failed. They had failed to stand up for the tenets of democracy during the Shah's reign, when corruption was rampant and freedom of expression and justice disappeared under increasingly tyrannical repression. After 20 years, she realized that the school's motto, this poem, was, in essence, a political statement:

> *Human beings are like parts of a body, created from the same essence,*
> *when one part is hurt and in pain, the others can not remain in peace and be quiet*
> *if the misery of others leaves you indifferent and with no feelings of sorrow*
> *you can not be called a human being.*

Another question comes to mind if we accept these stories as examples of caring. Do all forms of protest by health care workers constitute caring?

Fox's (1991) analysis of the Victorian nurses' strike in 1986 provides an answer to this question. The strike lasted 50 days and was a historical first within nursing in Australia. The primary cause of the strike was the current industrial award structure and wages. A similar dispute existed in the neighboring state of New South Wales at the time, but the dispute there was settled without recourse to strike action and without the human costs that are inevitably generated by strikes of this nature.

The argument has been put forward that nurses must care for themselves in order to be able to care for others (Johnson, Harrison, & McSkimming, 1992), and that the conditions under which nurses work are a vital factor in their ability to care for others. I doubt whether anyone would take issue with that argument. The crucial element is whether, in the course of achieving these conditions, the welfare of the recipient is protected. If a professional view of nursing is adopted, then there is no question that the ultimate "recipient" is the client and that caring for fellow nurses in terms of conditions of employment and the like is only the means to that end. That professional objective is sometimes lost sight of and the occupational view of nursing becomes dominant.

The conclusion that one draws from Fox's analysis of the Victorian strike is that, as the strike escalated, the ultimate objective of the welfare of the recipient, and even the welfare of the union's members, was lost sight of as the personalities and self-interests of major players dictated the choice of action. In New South Wales, the same outcome had been achieved without loss and suffering on the part of patients and relatives, without organized nursing becoming a house divided against itself, and without nurses being severely traumatized by the experience. In Victoria, all this and more was inflicted.

CONCLUSION

There is no question in my mind that what we were privileged to witness on our brief voyage can be classified as "engaged care," to use Benner and Wrubel's term (1991, p. 264). Analysis of these nursing situations has identified some of the directions we can take and some questions we need to explore in relation to the concept of caring in nursing at levels other than one-to-one. The challenge presented to us is how to identify "the knowledge, tact, craft and wisdom" embedded in stories such as these and "to extend and improve the skill of involvement and the practices" that go with these types of engaged care (Benner & Wrubel, 1991, p. 264).

In the words of Peter Ellyard (1988, as cited by Crawford, 1989, p. 46):

The future is not some place we are going to,
but one we are creating,
the paths to it are not found but made
and the activity of making them changes
both the maker and the destination.

REFERENCES

Benner, P., & Wrubel, J. (1991). Dialogue. *Image: The Journal of Nursing Scholarship, 23*(4), 264.

Boykin, A., & Schoenhofer, S. (1990). Caring in nursing: Analysis of extant theory. *Nursing Science Quarterly, 3*(2), 149–155.

Boykin, A., & Schoenhofer, S. (1991). Story as link between nursing practice, ontology, epistemology. *Image: The Journal of Nursing Scholarship, 23*(4), 245–248.

Campbell, A. (1984). *Professional care: Its meaning and practice.* Philadelphia: Fortress Press.

Courtney, R. (1987). Community practice: Nursing influence on policy formulation. *Nursing Outlook, 35*(4), 170–173.

Crawford, F. (1989, July). Educating for practice: Bringing thought and action together. *Proceedings of the Qualitative Research Conference* (pp. 46–52). Curtin University, Bentley, Western Australia.

Dunlop, M. (1986). Is a science of caring possible? *Journal of Advanced Nursing, 11,* 661–670.

Fox, C. (1991). *Enough is enough: The 1986 Victorian nurses' strike.* Sydney: University of New South Wales.

Gaut, D. (1986). Evaluating caring competencies in nursing practice. *Topics in Clinical Nursing, 8*(2), 77–83.

Hobson, W. (1992, July 4–5). Insights beyond the harem. [Review of *Daughter of Persia: A woman's journey from her father's harem through the Islamic revolution.*] *The Weekend Australian Review,* 5.

Johnson, K., Harrison, C., & McSkimming, S. (1992). An emphasis on caring. *International Association for Human Caring, 2*(4), 3.

Leininger, M. (1988). Leininger's theory of nursing: Cultural care diversity and universality. *Nursing Science Quarterly, 1,* 152–160.

McPherson, K. (1987). Health care policy, values, and nursing. *Advances in Nursing Science, 9*(3), 1–11.

Marek, P. (1990). Therapeutic reciprocity: A caring phenomenon. *Advances in Nursing Science, 13*(1), 49–59.

Mayeroff, M. (1972). *On caring.* New York: Harper & Row.

Milio, N. (1984). The realities of policymaking: Can nurses have an impact? *Journal of Nursing Administration, 14*(3), 18–23.

Morse, J., Solberg, S., Neander, W., Bottorff, J., & Johnson, J. (1990). Concepts of caring and caring as a concept. *Advances in Nursing Science, 13*(1), 1–14.

Morse, J., Bottorff, J., Neander, W., & Solberg, S. (1991). Comparative analysis of conceptualizations and theories of caring. *Image: The Journal of Nursing Scholarship, 23*(2), 119–126.

Noddings, N. (1984). *Caring: A feminine approach to ethics and moral education.* Berkeley: University of California Press.

Parker, R. (1990). Nurses' stories: The search for a relational ethic of care. *Advances in Nursing Science, 13*(1), 31–40.

Rawnsley, M. (1990). Of human bonding: The context of nursing as caring. *Advances in Nursing Science, 13*(1), 41–48.

Ray, M. (1989). The theory of bureaucratic caring for nursing practice in the organizational culture. *Nursing Administration Quarterly, 13*(2), 31–42.

Roach, M. (1987). *The human act of caring.* Ottawa: Canadian Hospital Association.

Sandelowski, M. (1991). Telling stories: Narrative approaches in qualitative research. *Image: The Journal of Nursing Scholarship, 223*(3), 161–166.

Schultz, P., & Schultz, R. (1987, April). *Nodding's caring and public policy: A linkage and its nursing implications.* Paper presented at the Ninth Annual Human Caring Research Conference, Menlo Park, CA.

Schuster, E. (1990). Earth caring. *Advances in Nursing Science, 13*(1), 25–30.

Street, A. (1992, July). *Being caring: Getting beyond the tyranny of "niceness" in health care.* Paper presented at the Fourteenth Annual Human Caring Research Conference, Melbourne, Australia.

Tschudin, V. (1992). *Ethics in nursing: The caring relationship* (2nd ed.). Oxford, England: Butterworth Heinemann.

Watts, R. (1990). Democratization of health care: Challenge for nursing. *Advances in Nursing Science, 13*(1), 37–46.

10

Toward Conscientization:
A Feminist Course Experience

Vera Regina Waldow

When women exercise their own power, they can build a caring environment. This chapter describes a feminist process used as a pedagogy strategy in a nursing course. The goal of the strategy was consciousness raising.

Education is a political and cultural activity that enables transformation through *praxis*—reflecting and acting on reality (Freire, 1973, 1985). When we reflect on our own praxis, we are able to effect change in such a way as to make meaning of a new reality. Freire wrote of *conscientização* (conscientization, meaning critical consciousness)—awareness of the sociocultural reality that shapes life, and the capacity to transform that reality (1985, p. 93).*

---

* The term *conscientização* translates to consciousness raising in English, but that term does not convey its real meaning, according to Freire. The term has appeared as conscientization in some of Freire's books. *Conscientização*, throughout this chapter, means the process by which human beings, not as recipients but as knowing subjects, perceive and understand the sociocultural reality that shapes their lives, and their capacity to take action against the oppressive elements of reality (Freire, 1985/ 1989).

The nursing profession in Brazil is seen as primarily a technical female activity that is unrecognized and lacks autonomy. Brazilian nurses face a conflict between the ideal role (direct care) and the real role (indirect care, meaning nursing management) (Nakamae, 1987). Brazilian nurses have been prepared for bedside care, but actually perform an administrative role.

Some studies (Almeida, 1986; Nakamae, 1987; Silva, 1986) have shown the work division within Brazil's nursing scenario. This division mirrors the social relationships within the capitalist/classist society of Brazil. The nursing schools still focus their curricula (based on a behaviorist model) on diseases, and medical models are still followed in most nursing curricula. Even in schools where the nursing curriculum has changed, there is no agreement between the new philosophy and what is actually emphasized by the faculty.

Two studies (Lopes, 1987; Loyola, 1987) have documented the transmission of oppressed behavior to nursing students. Power relationships are played out in the nursing schools and in the hospitals (Loyola, 1987).

Through education, individuals "become empowered to think about what they are doing, to become mindful, to share meanings, to conceptualize, to make varied sense of their lived world" (Greene, 1988, p. 12). There is an effort in feminism that is directed toward this empowerment. One of the methods used to increase women's consciousness is stimulation of consciousness raising, or activity identified with Freire's *conscientização*. By definition, *conscientização* comprises a sociocultural perspective and the perception of the contradictions of reality.

According to Stanley and Wise (1983), consciousness raising embraces different movement in consciousness: from lower to higher; from something that was not perceived before to something more concrete and perceived experientially; and so forth. Women's reality is based on and expressed by the language of experience.

Understanding of women's lives and delineation of the causes and consequences of women's oppression lead to approaches to social change. Chinn and Wheeler (1985), defending the need for a feminist perspective in nursing, said that feminism provides a personal, philosophic, and political means for analyzing the realities of women's lives as lived in patriarchal systems. Change would provide a chance to be different and an ability to accomplish what one chooses to do. Feminism is politically committed to such change, and a conception of feminist nursing praxis has been growing and will empower all women and nurses in the future (Chinn, 1989).

Teaching is a process of *empowerment to become*. Teachers should be persons who help others grow and who are dedicated to self-growth. Nursing educators can empower students and themselves to become real nursing professionals in a caring environment.

Wheeler and Chinn (1989) pointed out that "it is critical for women to come together and create woman-centered interactions and realities" (p. viii). Women are not accustomed to speaking up about their own feelings and realities Patriarchal and capitalist systems are very hostile toward stimulation of a woman's way of being. Instead, isolation, competitiveness, and "to have" are the norms.

Any sense of community and connectedness seems to be lost; there is a need to recapture the meaning of human kindness in a caring environment.

According to Moccia (1990), "caring *assumes* and *allows connection*" (emphasis added). Moccia called for the development of creative habits, the focus of which would be how we are connected rather than how we are different.

Connectedness means awareness of our own reality and experiences and those of others. It is a manner of consciousness that directs us to action, to caring. A caring environment implies an attitude of respect for others.

If we consider the universe to be an energy field, the community is a large human energy field in which interaction or exchange of matter and energy occurs continuously (Hardin, 1990). Caring is believed to be a necessary pattern of action. As a feminine attribute, caring means sensitiveness.

Education can enable people toward caring. Nurse educators who are aware of their potential for caring and of its power for change are able to become instruments of transformation.

DEVELOPING A COURSE BASED ON FEMINIST PEDAGOGY

I designed a course, the purpose of which was to reflect critically on nursing educators' practice. I took into account the history of nursing and its predominance of female practitioners, in order to achieve *conscientização* toward a future liberation of nursing. The course was developed as part of a Master's program in Nursing at the University of Santa Catarina, Brazil.

My goal throughout the course process was to stimulate reflection about nurses as women and about the world of nursing. The expected results were:

• Thinking more critically about ourselves as women and about our relationship to the world.

- Clarifying beliefs, attitudes, feelings, and meanings related to the teaching of nursing and to nursing in general.
- Benefiting from one another's knowledge, experience, guidance, and support.
- Disclosing our hidden power and becoming empowered to take effective action in order to improve ourselves and our praxis.

THE PARTICIPANTS

The course was organized to be a process of participation, interaction, and dialogue. Ten persons, including myself, participated in the discussions. Eight of the participants were faculty members of the Bachelor of Science Nursing Program (RN program). The other two were not teaching at the time but had taught in the past.

All the participants were Brazilians; only one was from the city where the course was held. Three were from cities nearby and the remainder were from different parts of the country.

STRATEGY

The classroom dynamics of the course were based on Wheeler and Chinn's feminist process (1989). These authors' suggestions on group process through the use of feminist forms of power were applicable to a teaching–learning experience. This type of approach, feminist pedagogy, is based on feminist praxis. Power is the main theme—power constructed and exercised by each individual toward a transformative praxis. Because the feminist process was a new proposal for the participants, meetings were planned in which the group could submit opinions and suggestions and define which items of this proposal would be utilized.

By consensus, the group made the following decisions.

Agenda

At every meeting, the agenda would be open for new topics or for modifications of topics suggested in a previous gathering.

Convener

The convener would be called "mediator" or "facilitator." Anyone could volunteer, at a meeting's closing, to mediate the next gathering. Every participant would then share the responsibility for mediating. The mediator would be responsible for opening the agenda, beginning the check-in, and starting the discussion of the day. The mediator would also observe the timetable established by consensus within the group, and would act as a reminder on time limitations.

If any participant felt the need to change to another phase, she would be free to suggest it to the group.

Check-in

In this phase, every member of the group would verbalize briefly her willingness to participate in the discussion as well as her expectations related to the gathering. Any participant's wish to not talk during this phase would be respected. The sharing of any feeling, event, experience, or circumstance with the group would be welcomed during check-in. The previous gathering would be summarized for those who were absent.

Rotating Chair

In this phase, the discussion would really begin. The chair would indicate whoever was to speak and the need to rotate to whoever wished to speak. The participant who was speaking was responsible for passing the chair to the next participant who raised her hand. Preference would be given to those who had not spoken yet or to someone who had not spoken recently.

Circling

The group would change to the circling phase when consensus was necessary. In the circling phase, every member would express her opinion about a specific issue. Decisions would be made by consensus. Sparking would be used if the group felt the need, whenever discussion became excited or a controversial issue was raised. Several persons could then talk in random order.

Principles of Unity

The existing principles of unity of the feminist process would be incorporated, with one addition as suggested during one of the meetings. The new principle facilitated an environment of support and respect for persons who had difficulty expressing themselves publicly.

Closing

The closing phase would be used at the end of every meeting. Each participant would state her criticism, appreciation, or affirmation in relation to the meeting.

My study consisted of reports on the discussions. The meetings were tape-recorded and the transcriptions of the discussions were subjected to qualitative analysis.

The course outline was submitted to the participants, who expressed their opinions and made some suggestions. (The final version appears in the chapter appendix.)

The course content consisted of a "start list" or guidelines for the main themes of the study. A variety of subthemes emerged and were later added to the main themes according to their analogy and appearance. The themes and subthemes were repeated in the course content, and comparison, contrasting, and aggregation of these themes as well as establishment of linkages and relationships among them and speculation on their meaning (Goetz & Le Compte, 1984), were part of the procedures.

The next section presents a sampling of the feelings and reactions of the participants, as expressed throughout the course. I selected statements that seemed to fit into the process of conscientization. Participants' criticisms, appreciation, and affirmations, expressed in the closing phase of the feminist process, are then summarized.

REACTION FEELINGS

Participants' feelings, comments, and opinions throughout the course process were denominated as reaction feelings. They included a series of statements in which the involvement of the participants in the process of reflection was perceived. Confusion and anxiety seemed to permeate all of the feelings that were verbalized, but, as the levels of these feelings varied, changes in the thinking processes were identified. These moments, considered as conscientization or consciousness raising times, were perceived as having ups and downs, highs and lows, advances and retrocessions.

Some of the participants said that they were in a process of change. Some seemed quite disturbed by conflicting feelings.

When the level of anxiety seemed to be disturbing, at least to me, we formally stopped the planned discussions in order to talk about our feelings. Meanwhile, during the regular sessions, these feelings emerged spontaneously, freely, and quite often.

No paraphrasing can explain and report human reactions accurately. Therefore, I give here the participants' voice transcriptions, the richest and truest testimonies of the reality they experienced at that time. The statements were extracted mainly from the check-in phase, and the closing phase, although throughout the discussions there were statements representative of particular reactions.

On Nursing Education

This reflection on education seems to be lacking. . . . this shows me what I did to my students—we do and continue doing. We are guilty. We have to change: we say one thing but we behave differently in practice.

I now realize how, as a teacher, I have failed to face the issue of women with my students. I can see how we let opportunities escape and now I am actually thinking of new roads . . . that I am going to travel now as a teacher. . . . I now recognize how negligent I have been about this matter all this time.

Why don't we discuss these values with our students? Why don't we work on how the students feel about all this?

We, as teachers, do not stimulate or encourage students' initiatives in organizing themselves politically.

Do our students really have much of a chance to exercise their critical faculties and to discuss issues during the semester?

It is something to think about, if we are really determined to change. We have to change our heads, to think and to put into practice what we think. We have to avoid saying one thing and doing another, and give the students, instead, conditions to feel secure and empowered to move ahead.

On the Nursing Profession

*I think that pessimism exists. We are usually full of regrets instead of look-
ing for and taking a stand. I think that now is the time to stop regretting
and to begin looking for a full stand, organizing as a profession in order to
conquer our place through competence and political action!*

*All this matter of the nursing profession used to seem quite natural to
me . . . now I need to think it over!*

*Now I am watching things, because I used to pass by them without really
seeing them. I used to pass by everything and I never saw what was really
happening. I don't know whether I was alienated!*

On Gender

Comments regarding gender and the role women are expected to play in
the eyes of the world were poignant.

*We were brought up not to ask. The submission of woman doesn't allow
this. Unfortunately, we are living in an extremely patriarchal country.*

Society places a heavy burden on women.

This is our stigma: being a housewife, a mother.

*Motherhood is extremely castrating for a woman. Why does it necessarily
have to be the woman who takes care of the children?*

*We don't need man's place, but rather, a place as human beings; there is a
place for all of us!*

On Feelings

Participants were searching for answers, for strategies, and for support.
Their feelings of excitement and confidence were permeated by feelings of
fear and insecurity. To some, the process of change, the road toward liberation, seemed to be lonely. They reported a need for attachment and support:

*Sometimes I feel very lonely in this position of having to solve the problems,
of being self-sufficient, me resolving, me doing, me fighting, me, me, me,
because I still couldn't have that . . . a group, to create a thing where*

one would be sustaining it. Except for moments like this. I think that what will emerge here are all the anxieties which will make us think, which will make us change our relationships with our families, with our colleagues, with work.

One of the participants, echoing what another had said, mentioned:

One of the things which bother me a lot is the question of feeling very lonely, isolated, you know? Because we always feel the need to have to identify ourselves, in thought, with the people we work with, to be intimate with the groups and to work together.

Nevertheless, despite the moments of anxiety, insecurity, fear, ambivalence, and loneliness, there was still hope. Two of the participants said, regarding the gender issue in nursing:

I think that we will show that we will make the unity . . . reveal ourselves . . . give strength . . . .
I second [her] words and I have taken the following as my motto: I will understand that I am a woman and by the fact that I am a woman I can get this, that, and that. I am holding firm to this thought and it's working!

CRITICISM

Several statements were gathered from the closings of the meetings. They are presented here as they occurred in the course development; that is, they follow the order of the content of the meetings.

A feeling of excitement was observed in the beginning. Comments referred to the atmosphere of the meetings and the flow of the discussions. Gradually, some of the comments pointed to what the discussions in the course were provoking—an opportunity for thinking critically, for learning, for growing, for listening to others, for getting somewhere.

The method in the course was perceived to be a way to facilitate expression of personal change and self-development. Change was described by some of the participants as already underway or envisioned as something to come next.

It is interesting to note that the statements in the first meeting were short summaries: "*Very interesting*"; "*I'm glad*"; "*I think we are getting somewhere*"; "*I lost the notion of time*"; "*It was good, it moved with a good pace*"; "*I* liked it. It went smoothly"; "I liked everybody's enthusiasm"; "I still haven't plucked up enough courage to speak." This last statement was made by a participant who had told the group about her difficulties in speaking. She seemed to get courage later on: she participated and narrated her own experiences, enriching the discussions like everybody else in the group, despite not being a talkative person.

In the subsequent closings, the criticisms became longer. Some indicated individuals' appreciation and affirmation as well as the group's development:

> I hope, from the bottom of my heart, that what is happening here with 10 people can happen with 10 more, led by each of us, which would amount to 100. I hope we can succeed in what we intend to do here in our group. I think that it is necessary to change. I believe in microrevolution. This kind of thing is a microrevolution, and we have to begin to think if we wish to get anywhere.
>
> I have enjoyed it very much. Every day I feel better, freer. I feel more like myself and I have better expectations all the time as we advance in our discussions. It is interesting, let us go to our microrevolution!

These were the views on individual growth and the group's growth:

> I love all this. It has been very helpful. We have internalized many things. We are growing.
>
> [The group] is in a phase of crescendo.
>
> I can see how far I would like to go.
>
> I am more and more convinced of the privilege we are having, of living this moment, of us being able to turn toward ourselves as women, doing as we wish, because we consider it important to invest in ourselves. These moments are proving to be very rich to me.
>
> I can feel that I am growing. We are going through transformation.
>
> This occasion is proving to be a time to reflect and think things through in a different way to redirect our practice. I see this as an exercise to prepare us for a new journey.

The importance of the group and the sharing of experiences were also points in the criticism:

> I realize from [the group's] accounts and everything else, how much more I need to do to get there. But I begin to see some shortcuts, some perspectives, some strategies and how to begin doing it also in practical terms. So, a good

thing remained from these meetings, which was learning from the other people's experiences, right?
I think that sharing our personal experiences has greatly affected me, since we feel a strong spirit of identification with our fellow nurses.

The participants referred to their sharing of certain problems and living experiences that were somehow similar, and to managing to bring to light certain events, limitations, and significant matters.

At the final closing, these were some of the participants' criticisms:

I found that our meetings were wonderful, that there was considerable growth. I felt it not only as far as I am concerned but also in the whole group. As a conclusion, I would like to quote a colleague of ours who, in defending her thesis, said something which caught my attention: "This subject cannot be finished with a period, it must be with a semicolon." We will continue.

Another participant agreed:

I think we grew and have gone ahead with the process of knowing ourselves, of knowing each other, which we had started last semester.
I also think that [the course—the feminist process] helped us to respect each other more, to accept each other, to understand, and to place ourselves in each other's place. I think it was an uncommon, a unique moment for us, and I'll take a lot of things forward in my life. So I hope we continue our search for values and beliefs which can support us in our forward journey and that it be a journey in which we can count on each other.
I also liked the experience very much. I think that there were moments when the discussions seemed to me very emotional and they brought out some reminders, incidents, experiences, one's life's passages, and the act of sharing the world of each other; yes . . . it was rewarding, very rich, and the proposal to continue this is very important, to go ahead together, united. It is as someone had said, like a helping relationship. I think we will need this support, this fellowship of sharing experiences, of friendship, yes?

Another participant, noting that much had already been said by the group, commented on the beginning of the course, the first meetings:

I was very concerned with this method [the Feminist Process] which I thought would be something complicated, boring, repetitive. And, you know what? It was something so natural, so pleasant, nothing like I had *imagined. Another thing was in relation to the coordination. We had all that discussion about the convener role and so forth and, in the end, we were always referring to the coordination but not with that old connotation anymore. I think that was due to the unity of the group. In relation to the process itself, I think that there was an involvement by the group. There was growth too, especially on my part, but on the part of the group as well. I think that there was something outstanding from each member, or something that had some affinity with something that one learned and in some way will always connect with that person. Lastly, I think that this was a delightful course, I am sorry that this is the closing, and semicolon!*

THE LITERATURE

Fasano (1979), reporting on students reactions to a women's studies course using consciousness-raising techniques, mentioned resistance to accepting sexism and oppression. Sensitivity and anger are also common. According to Fasano (1979), depression is encountered among nursing students who feel helpless after acknowledging sex discrimination.

The students' evaluations of the course reported by Fasano (1979) indicated that personal growth had been experienced and a more acute awareness of women and nursing's position in society had been achieved. Other items mentioned were changes in the students' plans for their future, and feelings of openness toward different options in life patterns and educational goals. The course was perceived as being helpful in providing frank discussion.

Feminist pedagogy has been noted in the literature as stimulating empowerment and a sense of community (Symonds, 1990). Dialogue, freedom, connectedness, wholeness, and integration have also been cited (Heding & Donovan, 1989).

Feminist pedagogy in patriarchal institutions can be perceived as a threat. The process for a move toward change cannot happen right away. Wheeler and Chinn (1989) observed that, when a community is created, it is easier to overcome isolation, fear, and frustration.

Weiler's study (1988) also addressed the challenge of feminist teaching methods, and reported on the tensions that emerge when putting them into practice.

The confrontation of self and the attempt to balance the "I" with the "we" may result in depression in women (Lerner, 1989). Acknowledgement of self-sacrifice and loss of self-esteem also accompany the unconscious awareness of self-betrayal. Actually, there is a realization that the personal is political, which questions and challenges the roles and rules defined for women. Consciousness raising and sociopolitical change lead to a feeling of depression in which the awareness of anger plays a critical part (Lerner, 1989).

Through consciousness-raising activities, women start to see reality differently, or, as stated by Stanley and Wise (1983), they experience a "new way of seeing the *same* reality" (emphasis added). Consciousness raising, or the spiral of feminist consciousness, is experienced differently, but, in general, it involves change and, consequently, conflict (Stanley & Wise, 1983).

Miller (1986) emphasized that "conflict is a necessity if women are to build for the future" (p. 125).

Conflict includes feelings of change, expansion, and joy, when it occurs in a productive way. Destructive conflict consists of a feeling that nothing can be changed or that there is an absolute impossibility of winning (Miller, 1986). In the process of conflict, women have a need for other people with whom they can share things and from whom they can receive support.

The best conflicts are those that lead to more and better connection rather than disconnection. This kind of conflict leads to growth, but both (or all) of the people involved have to be ready to enter into this form of conflict. (Miller, 1986, p. 140)

Lerner (1989) stated that depression is one form of emotional reaction associated with loss. She observed that the need for affiliation or the orientation toward relationships for emotional connectedness is a basic human need as well as a strength. The problem women face that predisposes them to depression is what happens in their relationships. According to some of the participants' reports, when their realities were disclosed, a sort of ambivalence in engaging in change resulted from their fear of losing the support of their relatives. They realized that a new way of being may not be welcome. A new journey toward transformation seemed exciting, but it was also scary. They reported some fear of rejection by their female peers; some had already experienced it. Miller (1986) noted that problems can arise when women begin to realize their differing experiences and perceptions. Women might fear losing connectedness and unity as well as the recreation of a situation of dominance–subordination. "Any difference can appear as threatening and as a signal that some people are 'better' or superior and others are lesser" (Miller, 1986, p. 136).

Meanwhile, women's groups based on feminism can benefit from discussing and overcoming their feelings, acknowledging and valuing differences. As asserted by Miller (1986), differences are a source of strength, and women "have a long history of learning to fear difference."

CONCLUSION

Feelings of insecurity and fear of facing the hostile male world can only be broken through the practice of ways of empowerment. Only by creating the habit of voicing our female language in a caring environment will we be able to get strength for change. A sense of community, a sharing of experiences and connectedness can be nourished in our everyday life by means of practice and action—that is, by praxis. Daily practice of "doing what we know and knowing what we do" will move women toward a new reality.

REFERENCES

Almeida, M. C. P. de (1986). *O saber da enfermagem e sua dimensão prática* (The nursing knowledge and its practical dimension). São Paulo: Cortez.

Chinn, P. L. (1989). Nursing patterns of knowing and feminist thought. *Nursing and Health Care, 10*(2), 70–75.

Chinn, P. L., & Wheeler, C. E. (1985). Feminism and nursing. *Nursing Outlook, 33*(2), 74–77.

Fasano, N. F. (1979). Credit for consciousness raising. *American Journal of Nursing, 16*(8), 3–6.

Freire, P. (1973). *Education for critical consciousness* (M. B. Ramos, Trans.). New York: Seabury.

Freire, P. (1985). *The politics of education: Culture, power, and liberation* (D. Macedo, Trans.). South Hadley, MA: Bergin & Garvey.

Freire, P. (1989). *Pedagogy of the oppressed* (M. B. Ramos, Trans.). New York: Continuum.

Goetz, J. D., & Le Compte, M. D. (1984). *Ethnography and qualitative design in educational research.* San Diego, CA: Academic Press.

Greene, M. (1988). *Dialectic of freedom.* New York: Teachers' College Press.

Hardin, S. (1990). A caring community. In M. Leininger & J. Watson (Eds.), *The caring imperative in education* (pp. 217–225). New York: National League for Nursing.

Heding, B. A., & Donovan, J. (1989). A feminist perspective of nursing education. *Nurse Educator, 14*(4), 8–13.

Lerner, H. G. (1989). *Women in therapy.* New York: Harper & Row.

Lopes, M. J. (1987). *O trabalho da enfermeira: Nem público nem privado—feminino, doméstico e desvalorizado* (The nurse's work: Neither public nor private—feminine, domestic and undervalued). Unpublished master's thesis, PUCRS, Instituto de Sociologia da Indústria, Porto Alegre, Brazil.

Loyola, C. M. D. (1987). *Os doces corpos do hospital: As enfermeiras e o poder institucional na estrutura hospitalar* (The sweet bodies of the hospital: Nurses and the institutional power in the structure of hospitals). Rio de Janeiro: UFRJ.

Miller, J. B. (1986). *Toward a new psychology of women.* Boston: Beacon.

Moccia, P. (1990). Deciding to care: A way to knowledge. In M. Leininger & J. Watson (Eds.), *The caring imperative in education* (pp. 207–215). New York: National League for Nursing.

Nakamae, D. D. (1987). *Novos caminhos da enfermagem: Por mudancas no ensino e na prática da profissão* (New ways for nursing: For change in the teaching and practice of the profession). São Paulo: Cortez.

Silva, G. (1986). *Enfermagem profissional—Análise crítica* (Professional nursing—Critical analysis). São Paulo: Cortez.

Stanley, L., & Wise, S. (1983). *Breaking out: Feminist consciousness and feminist research.* London: Routledge & Kegan Paul.

Symonds, J. M. (1990). Revolutionizing the student–teacher relationship. In *Curriculum revolution: Redefining the student–teacher relationship* (pp. 47–55). New York: National League for Nursing.

Weiler, K. (1988). *Women teaching for change: Gender, class and power.* South Hadley, MA: Bergin & Garvey.

Wheeler, C. E., & Chinn, P. L. (1989). *Peace and power: A handbook of feminist process* (2nd ed.). New York: National League for Nursing.

APPENDIX

Course Schedule

Date	Topics and Activities	Readings
9/18	Course outline discussion and methodology (feminist process)	Wheeler & Chinn[1]
9/25	Feminist process—discussion and practice	Wheeler & Chinn[1]
10/2	Feminist process practice	Wheeler & Chinn[1]
10/9	Hidden curriculum and nursing education	Giroux[2]; Pitts[3]
10/16	Hidden curriculum and nursing practice	Loyola[4]
10/23	The issue of oppression (first reaction paper due)	Freire[5]
10/30	Women's issues: feminism, ideology, concepts	Westkott[6]; Ramazanoglu[7]
11/6	Women's oppression and nursing	Roberts[8]
11/13	Women's issues and nursing: power, political action	Sarti[9]; Lopes[10]
11/20	Nursing education in a feminist dimension	Hedin[11]; Ryan[12]
11/27	Nursing education: suggestions, alternatives	Hedin & Donovan[13] (suggested); Wheeler & Chinn[1]
12/4	Closing (final appreciation, criticism, and affirmation)	

[1] Wheeler, C. E., & Chinn, P. L. (1989). *Peace and power: A handbook of feminist process* (2nd ed.). New York: National League for Nursing.

[2] Giroux, H. (1983). Schooling and the politics of the hidden curriculum. In *Theory and resistance in education: A pedagogy for the opposition* (pp. 42–71). South Hadley, MA: Bergin & Garvey.

[3] Pitts, T. P. (1985). The covert curriculum: What does nursing education really teach? *Nursing Outlook, 33*(1), 37–39, 42.

[4] Loyola, C. M. D. (1987). *Os doces corpos do hospital: As enfermeiras e o poder institucional na estrutura hospitalar* (The sweet bodies of the hospital: Nurses and the institutional power in the structure of hospitals). Rio de Janeiro: UFRJ.

[5] Freire, P. (1989). *Pedagogy of the oppressed* (M. B. Ramos, Trans.). New York: Continuum.

[6] Westkott, M. (1983). Women's studies as a strategy for change: Between criticism and vision. In R. D. Klein & G. Bowles, *Theories of women's studies* (pp. 210–218). London: Routledge & Kegan Paul.

[7] Ramazanoglu, C. (1989). Feminism as contradiction. In *Feminism and the contradictions of oppression* (pp. 5–23). London: Routledge & Kegan Paul.

[8] Roberts, S. J. (1983). Oppressed group behavior: Implications for nursing. *Advances in Nursing Science, 5*(7), pp. 21–30.

[9] Sarti, C. (1988). Feminismo no Brasil: Una trajetória particular (Feminism in Brazil: A particular trajectory). *Cadernos de Pesquisa, 64*, 38–47.

[10] Lopes, M. J. (1987). *O trabalho da enfermeira: Nem público nem privado—feminino, doméstico e desvalorizado* (The nurse's work: Neither public nor private—feminine, domestic and undervalued). Unpublished master's thesis, PUCRS, Instituto de Sociologia da Indústria, Porto Alegre, Brazil.

[11] Hedin, B. A. (1989). With eyes aglitter: Journey to the curriculum revolution. *Nurse Educator, 14*(4), 3–5.

[12] Ryan, M. (1989). Classrooms and concepts: The challenge of feminist pedagogy. *Feminist Teacher, 14*(4), 39–42.

[13] Hedin, B. A., & Donovan, J. (1989). A feminist perspective of nursing education. *Nurse Educator, 14*(4), 8–13.

PART III

ETHICS/RESEARCH METHODOLOGIES

11

The Ethic of Care: Nursing's Excellence for a Troubled World

Sara T. Fry

INTRODUCTION

The need for human caring *is* universal. At the present time, many countries of the world are engaged in armed conflict. Many others are besieged by drought, poverty, hunger, and natural disasters. HIV infection occurs throughout the world and those suffering from AIDS are placing a heavy demand on available health care services in many countries. In all of these events, real people exist who experience the need for human caring.

While all people express human caring differently, according to their culture and human resources, the health professions have a social mandate to provide human caring in response to health needs. The nursing profession, in particular, offers human caring as its excellence to all people with health needs. Nursing understands human caring to be an involvement with others and a concern with how they experience their world.

This conference on *Human Caring: A Global Agenda*, hosted by the International Association for Human Caring and the Royal College of

Nursing, Australia, attests to the fact that the phenomenon of human caring is of particular concern to all nurses. Nurses are interested in the various cultural meanings of caring, educational preparation for human caring, and the costs of providing human caring. Thus, the goals of the conference are to increase our knowledge of caring and to assist us in gaining new insights about caring as nursing's special excellence.

In light of these goals, this presentation provides an overview of the concept of human caring, reviews several definitions of caring, and discusses several models of caring. I will also raise a few questions about the ethic of care and care-ethics theories. My intent is to demonstrate why any theory of human caring needs to be a *practical* ethic if it is to be useful to the practice of nursing. I hope that my comments will stimulate our thinking about human caring and provide an appropriate background for the other presentations of the conference.

CONCEPT OF HUMAN CARING

The concept of human caring has several important attributes. It is the way that humans relate to the world and to each other; it supports caring behaviors and is often identified with moral and social ideals (Griffin, 1983). Human caring also expresses itself in activities or behaviors and is usually associated with certain attitudes and feelings. Human caring is a moral concept when caring is directed toward human needs and is perceived as a duty to respond to need.

These attributes of human caring are contained in definitions of caring. Leininger, for example, defined caring as "those human acts and processes that provide assistance to another individual or group based on an interest in or concern for that human being(s), or to meet an expressed obvious or anticipated need" (1984, p. 46). Other definitions of caring also emphasize that caring is a motivation to protect the welfare of another person or to help that person grow and actualize himself (Gaylin, 1976; Mayeroff, 1971).

MODELS OF HUMAN CARING

Models of human caring emphasize the various attributes of the concept (Fry, 1991). A Cultural Model of Caring relates caring to cultural beliefs, practices, and human survival (Leininger, 1984) and has provided the conceptual framework for several studies of human caring among different cultural groups (Boyle, 1984; Dugan, 1984; Wang, 1984).

A Feminist Model of Caring relates human caring to the feminist perspective of moral development (Gilligan, 1977) and is often understood as an attitude that can be learned and nurtured through educational processes (Noddings, 1984). When fully developed, an attitude of human caring will tend to result in ethical behavior and choices.

A Humanistic Model of Caring relates human caring to a moral obligation or duty to be caring (Pellegrino, 1985). This model of caring is supported by a philosophy of moral commitment toward protecting human dignity and preserving humanity (Gadow, 1985; Gaut, 1984; Ray, 1987). It often takes the form of respect for persons or an attitude of Christian love toward others (Frankena, 1983).

An Obligation Model of Caring emphasizes compassion, doing good for others, and medical competence, and is directed toward the good of an individual. One is obliged to be caring in order to produce some good or to create some benefit for another individual.

A Covenant Model of Caring emphasizes the presence of fidelity in relationships. Fidelity between persons stems from the covenant made between persons when they stand in particular relationships to one another: mother and child, teacher and student, nurse and patient. Nurse caring, then, involves compassion, doing for others, respect for persons, and the protection of human dignity.

All of these models of caring are important because they indicate that moral caring requires certain actions and judgments on the part of the one who cares. Human caring is more than just a sentiment, an ideal, or a striving toward some state of affairs. Human caring as moral action requires clarity about the motivations or reasons for one to care (Fry, 1990). While it is helpful to think about the moral foundations for human caring as being basically obligation-driven or covenant-driven, it is more important to carry out caring in human relationships. Thus, a model of human caring should be linked with traditional ethical approaches in order to provide a *practical ethic* for health care practices (Fry, 1991).

A PRACTICAL ETHIC OF HUMAN CARING

A practical ethic of human caring will provide adequate guidelines for nursing actions under a wide variety of human care situations if it is not defined too narrowly. When used in conjunction with traditional ethics, it will be possible to distinguish "good" caring actions from "bad" ones. Traditional ethics theories and their focus on principles have their faults (Degrazia, 1992), but they do provide a structured approach to consider the types of moral concerns that nurses confront on a daily basis. They also provide a common language and understanding about moral relationships that nursing needs to be aware of if it wants to be taken seriously in discussions about the ethics of health care relationships. There is no particular virtue to developing a care-ethic language that has meaning only for nurses!

A practical ethic of human caring will also recognize a distinction between caring for and caring about. It is desirable for nurses to both care for and care about their patients, but nursing's excellence in a troubled world is clearly caring for. All the presentations of this conference will indicate how nurses care for others and will help generate new levels of understanding about the phenomenon of human caring and its moral dimensions, worldwide. To these possibilities, we should now turn.

REFERENCES

Boyle, J. (1984). Indigenous caring practices in a Guatemalan colony. In M. M. Leininger (Ed.), *Care: The essence of nursing and health* (pp. 123–132). Detroit: Wayne State University Press.

Degrazia, D. (1992). Moving forward in bioethical theory: Theories, cases, and specified principalism. *The Journal of Medicine & Philosophy, 17*(5), 511–539.

Dugan, A. B. (1984). Compadrazgo: A caring phenomenon among urban Latinos and its relationship to health. In M. M. Leininger (Ed.), *Care: The essence of nursing and health* (pp. 183–194). Detroit: Wayne State University Press.

Frankena, W. K. (1983). Moral-point-of-view theories. In N. E. Bowie (Ed.), *Ethical theory in the last quarter of the twentieth century* (pp. 39–79). Indianapolis: Hackett.

Fry, S. T. (1990). The philosophical foundations of caring. In M. M. Leininger (Ed.), *Ethical and moral dimensions of care* (pp. 13–24). Detroit: Wayne State University Press.

Fry, S. T. (1991). A theory of caring: Pitfalls and promises. In D. A. Gaut & M. M. Leininger (Ed.), *Caring: The compassionate healer* (pp. 161–172). New York: National League for Nursing.

Gadow, S. A. (1985). Nurse and patient: The caring relationship. In A. H. Bishop & J. R. Scudder (Eds.), *Caring, curing, coping: Nurse, physician, patient relationships* (pp. 31–43). Birmingham: University of Alabama.

Gaut, D. A. (1984). A philosophic orientation to caring research. In M. M. Leininger (Ed.), *Care: The essence of nursing and health* (pp. 17–25). Detroit: Wayne State University Press.

Gaylin, W. (1976). *Caring*. New York: Avon.

Gilligan, C. (1977). In a different voice: Women's conceptions of self and of morality. *Harvard Educational Review, 47*, 481–517.

Griffin, A. P. (1983). A philosophical analysis of caring in nursing. *Journal of Advanced Nursing, 8*, 289–295.

Leininger, M. M. (1984). *Care: The essence of nursing and health*. Detroit: Wayne State University Press.

Mayeroff, M. (1971). *On caring*. New York: Harper & Row.

Noddings, N. (1984). *Caring: A feminine approach to ethics and moral education*. Berkeley: University of California Press.

Pellegrino, E. (1985). The caring ethic: The relation of physician to patient. In A. H. Bishop & J. R. Scudder (Eds.), *Caring, curing, coping: Nurse, physician, patient relationships* (pp. 8–30). Birmingham: University of Alabama Press.

Ray, M. A. (1987). Technological caring: A new model in critical care. *Dimensions in Critical Care Nursing, 6*(3), 166–173.

Wang, J. F. (1984). Caretaker–child interaction observed in two Appalachian clinics. In M. M. Leininger (Ed.), *Care: The essence of nursing and health*. Detroit: Wayne State University Press.

12

The Interdisciplinary Meanings of Human Caring

Janet M. Lakomy

*T*he concept of caring continues to receive increased attention and emphasis in health care, nursing, and nursing research. Caring has been posited as the essence of nursing (Leininger, 1981, 1984; Noddings, 1984; Watson, 1979, 1985). In addition, caring has been addressed by and has importance to many disciplines, as reflected in the varied meanings of human caring acknowledged by psychoneuroimmunology, sociobehavioral sciences, anthropology, fine arts, humanities, including philosophy and ethics, and theology. As illustrated later in the chapter, the meanings of caring have suggested both diversity and a universal theme. In order for nursing to truly be accountable to society in all its human conditions and needs for healing, a deep interdisciplinary understanding of the nature and meanings of human caring from an interdisciplinary perspective is imperative.

RESEARCH QUESTIONS

The purpose of this study was to discover and create the meanings of human caring through the development of a guide to the caring literature within a selected interdisciplinary perspective. Thus, three research questions were formulated for this study:

- What is the meaning of human caring within a selected disciplinary focus?
- How does one understand the meanings of human caring from a selected interdisciplinary focus?
- From a selected interdisciplinary focus, how does one access the caring literature?

SIGNIFICANCE OF THE PROBLEM

The scientific base of the helping professions has shifted from biomedical science to the human sciences and subsequently includes humanities, social sciences, and ethical and metaphysical perspectives relevant to the human condition and human caring. At present, much of the historical evolution and theoretical underpinnings of human caring are inaccessible to the majority of the nursing profession as well as other helping professionals. The rich resources in the humanities are not organized for retrieval for a variety of users—specifically, health care professionals. In addition, knowledge on human caring is not presently retrievable through current biomedical taxonomies. More refined, sensitive taxonomies are needed to increase access, retrieval, and integration of human caring for use in practice, education, and research.

RATIONALE FOR SELECTING DISCIPLINES FOR CARING LITERATURE

In exploring the knowledge base for human caring, multiple frames of reference of caring knowledge were encountered from various perspectives. Nine disciplines were selected to participate in the discovery and identification of the exemplary human caring literature. Exemplary literature denoted classical, foundational, and representative works, including articles, books, and monographs on human caring. The nine disciplines were: psychoneuroimmunology, fine arts, sociobehavioral sciences, anthropology, humanities, including philosophy and ethics, theology, and nursing.

Psychoneuroimmunologists contributed insights about caring relative to how the person was structurally, mentally, and functionally affected during and after experiencing caring. Researchers in psychoneuroimmunology have concluded that social support networks, positive relationships, and a sense of control by individuals have had a positive and activating effect on the immune response (Ader, 1981; Cohen & Syme, 1985; Rodin, 1986). Psychoneuroimmunologists continue to do much research on how the immune response could be activated through interventions and experiences such as caring. Thus, a possibility exists for the person who has experienced caring to activate his or her immune system when experiencing stressors in life in order to potentiate and enhance his or her total well-being.

Fine artists have provided persons with captured illustrations and works of art that portray individuals' caring with one another. Works of art, such as still life, fruit, and flowers portrayed a celebration with nature, being, and existence. When a portrayed "caring" work of art was experienced by another person, this person could transcend the art and experience the healing power of caring. When individuals viewed art, they were able to experience the colors, designs, background, and emotions as caring. The viewer could perceive art from many different dimensions and allow it to remain suspended if desired. Through the artist's work, the healing power of caring could emerge and the viewer could transcend the work and experience caring at a higher and deeper level.

Sociobehavioral scientists contributed insights on caring relative to how the caring person thinks, learns, behaves, and relates to others. In everyday life and coping situations, persons are constantly confronted with stressors. A positive and productive method of coping with stressors can be experienced through caring with self and caring with one another. Lazarus and Folkman (1984) documented that, through coping, stressful transactions could be mastered. Emotional states contributed to health and illness. Thus, emotions and mental states were significant both in susceptibility to disease and recovery from disease. A distinct possibility existed that within one's mind was a power capable of exerting forces that could either enhance or inhibit the progress of disease. Thus, the person's active and positive participation could influence not only the onset of disease, but the outcome of treatment and the person's quality of life.

Anthropologists contributed insights on caring relative to how the person has evolved culturally, through cultures' symbols, values, meanings, and artifacts. This study focused on the following four cultural groups: Caucasians, Blacks, Mexican Americans, and American Indians. These cultures were selected because they represented dominant cultural groups in the

United States. Each culture brought to the community a group of beliefs, values, symbols, and artifacts that represented the culture's existence within society. Thus, in the process of caring with and being cared for by these people, one must be cognizant of their culture, beliefs, and values.

Humanities depicted the person's inner spirit through various modes of expression (film, literature, music, and drama). Scholars in the humanities have focused on "being," knowing, and interrelationships between the one caring and the one being cared for.

Philosophers contributed insights into caring by asking: What is the being of caring and what is caring as such? Philosophers have provided the foundation for relationship, person, and "eros" within caring. Within philosophy, caring has been approached and addressed through the ontology of caring, the essence of being, the relations among persons, and their required developmental growth process. Thus, caring involved self-awareness, positive relationships among persons, and a developmental growth process by those experiencing caring.

Ethicists contributed insights on caring by their evolution from classical or principle-based ethics to the work of Noddings (1984), *Caring: A Feminine Approach to Ethics and Moral Education*. Ethics contributed the locus for care by the rules, principles, and experiential responses that served as norms for appropriate professional behavior. Traditionally, ethics has been defined as an inquiry into rules and principles of morality, of right and wrong conduct, of virtue and vice, and/or of good and evil as they related to conduct. Within the norms of nursing, caring was seen to subsume the moral/ethical imperatives. Thus, the locus of nursing ethics is caring. One must ask, what moral/ethical obligations are involved in nursing as the professionalization of human care? The locus for the rules and principles that serve as norms for appropriate professional behavior is caring (Roach, 1984).

Theologians contributed insights into the person's relationship with the divine, into the mystery of the human person, and into human history. From the theological perspective, caring was epitomized in God, the covenant. When one was not faithful to the covenant, caring disappeared.

In the Christian tradition, Jesus was a caring, loving, and compassionate person, and the norm and inspiration of human caring relationships became a commandment of love. In the early Christian church, nursing was a unique kind of human caring. Through the refinement of a call, nursing developed as a commitment to make the healing presence of a higher power experienced in a suffering world (Roach, 1984).

Nursing scholars, such as Benner (1984), Gaut (1981, 1983, 1984), Leininger (1980, 1981, 1984), Patterson and Zderad (1976), Ray (1981, 1984), Watson (1979, 1985), and others, have contributed various insights on caring. Caring has been posited as the essence of nursing; the attributes that describe nursing have care as their locus (Roach, 1984). Leininger (1978) presented the thesis that caring was the most unifying, dominant, and central intellectual and practice focus in nursing. Nursing was the discipline most directly and intimately involved with caring needs and behaviors. The four most common constructs of caring behaviors and processes were: concern for, respect, compassion, and attention (Leininger, 1986). "There can be no curing without caring, but there may be caring without curing" (Leininger, 1980, p. 8).

In discovering and creating the meanings of human caring through the development of a guide to the human caring literature, an interdisciplinary framework was imperative. To avoid or eliminate a reductionist view of the discovered and created meanings of human caring, nursing needed to search for an integral humanism for the unification of the caring knowledge.

There was a rich resource of knowledge on human caring in the humanities; however, it was not retrievable through the biomedical taxonomies. More refined, sensitive taxonomies on human caring needed development to increase access, retrieval, and integration for use in practice, education, and research. Through the discovery and creation of the meanings of human caring, a guide to the caring literature has the capacity to make an impact on the health care delivery system and on health care policy today and in the future.

METHODOLOGY

Hermeneutics, the understanding and interpretation or explanation of texts (Ricoeur, 1981), was the methodology selected for this study. The nineteenth-century Romantic hermeneutics held that explanation was not the goal of hermeneutic investigation, but rather understanding was achieved through the interpretation of the text, discourse fixed by writing, and meaningfully oriented behavior (Ricoeur, 1981). The reconstruction of hermeneutics, in the late nineteenth century and continuing into the twentieth century, brought understanding and explanation back into the hermeneutical circle (Klemm, 1983).

Ricoeur's hermeneutical theory is a dialectical model of textual interpretation based on discourse and the combination of understanding and explanation (Klemm, 1983). For Ricoeur, "what it means to be human" is the overall philosophical intention (Ricoeur, 1976). Ricoeur's central idea is that the text is discourse that has been fixed by writing. Discourse refers to a description, expression, or representation of the world. Realized as an event, discourse is understood as meaning. Thus, the medium through which one understood oneself was through text (Ricoeur, 1981).

Gadamer claimed that hermeneutics is both ontological and universal. Hermeneutics is ontological because, in the world, our primordial mode of being is understanding. The genuinely open interpreter begins the hermeneutical conversation of the text by listening and allowing the text to assert its viewpoints (Gadamer, 1976). Through understanding, meaning comes into being. Finally, the medium of all understanding and all tradition is language, and language is the medium in which we live (Gadamer, 1975).

The modified hermeneutical strategies comprised the methodology developed for the study. The perspectives from Ricoeur's and Gadamer's philosophical hermeneutics underlaid the hermeneutical design and strategies used in this study.

RICOEUR'S PROCESS OF HERMENEUTICAL ANALYSIS

Ricoeur's hermeneutical analysis consists of the following process:

1. *Initial reading of the text.* The investigator begins with a "naive" understanding of the text as it is. Thus, the investigator perceives a first gleaning of the text's meaning. During the first reading, the integrity of understanding and explanation begins. Initial impressions can then be assessed, corrected, and deepened by recourse to the objective structure of text. Hence, the meaning of the text-work is constituted by the investigator as it immediately presents itself, without questioning whether the appearing text-world is the "true" one (Klemm, 1983).

2. *Distanciation.* This condition of interpretation requires not projecting oneself and one's own beliefs and prejudices on the text. Thus, in order to discern the immanent design in the text, the investigator becomes a detached, reflexive subject who brackets the referential intention of the text (Klemm, 1983). For the investigator, only by losing oneself will one find oneself (Ricoeur, 1981).

3. *Structural analysis.* The text is reread from a critical investigator's perspective. Structural analysis is the process of hermeneutical

explanation or interpretation and understanding of the text. The unit of analysis in hermeneutics is the sentence, followed by the paragraph, the section, the chapter, and then the whole of the text. Meaning is expressed in sentence units. The function of structural analysis leads the investigator from surface semantics to in-depth semantics. After in-depth semantics and interpretation, engagement in explanation and participatory belonging at a higher level are possible (Ricoeur, 1976).

4. *Identification of the metaphor of the text.* A metaphor is contextual, a momentary creation of language that is not found in the dictionary and that creates new meaning. In order to understand the metaphor, the key is to understand the text (Ricoeur, 1981). Thus, the hermeneutic interpretation is a dialectical discourse between the text in its projection of the human caring work and the meaning and contextual reference of the work.

5. *Appropriation.* This term means attunement with the metaphor, the world of text, and the projection of the imagery of the world that is projected in front of the text. Appropriation is the end of the hermeneutical process, a proposed world, an understanding at and through a distance; it means "to make one's own what was initially alien." The meaning is not behind the text as a hidden intention is. Instead, the meaning is in front of it as that which the work unfolded, discovered, disclosed, and revealed. To understand the text is to understand oneself in front of the text. To understand oneself in front of the text is to let the work and the world enlarge the horizon of the understanding that one has of oneself (Ricoeur, 1976, 1981). Hence, appropriation is what it means for one to be human through a hermeneutical encounter with the text. Appropriation occurs when one can see oneself reflected in text so that one can say, "I understand my own authentic being through this text-world" (Klemm, 1983).

DATA GENERATION

Sixteen experts were interviewed regarding the specific disciplines' knowledge base on human caring. A nonstructured, tape-recorded interview was conducted. The interview focused on the expert's meanings of caring and the disciplines's exemplary literature and knowledge base on human caring. The compiled bibliography was assessed by a second panel of nursing experts for face and content validity. The nursing experts had expertise in nursing and one or more disciplines. In addition, a literature search (Medline, Psychological Abstracts, Dissertation Abstracts, and Nursing and Allied Health) was done to identify additional literature on human caring. Finally, books, monographs, and articles on human caring not accessible through the literature searches were identified by the interdisciplinary experts and myself and included in the bibliography.

In discovering and creating the meanings of human caring, the best available exemplification of human caring from a work of literature was selected based on preestablished investigator criteria. Tolstoy's *The Death of Ivan Ilyich* (1981) was the work of literature selected for analysis. The Tolstoy work: exemplified representative ideas of human caring, main features of human caring, and organizing principles of human caring; reflected the essence of human caring; was a descriptive and contextual story of human caring; portrayed caring and noncaring situations and experiences; permitted all nine disciplines to provide a lens to discover and create the meanings of human caring from an interdisciplinary focus; and centered on the one being cared with, the one caring, or both. From the analyzed meanings of human caring in this work, the experts' meanings of caring, and the meanings of caring from the literature, an original portrait of caring emerged (Smerke, 1988). In discovering and applying each discipline's foundations on the conceptual and theoretical meanings of human caring, one (or more) representative work(s) of caring literature was (were) selected. The selected representative literature elucidated the discipline's foundations on the conceptual and theoretical meanings of human caring and provided the investigator with a disciplinary lens through which to understand and illuminate the portrait of caring from one or more selected disciplinary foci. The representative literature was interplayed with the portrait of caring. Each discipline shed light and insight onto the portrait of caring through the representative literature. Thus, through the interplay between the representative literature and the portrait of caring, an illuminated portrait of caring emerged with an interdisciplinary focus. The illuminated portrait of caring then provided the framework for the guide to the caring literature.

The Ethnograph software program was used to assist with data manipulation tasks (Seidel, Kjolseth, & Clark, 1985). The text from the interviews and the significant statements from the work of literature selected for the analysis were numbered so that the emergent themes from the text could be sorted. The unit of analysis for this study was the text of the interviews and selected sentences from the work of literature. Through a hermeneutical analysis, the meanings of human caring were grounded and expanded.

FINDINGS AND DISCUSSION

The study had three major outcomes: theoretical contribution, original and creative contribution, and enduring scientific contribution. This discussion will focus on the enduring scientific contribution.

Table 12–1 lists the interdisciplinary meanings of caring that emerged from the literature. A synopsis of the interdisciplinary meanings of caring, with further elucidation of the varied meanings, follows.

The meaning and experience of caring with the *person* are conveyed in the philosophical, fine arts, and nursing literature. When a nurse is caring, he or she has an understanding and love for humanity, utilizes a humanistic approach, has a love of self and others, allows the person the freedom to be human, promotes and sustains the human qualities of the person, has an understanding of reality and of the meaning of life and death, and promotes the person's full potential.

Relationships was discovered as another meaning of human caring within the literature from anthropology, psychoneuroimmunology, philosophy, sociobehavioral sciences, theology, and nursing. In a caring relationship, the nurse expresses the authentic use of self; develops a friendship and companionship; establishes covenants; provides social support and support systems; builds communities; fosters family relationships and social integration; develops interpersonal, interconnected, mutual, and interrelated associations; recognizes the uniqueness of the other person; portrays an existential presence by being sensitive, supportive, and available; and utilizes the I–Thou relationship.

Dialogue is portrayed as caring from the literature in sociobehavioral sciences, philosophy, ethics, and nursing. The caring nurse listens and communicates with the person.

Healing is conveyed in the literature from the disciplines of psychoneuroimmunology, ethics, fine arts, philosophy, sociobehavioral sciences, theology, and nursing as caring. The person experiencing caring can potentiate the self-healer from within through holistic and transcendental approaches,

Table 12–1
Interdisciplinary Meanings of Human Caring

Person	Environments
Relationships	Experiential process
Dialogue	Caring behaviors
Healing	Economics
Choices	

such as journal writing, touch, music, laughter, and imagery; and healing has the capacity to instill faith and hope within the nurse and the person.

A caring nurse allows the person *choices*. This meaning of caring is conveyed in the literature from ethics and nursing. Choices focus on professional value, personal value, understanding the meaning of values, and moral decision making.

The fine arts and nursing literature describes caring as being concerned and attentive to *environments*. The caring environment is supportive, protective, and corrective.

The literature from the fine arts, humanities, ethics, theology, and nursing conveys caring as an *experiential process*. The caring process provides the catalyst for human growth and development and for self and group actualization. The caring process is described as a celebration of life, with the nurse being compassionate, enabling, adaptable, accessible, available, patient, open, and genuine with the person. The person experiences a new level of awareness and understanding, an awakening, renewed understanding, transformation, transcendence, illumination, and a sense of control. Through the caring process, the nurse lives in the present moment and gives information, carries out procedures, does extra things for the person, and promotes the health of the person.

Many *caring behaviors* are described in the psychoneuroimmunology, philosophy, sociobehavioral sciences, fine arts, and nursing literature. Some of the caring behaviors include: the caring nurse conveys a gentle and tender hand when holding hands; facilitates mind–body interactions; and demonstrates respect, empathy, sharing, sympathy, kindness, concern, nurturance, and forgiveness for the person. In addition, the caring nurse portrays a nonjudgmental manner; demonstrates honesty, hope, and courage; and is considerate, friendly, spontaneous, willing, attentive, protective, and sensitive to the needs of the person. The person experiencing the caring displays relaxation, tranquillity, balance, peacefulness, security, happiness, and comfort.

Finally, caring conveys *economics* from the literature in anthropology and sociobehavioral sciences. The cared person experiences financial security. Thus, seven major themes for human caring emerged from the hermeneutical analysis (see Table 12–2).

Enduring Scientific Contribution

The enduring scientific contribution was the interdisciplinary guide to the caring literature. The meanings of human caring were not discipline-

Table 12–2
Major Themes of Human Caring, and Disciplines Sharing the Meaning

Themes	Disciplines
Essence of person/being	All nine
Relationships/encounters	All nine
Decisions/choices/judgments	Ethics and nursing
Genuine dialogue	Fine arts, humanities, philosophy, theology, and nursing
Experiential process	Fine arts, humanities, ethics, theology, and nursing
Healing modalities	All nine
Human/economic resource exchanges	Anthropology, ethics, and nursing

specific; rather, the meanings spanned the disciplines. Thus, a user accessing information of caring is now able to generate an interdisciplinary perspective on some aspect or meaning of human caring as well as a listing of books, articles, or monographs on human caring from one discipline.

The framework for the guide has a five-level structure. The overarching term for level one of the caring knowledge base is human caring. Level two has two divisions: caring and noncaring. Level three of the guide represents the seven major themes for the meanings of human caring (see Table 12–2). The fourth level of the guide represents the meanings of caring that connote the process, action, or method involved in the experience or fulfillment of the major themes of caring at level three. Finally, level five represents the characteristics of the meanings of human caring from level four.

The arrangement of the themes of human caring was not in any hierarchical or given order. The themes were placed in the order in which they occurred during the literature analysis.

The characteristics at level five were not mutually exclusive for a given division. In addition, several meanings expressed at level four had no identifying characteristics at level five.

If the user selected a key word that was located under several divisions, the computer would direct the user to specify which division he or she was interested in or would allow the user to select both divisions. Then the computer would generate the requested bibliography. The themes, divisions, and characteristics of caring are all acceptable key words by which to access the literature from an interdisciplinary perspective.

Levels Three, Four, and Five of the Framework

Each of the levels within the guide is discussed here with the corresponding descending levels. One of the major themes of the meanings of human caring was *essence of person/being* (Table 12–3). At level four there were six divisions of essence of person/being: center, freedom, moral ideal, love, consciousness, and wholeness/uniqueness. All of these were processes or methods that could promote and enhance the essence of the person. At level five, center had the following characteristics: heal, interpenetration, and balance. Freedom had liberation as its characteristic at level five. Protection, enhancement, and preservation were meanings of moral ideal at level five. Love had the following characteristics: acceptance, liberation, joy, self-fulfillment, union, transformation, and forgiveness. There was no level-five characteristic for consciousness. Wholeness/uniqueness had the following characteristics at level five: body/mind/soul, integration, and full potential.

The second major theme of the meanings of human caring was *genuine relationships/encounters* (Table 12–4). There were eight divisions for this theme at level four: transpersonal caring, authenticity, I–Thou, flash, social networks, friendship, family, and presence. As shown in Table 12–4, each of these divisions had several characteristics at level five.

The third major theme for the meanings of human caring was *decisions/choices/judgments*. Two divisions existed at level four: principle-based ethics and experiential-based ethics, the ethics of caring. Table 12–5 shows the characteristics of each.

Table 12–3
Interdisciplinary Guide: Major Themes

Level Three Theme: Essence of Person/Being	
Level Four	Level Five
Center	Heal; interpenetration; balance
Freedom	Liberation
Moral ideal	Protection; enhancement; preservation
Love	Acceptance; liberation; joy; self-fulfillment; union; transformation; forgiveness
Consciousness	
Wholeness/uniqueness	Body/mind/soul; integration; full potential

Table 12–4
Interdisciplinary Guide: Major Themes

Level Three Theme: Genuine Relationships/Encounters	
Level Four	Level Five
Transpersonal caring	Intersubjectivity; respect; availability; mutuality; unique self; reciprocity; sensitivity
Authenticity	Connection; selflessness; helping; presence; joy; warmth; concern; compassion; comfort; empathy; sensitivity
I–Thou	Mutuality; immediacy; directness; participation; presentness; collaboration; intensity; genuine meeting; ineffability; authenticity
Flash	Authenticity; divine reality; genuine; spiritual experience; mutuality; reciprocity; communion
Social networks	Caring exchanges; affiliation; social ties; social bonds; caring communities; friendship; nurturance; transcendence; social support; social integration; affiliation
Friendship	Free expression; symbiosis; open sharing; companionship; tenderness
Family	Interconnection; belonging; warmth
Presence	Unmasked; hopeful; tenderness; openness; generous; covenant

Table 12–5
Interdisciplinary Guide: Major Themes

Level Three Theme: Decisions/Choices/Judgments	
Level Four	Level Five
Principle-based ethics	Beneficence; justice; autonomy; duty; obligation; cause; basic truth
Experiential-based ethics/ethics of caring	Goodness; character; moral support; virtues; desire; trust; right; decisions; values; intuition; compassion; understanding

Table 12–6
Interdisciplinary Guide: Major Themes

Level Three Theme: Genuine Dialogue	
Level Four	Level Five
Listening	Hearing
Silence	Self-knowledge
Communication	
Talking	
Self-expression	
Outcome of dialogue	Affirmation; acceptance; awakening; warmth; courage; liberation; understanding

Table 12–7
Interdisciplinary Guide: Major Themes

Level Three Theme: Experiential Process	
Level Four	Level Five
Transcendence	Time; present moment
Illumination	
Transformation	Becoming
Revelations	
Growth/development	Celebration of life; control; gratification of needs
Hunger	Respect; warmth; relationships
Moral/ethical	Look; interconnectedness; bonding; actualization
Reflection	
Knowledge/awareness/ understanding	Awakening; perception; realign self; realization; information; cognizant; explanatory model
Affective experiences	Being accessible; joy; courage; doing extra things; tranquillity; being available; considerate; sympathy; being open; kind; beauty; being with; gentle and tender hand; enabling; willingness; hope; being genuine; holding hands; fun; peace; engagement; forgiveness; dignity; excitement; relaxed; happiness; alternating rhythms; secure; spontaneity

The fourth major meaning of human caring was *genuine dialogue* (Table 12–6). Genuine dialogue had six divisions at level four: listening, silence, communication, talking, self-expression, and outcome of dialogue. There were no characteristics at level five for communication, talking, or self-expression. Listening, silence, and outcome of dialogue had the characteristics shown in Table 12–6.

Experiential process was another major theme of the meanings of human caring. As shown in Table 12–7, there were ten divisions at level four for the theme: transcendence, illumination, transformation, revelations, growth/development, hunger, moral/ethical, reflection, knowledge/awareness/understanding, and affective experiences. Illumination, revelations, and reflection had no characteristics listed at level five. The level-five characteristics for the remaining divisions are listed in Table 12–7.

Another major theme, *healing modalities,* had ten divisions: touching, enabling actions, technical competence, imagery/visualization, self-healer, outcome of healing, music, holistic/transcendental methods, centering, and humor/laughter (Table 12–8). Imagery/visualization, self-healer, music, holistic/transcendental methods, centering, and humor/laughter had no characteristics at level five. The characteristics for the remaining divisions are listed in Table 12–8.

The last level three theme for the meanings of human caring was *human/ economic resource exchanges.* Social networks, interpersonal relations, food, housing, and supportive exchanges were the divisions at level four. Social

Table 12–8
Interdisciplinary Guide: Major Themes

Level Three Theme: Healing Modalities	
Level Four	Level Five
Touching	Engagement; enablement; caresses
Enabling actions	Instilling faith; instilling hope; journal writing
Technical competence	Facilitating modalities; enhancing interventions
Imagery/visualization	
Self-healer	
Outcome of healing	Harmony; renewal of self
Music	
Holistic transcendental methods	
Centering	
Humor/laughter	

networks, interpersonal relations, food, and housing had no characteristics at level five. Supportive exchanges had the following characteristics at level five: instrumental, social, and personal.

CONDUCTING A SEARCH WITHIN THE CARING LITERATURE

A generated list of acceptable key words is made available to enable the user to begin his or her search on caring. The list of key words is arranged alphabetically, but is cross-referenced for easy retrieval of other related meanings. The user is able to search for more than one key word at a time, to join key words together, and to do multiple key-word searches to obtain a broader scope on a particular area of interest. After the user has completed the search, the computer prompts the user to respond to whether the user wants a broader search, a narrower search, or another search, or prefers to quit the search process. For example, if the user selects a word at level five and the computer completes the search, the computer asks whether the user wants to search at level three. If the user agrees with this option, the appropriate key words for level three appear on the screen, and the user selects the appropriate words. The option to quit the search or perform another search would also be available to the user.

EXAMPLE OF SIMULATED SEARCH FOR THE MEANING OF HUMAN CARING

A user was very concerned in clinical practice with communication skills among the staff and with the clients and families. She was interested in obtaining articles, books, research studies, and any other information that discussed the process and potential results of communication with clients, families, and peers. She began with the list of preestablished key words for the human caring literature. Because she was interested in communication, she began under C for communication. She found that communication was an acceptable word, so she typed COMMUNICATION into the computer. She was given the following possible searches on DIALOGUE: COMMUNICATION or ALL LITERATURE. She selected ALL LITERATURE because she wanted to get as much information as possible. The search provided the user with an interdisciplinary bibliography on dialogue.

IMPLICATIONS

Several implications were developed for this study. The guide to caring literature will provide easier access, retrieval, and integration of the caring literature for use in practice, education, and research. In addition, investigators need to continue to glean the emerging meanings of human caring from an interdisciplinary perspective. Finally, an interdisciplinary theoretical knowledge base emerged from the study for use in human caring research.

In summary, there were three major outcomes: a theoretical contribution, an original and creative contribution, and an enduring scientific/scholarly contribution. The framework to the guide to the caring literature will increase access, retrieval, and integration of the caring literature for use in practice, education, and research.

CONCLUSIONS

Meanings of human caring were not discipline-specific; rather, they spanned across the disciplines. Seven major themes emerged as the meanings of human caring. Transforming love was the interdisciplinary meaning of human caring, and meanings of human caring continue to emerge. In discovering and creating the meanings of human caring, it is imperative that investigators do not stifle the emergent meanings of human caring from an interdisciplinary perspective by applying a constricting definition to caring.

REFERENCES

Ader, R. (1981). *Psychoneuroimmunology*. New York: Academic Press.

Benner, P. (1984). *From novice to expert*. Menlo Park, CA: Addison-Wesley.

Cohen, S., & Syme, S. (1985). *Social support and health*. New York: Academic Press.

Gadamer, H. (1975). *Truth and method* (G. Barden & J. Cumming, Trans.). New York: Seabury.

Gadamer, H. (1976). *Hegel's dialectic* (P. Smith, Trans.). New Haven: Yale University Press.

Gaut, D. A. (1981). Conceptual analysis of caring: Research method. In M. Leininger (Ed.), *Caring: An essential human need* (pp. 17–24). Thorofare, NJ: Slack.

Gaut, D. A. (1983). Development of a theoretically adequate description of caring. *Western Journal of Nursing Research, 5*(4), 312–324.

Gaut, D. A. (1984). A theoretic description of caring as action. In M. Leininger (Ed.), *Care: The essence of nursing and health* (pp. 27–44). Thorofare, NJ: Slack.

Klemm, D. (1983). *The hermeneutical theory of Paul Ricoeur*. East Brunswick, NJ: Associated University Press, Inc.

Lazarus, R., & Folkman, S. (1984). *Stress, appraisal, and coping*. New York: Springer.

Leininger, M. (1978). *Transcultural nursing: Concepts, theories, and practices*. New York: Wiley.

Leininger, M. (1980). Caring: A central focus of nursing and health care series. *Nursing and Health Care, 1*(3), 135.

Leininger, M. (1981). *Caring: An essential human need.* (pp. 1–16). Thorofare, NJ: Slack.

Leininger, M. (1984). *Care: The essence of nursing and health.* (pp. 1–26). Thorofare, NJ: Slack.

Leininger, M. (1986, April). *Humanistic care: History, meaning and power.* Paper presented at the Eighth National Caring Conference, San Francisco.

Noddings, N. (1984). *Caring: A feminine approach to ethics and moral education*. Berkeley: University of California Press.

Patterson, J., & Zderad, L. (1976). *Humanistic nursing*. New York: Wiley.

Ray, M. A. (1981). A philosophical analysis of caring within nursing. In M. Leininger (Ed.), *Caring: An essential human need* (pp. 25–36). Thorofare, NJ: Slack.

Ray, M. A. (1984). The development of a classification system of institutional caring. In M. Leininger (Ed.), *Care: The essence of nursing and health* (pp. 95–112). Thorofare, NJ: Slack.

Ricoeur, P. (1976). *Interpretation theory: Discourse and the surplus of meaning*. Fort Worth, TX: The Texas Christian University Press.

Ricoeur, P. (1981). *Hermeneutics and the human sciences* (J. Thompson, Trans.). Cambridge, England: Cambridge University Press.

Roach, S. (1984). *Caring: The human mode of being, implications for nursing* (monograph). Toronto, Canada: The University of Toronto.

Rodin, J. (1986). Aging and health: Effects of sense of control. *Science, 233*, 1271–1276.

Seidel, J., Kjolseth, R., & Clark, J. (1985). *The Ethnograph: A user's guide*. Littleton, CO: Qualis Research Associates.

Smerke, J. (1988). *The discovery and creation of the meanings of human caring through the development of a guide to the caring literature*. Ann Arbor, MI: Unpublished doctoral dissertation.

Tolstoy, L. (1981). *The death of Ivan Ilyich.* New York: Bantam Books.

Watson, J. (1979). *Nursing: The philosophy and science of caring.* Boston: Little, Brown.

Watson, J. (1985). *Nursing: Human science and human care.* Norwalk, CT: Appleton-Century-Crofts.

13

Experiencing the Mystery in Cross-Cultural Research on Care

Agnes M. Aamodt

*I*n the Maori language, there is a phrase *Tihe Mauriora* (Hulme, 1984), literally meaning "sneeze of life." It is used by the Maori at the beginning of formal speeches to say "I salute the breath of life in you," symbolizing the secret and mysterious power of people, birds, land, forest, water, and air. For me, this secret and mysterious power captures the essence of what I have sometimes experienced in my field studies of conceptualizations of care. And so I say to you, "*Tihe Mauriora*: may your breath bring you power from all that is secret and mysterious in your clinical nursing research and practice."

The purpose of this chapter is to éxamine the mysterious and perplexing as I describe, analyze, and label concepts in clinical nursing research. I have asked myself (Aamodt, 1992): What realities in care of the human conditions are not acknowledged in our current nursing theories? What meanings and/or labels of human response and care can be added to the lexicon informing nursing knowledge? Beginning answers to these questions can be found within the substance of this chapter. Always guiding my writings are two overall questions that give direction to my research program, whatever my focus:

1. What characteristics of care promote human responses for quality human experience?
2. Where is the whole of the meanings in folk theories from which we can generate constructs to use in the development of nursing theories?

Implicit in these two questions is a query into the processes of discovering nursing and scientific concepts among the culturally relevant domains of meaning imbedded in the folk theories carried by collective members of a cultural group. My intent is and has been to identify selected concepts from within these domains of meaning for eventual use in the generation of nursing theory. To say it another way, I look to the real world a cultural group lives in for meanings to label—for example, the real world of holding a head to sip water, calling a support group together for a child about to be told his diagnosis is cancer, or watching over a father or mother with a child in crisis from a high fever or an overdose of a drug. In this real world, I hope to find ideas to give a name to and to link one with another in order to build nursing theories for practicing nurses in multicultural settings. To me, there is a need to passionately search beyond our current nursing theories for shapes, colors, sounds, and smells to fill in some of the clear spaces or empty categories and expand our present worldview of knowledge.

As I plan for my research, experience field work, and review the stories of my informants, I find myself asking: Where do the themes or patterns come from? When did I know? Where was I? What feelings, odors, movements, sounds can I talk about? What changed? In other words, what aroused the fire and kindled the emergence of the label of "watching" from a story as simplistic as recounting what happened when a child felt dizzy after chemotherapy? What was it that, in hindsight, appeared perplexing and somewhat mysterious? We all know that we are a part of every event we experience. In both qualitative and quantitative research, the researcher is, in the final analysis, the tool or instrument responsible for the direction and final outcome of the generalizations that emerge as data are raised to a different level of abstraction. What can we say about the humanistic and scientific processes experienced in research?

An assumption underlying what I attempt to analyze here is that the mystery in the nonlogical, the unstructured, and the whimsical can show nurse scientists an important part of what they see as truth in their research. The process is something we have all experienced as ideas shoot through our brains before we can write them down. Pearce (1971) wrote about the mind and reality and a mode of thinking we can develop in ourselves suggestive of early childhood. Because we are all a part of every event we experience, we are so much a part of the research process that we cannot really separate our discoveries from ourselves. Here is the setting of the mystery: What is logical about the nonlogical? Pearce told us about autistic thinking or A-thinking, a creative will-o'-the-wisp process as opposed to a logically reasoned view. This kind of dream-world left-handed thinking is what my analysis is about. The A-thinking of Pearce recognizes a kind of thread remaining intact between a logically reasoned thought and a grasp of insight coming with an explosive force only after we have reached a saturation point of rigorous logical thinking. Crucial to this process is remembering that when the "truth" of light happens to us, it is preceded by and comes out of this serious work that is logically reasoned thought. A new possibility is recognized that is more than the sum of the parts.

Six field settings focusing on care and caretaking in different cultures provide data for this analysis:

- Papago children as they learn about health and healing on the Tohono O'odham Reservation.
- Norwegian American women in western Wisconsin, in the United States, as they take care of neighbors.
- Preschoolers caring for mothers.
- Elderly women caring for themselves in a nurse–client encounter.
- Children viewing care during cancer therapy.
- Men viewing care at a time of crisis.

In each field of experience, I was looking for patterns or themes in what my informants said and did, for eventual use in conceptualizations of care. For example, I asked myself: What could it mean when Buddy, aged 13 years, talked about the decisions he and his nurse made prior to an IV injection?

> *You see we can't get any blood or anything up there [pointing to his upper left hand] because it won't work so we use these veins [pointing to his right hand] but we (that is, the nurse and I) forgot, used the left hand, and it hurt.*
>
> *(Buddy, 13 years)*

For me, this little vignette eventually became a part of "watching," a pivotal construct for care phenomena from the view of children with cancer. At another time, other primitive constructs or conceptualizations of care emerged from similar kinds of vignettes: "so this is it," "working on acceptance," "the pits of dependency is not being able to scratch yourself when you itch," and "not thinking."

For the purpose of this chapter, I have identified five patterns of behavior of myself as field worker/ethnographic researcher that link in my thinking to the mystery in how I chose (and choose) labels such as "watching" in the culture of childhood, "neighboring" in a Norwegian American system of care, and "the pits of dependency" and "working on acceptance" as elements in a system of self-care of the elderly. The patterns of behavior I discuss in this chapter are:

1. Feeding my unconscious and allowing for changes in myself.
2. Waiting in the booming, buzzing confusion.
3. Looking for what I hear and see.
4. Seeing and hearing what I have seen and heard repeated.
5. Learning what appeals to me, what I like.

FEEDING MY UNCONSCIOUS AND ALLOWING FOR CHANGES IN MYSELF

When I could let flies walk across my wet forehead in the hot summer sun on the Papago Indian Reservation; when I could pick up a formula bottle from a sandy floor and wipe the nipple on the back of my skirt before I gave it back to a baby; when I lived as a member of my Papago Indian family; and when I felt questions from my non-Papago friends in the city hit me like a stream of bullets because they made no sense, I knew I was becoming more and more like a Papago Indian.

Ethnographic research demands a field worker with open eyes, open ears, a resilient cognitive and affective system, and a readiness for changing sensual experiences. I was looking for a new frontier of how human beings experience health care, especially cross-cultural care, and I knew that my own ways of cleanliness, eating, sleeping, and decision making would be under attack consciously and unconsciously. My elaborate conceptualizations from nursing and Norwegian-Lutheran traditions, whether I willed it or not, were going to color how I viewed this new world. Indeed, I would not be going into the field with the *tabula rasa* of Thomas Aquinas and John Locke. In other words, my intellect was not a clean slate or a blank sheet of paper. I had been fed on conceptualizations of anthropology—unity versus diversity in the name of culture, linguistic domains of meaning informing human experiences and the collective conscious and unconscious, and, in nursing, theories including health, environment, disease, patients, and care as crucial constructs. To me, research has one great mystery: How does previous and present knowledge influence my work? What happens to one's self? What changes occur as one confronts the many patternings observable during a research experience?

WAITING IN THE BOOMING, BUZZING CONFUSION

True ethnographic field experience calls for moving from one's own environment, where meanings are somewhat clear and responses of laughter, crying, and fear are spontaneous, to a new set of meanings where reality is based on a different set of symbols and when to laugh, cry, or be afraid is not known. How I learned to respond to "flies," "dirt," and "senseless questions" told me about the similarities and differences of "my" symbolism and "their" symbolism.

The intent of ethnography is to learn the story of the people from their view. What did it mean when I heard children with cancer say, "It's the dying that's hard" or "The way I take care of my mother is to wake her up and then let her sleep ten minutes longer." For me, the first two to three months of any field work is a time of ambiguity, uncertainty, and confusion. Life is truly a conundrum, a riddle, a time of making mistakes, of false assumptions, and of hearing, seeing, and appreciating a minuscule amount of what is going on. The experience of visiting a family or starting a new job is similar. I continually asked, "What are the rules?" Five months into my research with the Papago, I was asked about an accident scene at which I had helped on my way into the village. Later, a consultant said to me, "To be asked about a villager you have seen outside the village by a villager inside a village means you have been accepted—at least by the person asking the question." This meaning of my simple act had not occurred to me. Waiting for the confusion to settle into patterns is one way of learning the insider's view. To allow the confusion to be resolved too soon makes one vulnerable to adopting patterns from a cognitive map held prior to entering the field. Waiting for the new symbols to arrange themselves and tolerating the booming, buzzing confusion often makes me feel sick to my stomach and lonesome, with a yearning for something familiar. I breathe more easily when what I see and hear makes sense to me. Pearce (1971) spoke of *metanonia*, a Greek word for a "fundamental transformation of the mind," a reshaping of concepts. Thus, when patterns make sense, I have been making decisions about what I will be seeing and hearing. About three months into my field work, my field notes usually do indeed reflect this and beginning conceptualizations slowly appear, for example, "watching," "neighboring," and "not being able to scratch."

LOOKING FOR WHAT I HEAR AND SEE

Whether I'm helping to cook for the *kokoi* (those who have gone on) on All Souls' Day among the Papago Indians, eating with a group of Norwegian women, or lying on a water bed talking to a child with cancer, I listen and look for snatches of meaning, for what makes sense. Where my ideas come from, however, continues to be a mystery to me.

Two stories will illustrate this pattern. One at a time, a group of students and I were discussing their previous week's field experience. An elderly woman had said during a nurse–client encounter, "I've had hypertension, headaches, swollen feet, diarrhea. Friends, nurses and doctors keep asking me if I'm accepting how I feel and what I have to do for it, and I say 'Not really, but I'm working on it.'" In our discussion of this vignette, we were tossing around alternative ideas. What was being conceptualized? In an almost explosive moment, we had it—"working on acceptance." For us, "working on acceptance" became a primitive concept with possibilities for nurse researchers with an interest in conceptualizations of acceptance/nonacceptance and compliance/noncompliance. In a short moment, we had changed the meaning from an absolute label ("accepting") to a process-oriented label ("working on acceptance") that truly represented, from our view, a sense of self-care from a client's view.

The second story of looking for what I hear and see comes from the Norwegian American research in Wisconsin. I was searching in my field experiences, my interviews, and my written field notes for some kind of focus on a caring pattern of behavior. One afternoon, while helping a favorite aunt of mine with a jigsaw puzzle, we talked about how her days went, living in a rural used-to-be-farming community now occupied by families who worked in town. Aunt Inga said to me, "I miss my neighbors so, I really miss my neighbors so! I used to see them driving by to town, when their lights went off and on, and when the kids walked to school." As we sat together, I knew I had found what would work for a focus of care—neighboring. Care of neighbors by neighbors unveiled a host of primitive conceptual categories of care: "visiting," "checking on," "being there," "fixing coffee," and "praying with." In both examples, the instant of insight was what I had waited for, and I knew when I had it: "working on acceptance," in a conversation with co-field workers, and "neighboring," in the reminiscences of an informant.

SEEING AND HEARING WHAT I HAVE SEEN AND HEARD REPEATED

What is really the same but becomes apparent in a different form or context? After I've identified a label that is interesting to my research question, I look to a range of examples to provide elaboration of the concept. This becomes both perplexing and mysterious. In the cancer study, we generated a label of human response ("so this is it") and then began to discover a range of variations that fit with the label. As the meaning for the concept "so this is it" grew, it became alternately a time when a diagnosis of cancer was made after months of feelings of fatigue, restlessness, and pain, a time of dizziness and nausea following chemotherapy and feeling "worse than you've ever felt," and a time when a decision was made to not do chemotherapy anymore. "So this is it" was designated a first stage in our model (Aamodt, 1992) of cyclical responses of care during chemotherapy. The fact of its repetition in different settings helped us (the researchers) to understand the notion of cyclical responses as our model developed.

"Nurses as friends and enemies" suggests another label perplexing to me in my field experience. To be a friend and enemy at one and the same time represented some of the complexities in relationships of care providers and care receivers. To the children with cancer, nurses gave hugs, told jokes, rubbed backs, and were generally comforting. The relationships of nurses and patients became tangled into a hodgepodge of not well understood complexity when nurses were also linked with giving "garbage," that is, inserting needles for chemotherapy and attending to other hurtful procedures. Thus, the behaviors became a series of perplexing opposites, difficult to identify and difficult to label. For me, recognizing and describing the context is as much a time of invention by the researcher as recognizing the thread that continues from one context to another.

LEARNING WHAT APPEALS TO ME, WHAT I LIKE

I have recounted several examples of so-called insight that occurred after moments of, or perhaps within the context of, the booming, buzzing confusion of children and adults caring for each other and themselves—neighboring, working on acceptance, and being there. In my own work—and I dare say in all research, qualitative and quantitative—what appeals to researchers must come forth someplace in the analysis. The creative experience demands something that is satisfying to the inventor. I knew I liked "working on acceptance" because it was neither "yes" or "no." I liked "friends and enemies" because of the ambiguity it represented. Nurses cannot be either just friends or just enemies. We are more complex than just a simple friend or enemy in relation to our patients. What is the whole that represents a sense of these opposites? I like that kind of a question. I liked "so this is it" because to me it represented a moment of truth to the patient—"so that's what I've got," "so that's the way it hurts," "so that's what it's like to know that I will die soon." I liked "watching," another concept from the world of children, because it spoke from the child's view and the manner in which children attend to the world around them when parents, siblings, nurses, doctors, and friends touch them, prod them, laugh with them, talk to them, tell them. I like the idea that the experience of chemotherapy, or any treatment, can generate a sense of an expert in all of us. I especially like times when clients have something to say to nursing.

To me, the greatest mystery in "What do I like?" comes from how in the world it happens anyway. Pearce's (1971) notions of the experience of autistic or A-thinking, where the spirit bloweth and a sense of the whole emerges from a kind of dream world of left-handed thinking, tells us some of the "how." Nursing research will surely capture breakthroughs of luminous and awesome qualities as we pursue the mystery and perplexity in what appeals and what we like. If I were to guess at what I might find out in the next 50 years of my research, I would say I will have an increasing fondness for the interrelationships in the ideas of biochemistry, cultural diversity, and caretaking. My studies might take the form of masculine conceptions of care, self-care and survivors of chronic illness among American Indians, and "so this is it" in the world of sleep—all of these influenced by my unconscious processes and autistic dreamlike thinking.

CONCLUSION

I have attempted to describe how we can think about clinical nursing research and how we use ourselves as crucial tools or instruments in collecting, analyzing, and writing about our experience. We need to look beyond the patterns of behavior of field work I have described—feeding and listening to the unconscious, waiting through the booming, buzzing confusion for what we see and hear, looking for repetition in all the ambiguity, and then listening to ourselves as we follow what we like. We need to keep asking where moments of left-handed dream-world thinking will take us in our pursuit of the truths of nursing.

Tihe Mauriora. Look to your sneeze of life, to the stories you hear from yourself and others in that never-never land where you will find a secret power like that of the Maori.

REFERENCES

Aamodt, A. (1992). Toward conceptualizations in nursing: Harbingers from the sciences and humanities. *Journal of Professional Nursing, 8*(3), 184–194.

Hulme, K. (1984). *The bone people.* New Zealand: Spiral/Hodder & Stoughton.

Pearce, J. C. (1971). *The crack in the cosmic egg.* New York: Washington Square.

14

Use of Narrative in Human Caring Inquiry

Toni M. Vezeau

Nursing has been increasingly characterized as art, in connection with aesthetic relationship and caring. Aesthetic methods of inquiry, such as narrative, have been suggested to study caring (Watson, 1985, 1988; Webster, 1990; Younger, 1990), because they are consistent with an holistic perceptual approach toward the understanding and appreciation of a unique person or event (Carper, 1978; Charon, 1986; Tisdale, 1986). However, particular persons and events have not been the typical concern of nursing inquiry, because individual accounts do not lead to generalizable knowledge. Both aspects of knowledge, general and particular, are essential in order for caring to be present in provider, client, and environmental relationships. The purpose of this chapter is to offer an alternative approach, fictional narrative, to explore human experiences within the framework of human care nursing.

Narrative is endorsed here as a method of exploration for nursing inquiry, but there are serious problems. The term *narrative* has been used interchangeably with story and interview (Churchill & Churchill, 1987; Long, 1986; Parker, 1990). Narrative has been an umbrella term that is inclusive of all storied forms of communication. This chapter takes the position that each storied form of inquiry, such as paradigm cases, journals, "telling your story" by clinical nurses, and qualitative interview, is unique. Although certainly related and valuable, the motivation, style, and outcome are significantly different.

WHAT IS NARRATIVE?

Narrative makes a world in which to meet for sharing personal realities, framed in often simple language (Lopez, 1980). Narrative is not simply an expression of ideas; at its heart, it is a form of inquiry. Narrative inquiry is intended to enlarge rather than narrow the vision about a particular experience. The storyteller contributes metaphors to extend understanding past the literal connection by asserting the human meanings of events. The readers bring reflection and openness in allowing the "shock of recognition" (Preston, 1987; Younger, 1990). Narrative in its use of metaphor demonstrates a profound weaving of human context and human responses that is a solid base for knowledge development in human care nursing.

Description of the Term

To clarify what is meant by narrative is essential to this discussion. We all know what stories are. Since our earliest memories as children, we have received others' realities and expressed our own through them. Narrative is a representation of a personal reality, editorialized and discrete, as all information is. Most often, narrative does not try to answer specific questions; the object is exploration. The usual outcome is not certainty about a phenomenon, but the discovery of salient questions about the phenomenon that were not envisioned prior to the narrative.

Narrative is greatly different from scientific inquiry. Traditional science views the particular, the part, as the cleanest and simplest aspect to study. The part is distinctly measurable. However, the part is not thought to have value in itself; its value is contingent on what can be generalized from many like parts. Traditional science values the general, the typical, and the most common, specifically because the part cannot be trusted to yield reliable and valid truth. Narrative reverses this figure–ground relationship by valuing the part for its own personal truth. In a sense, narrative tests the conventional wisdom, the theory, about a type of experience by presenting a particular situation. The teller and audience both determine consonance and dissonance between the unique and the experience of the universal.

It is important to understand that narratives are not solely particular instances. Narratives can be deconstructed for particulars—facts, style, scenery. Narratives can also be appreciated as a whole in which meanings and feelings are experienced. In most narratives, these two stances toward story are simultaneous but the particular instance is emphasized in the figure–ground appreciation of the phenomenon.

SIMILARITIES AND DIFFERENCES AMONG NARRATIVE FORMS

Nursing has a history of inquiry and it includes narrative approaches that develop personal knowledge rooted in clinical practice (Boykin & Schoenhofer, 1991). Stories are the way patients have informed us about their experience of health and transition. Stories have also been an essential method to convey nurses' knowledge of individuals to each other. Nursing is no stranger to narrative; it has always been a part of how we have explored the shared world of our patients.

But are all types of narratives the same? In the past few years, narrative and story have been frequent topics examined in nursing conferences and journal articles. Discussions have included mixtures of interview findings and poetry—each treated as similar data. Discrimination among different types of story is important if we are to use them as inquiry that develops nursing knowledge and cultural health information.

Narrative styles are almost endless, but the primary ones that nursing has used in inquiry are: journals, hermeneutics entailing patient-as-text, interviews, paradigm cases, "telling your own story," and fictional narrative. Each of these forms has important aspects to attend to and cannot be equated. To lump all under the rubric "story" denies the unique potential of each to enhance understanding of our world.

Similarities

When they are listed here as categories—journals, patient-as-text, interview, paradigm cases, "telling your story," and fiction—it is easy to see that they differ from each other. There must be similarities among them, however, for they are all considered story.

Dorothy Parker once stated, "Anything twice told is fiction." A story about an actual occurrence is representational; it is not the lived event. The teller edits the event in the telling. Certain details are brought to the fore; others are deemed peripheral to the meaning and development of the story and are dismissed. Temporal ordering takes place to make sense, to make relational, disparate aspects of a story. There is a configuring of events into a whole unit of understanding. The thrust of storytelling is to effect reasonableness in a string of events that may be based in reason, as well as emotion, bodily sensations, intuition, and imagination.

Compared to most other forms of inquiry, narratives do not remain the same. They are not static. Each encounter with a story—in our journals, our patients, interview data, patient's stories—the narrative becomes reinterpreted through the evolving lens of our life experience. The exception to this may be the use of story in paradigm cases—individually, readers decide the allegiance to the predetermined meaning put forth and the latitude to use one's imagination.

Probably one of the most important attributes of this genre of inquiry as it concerns nursing is the capacity of stories to help heal.

> Storytelling may set the stage for recovery, and, as nurses, we need to appreciate its value. . . . I believe nurses need to stay with the anxiety engendered in them by the stories they hear; they should not escape behind assessment guides or history-taking activities. Storytelling is more than entertainment or socializing. Storytelling helps patients find meaning in their experiences and gives them the opportunity to reconstruct their lives. Storytelling promotes healing. (Bartol, 1989b, p. 565)

Stories can create a harmony, a sense of congruence between the self and world, which is a primary aspect of Watson's (1988) description of health in her theory of caring. Harmony develops not only for the patient, but for the caregiver as well (Hillman, 1983). All narrative forms allow us to live in our world as engaged mortals, mediating risks and untoward events with the hope and healing that are within our power to evoke.

Differences

Although similar enough to be included in the same genre, the narrative forms presented have important differences. Nursing needs to appreciate these differences so that the term narrative does not remain so generic that it is meaningless.

Intimacy and Distance.   Much of the difference among the forms lies in the play of intimacy and distance (Bartol, 1989a, 1989b; Boykin & Schoenhofer, 1991; Churchill & Churchill, 1987). Intimacy refers to one's standing in the lived experience, fully engaged; distance is one's capacity to lean back, as if to view it from the outside.

Journals represent the most subjective, and therefore intimate, narrative form in which distance is the reflective posture a person takes to his or her own lived experience. Viewing a patient as text requires intimacy but implies much more existential distance. Paradigm cases involve the most distance among narrative forms because both the patient and the nurse are held up for public consideration.

Intimacy (the degree of subjectivity) within interview data, as an example, depends on a number of aspects: the degree of adherence to a schedule of questions, the setting, the personal distance the informants have put between themselves and the experience, and, especially, the quality of the relationship with the interviewer. Interview data may not greatly reflect the subjective state of the informant; the fact that interview was used to secure meaningful content does not necessarily guarantee the results hoped for by the researcher. Nurses must be careful not to overgeneralize data that are sought essentially by strangers in an artificial context. Even though an inquiry may involve a type of narrative, no assumptions can be made regarding the degree of subjectification and objectification toward the phenomenon.

Point of View.   Nonfiction and fictional narratives are dissimilar for the point of view they represent. The point of view in fiction is often variable. In nonfiction, the point of view is inseparable from the teller; in many cases, the story is the point of view itself. Fiction writers choose a point of view that is central to the meaning of the story and becomes the linchpin holding together characters, context, and meaning.

The significance of this point is that, in nonfiction narrative accounts, nurses cannot attribute the point of view of an informant as necessarily true for anyone else. Generalizability of qualitative inquiry contradicts this point by positing the transferability of one's story for others in a similar context (Lincoln & Guba, 1985).

Claim to Truth.   Truth claims among narrative forms differ. Perhaps the widest chasm is between nonfiction (journal, patient-as-text, interviews, paradigm cases) and fiction. Paul Ricoeur (1985) in his examination of narrative makes this important distinction.

I am reserving the term "fiction" for those literary creations that do not have historical narrative's ambition to constitute a true narrative. If we take "configuration" and "fiction" as synonyms we no longer have a term available to account for the different relation of each of these two narrative modes to the question of truth. What historical narrative and fictional narrative do have in common is that they both stem from the same configuring operations. . . . On the other hand, what opposes them to each other does not have to do with the structuring activity invested in their narrative structures as such, rather it has to do with "truth-claim." (p. 3)

With nonfiction there is a "true" version. The degree of belief in the story expected from the reader differs among the forms. In journals and interviews, the teller's personal truth is what is sought. An allegiance to historical facts frames the story for the teller and the audience. The facts are addressed first by the teller and narratively "smoothed" so that often the story has a seamless appearance (Spence, 1982). There is sureness, clarity, and homogeneity within a personal story in terms of what an experience means (Robinson, 1990, p. 1173). Historically based stories, in part, aim to convince the listener and to control the interpretation of the event. The meaning is prescribed as well as described, because the teller is also the protagonist of the story. In paradigm cases, truth is determined in terms of "true for the profession in this situation."

Fiction presents a parallel world which, prior to the reading, is not a shared environment of a lived historical event. There may be no referent, no actual occasion, for comparison. Fiction stands alone. Writers of fiction cannot claim truth; they create a place in which readers can perhaps find their own.

FICTIONAL NARRATIVE AS AN AESTHETIC MODE OF NURSING INQUIRY

I wish to clarify my inclusion of fictional narrative as a storied form of inquiry for nursing. This is where my own work has gone and I believe it is a more common activity than is generally known. Nurses create fiction—stories that have a base in our experiences as nurses—not for historical representation, but as a vehicle to explore the possibilities of meaning with a lived event.

Storytellers undergo very personal epistemological processes as they pursue a story. Tellers learn to live the lives of others, as they imagine them, to learn the exterior landscape of the context—the sights, sounds, and smells—as well as the interior landscape of the experience. The storyteller learns what personal truths can be found in certain human conditions based on profound reflection and imaginary living. An authentic story comes about when the teller's knowledge base demonstrates the breadth and depth of the human condition in a specific context.

The writing of fiction is active inquiry. If there are other outcomes—entertainment, catharsis, fear—these are secondary to facing an initial question or problem. Tellers develop a story to discover what is on the other side. They want to live in that place a bit longer until they know more—not all, but more. The process of living in the story, of questioning, is the primary goal of telling a story.

I have spoken to the differences that fiction has with nonfictional narrative forms of inquiry. However, because very little fiction is being shared within scholarly arenas, as I am proposing here today, I want to clarify my ideas about why fiction belongs within accepted nursing inquiry.

Nursing is attempting to define itself as science. Although it has been acknowledged that clinical nursing can also be an art, it is nursing as science that is credentialed and funded. Creative writing as inquiry is distinctly unscientific, and, since "scientific" is presently equated with "scholarly," creative fiction is generally considered unscholarly.

For all that has been written about aesthetic knowing (Benner & Wrubel, 1989; Carper, 1978; Watson, 1985), there has been little aesthetic inquiry encouraged or published. As stated in the introduction to this chapter, there is a need for nursing as a profession that cares for individuals to develop a path of inquiry that uses aesthetic knowing of individual situations.

The writing of creative fiction is essentially experimentation with unique circumstances:

> It [is] a heuristic device, a thought-experiment. Physicists often do thought-experiments. Einstein shoots a light ray through a moving elevator; Schrodinger puts a cat in a box. There is no elevator, no cat, no box. The experiment is performed, the question is asked, in the mind. Einstein's elevator, Schrodinger's cat, my [characters], are simply a way of thinking. They are questions, not answers; process, not stasis. One of the essential functions of . . . fiction, I think, is precisely this kind of question-asking: reversals of a habitual way of thinking, metaphors for what our language has no words for as yet, experiments in imagination. (Le Guin, 1989, p. 9)

While fiction may be sparked by events at the bedside, the nurse writers use imagination and their wealth of engagement with others in health care settings to communicate context and meaning. However, creative fiction has been an underground pursuit among nurses.

Outside of nursing, the journal *Literature and Medicine* has looked at narrative as aesthetic inquiry for over a decade. Initially, the journal was not only discussion about narrative's link to healing but it also presented original creative works. Through the decade, however, the focus has changed. Many contributors have taken a utilitarian view toward fictional literature. There is a call to develop a specific method of analysis and a specific theoretical stance to literature in its relation to healing. The call is for a more scientific approach to literary arts. Currently in the journal, fictional narrative is not viewed as a process of inquiry, or as exploration for the furthering of personal knowing, but as another source for generalizable knowledge.

There is a niche to be filled here that nursing can view as an opportunity: the exploration of the particular in aesthetic inquiry. The thrust of narrative inquiry in nursing can probe the process and product of writing about our patients and our practice for enhanced personal knowing, without a singular focus on the development of precise methodology.

As process, aesthetic inquiry through narrative has benefits to offer nursing. Fictional narrative improves the recognition of the ambiguity of words and symbols that is the heart of nursing practice. Prolonged contact with fiction, reading or writing, will create enthusiasm for and appreciation of uncertainty. Bartol (1986) stated:

> *Creative literature has a humanizing effect. It helps develop sensitivity to the complex psychological and physical components of human behavior in health and illness. It wakens us from the numbness that all too frequently accompanies routine. At the very least, it points to the ambiguity we need to learn to tolerate in nursing. . . . Creative literature can assist us in gaining this necessary vision. (p. 23)*

This view is fundamental for caring in nursing within a global environment. Caring depends on knowledgeable caregivers—knowledge based not only on the general situation but on the aesthetic knowledge of individuals as well. Tolerance for ambiguity cannot be learned in scientific approaches to inquiry; that is contradictory to the intent of science. Aesthetic inquiry, based in nursing practice and other arts, can.

The stance of the nurse writer in fictional narrative is different than in other forms of narrative inquiry. Writing requires a prolonged engagement in a certain frame of mind that constantly, consciously, shifts figure–ground relationships. The writer attempts to maintain an extreme openness and reverence for the particular because the particular makes more sense within an individual context. The general, the theoretical becomes fairly incomprehensible; the writer of fiction cannot get a hold on it.

Differing from much scientific inquiry, the writer remains fully attached to the phenomenon, but not the product, which evolves as the writer understands more.

> When you write, you lay out a line of words. The line of words is a miner's pick, a woodcarver's gouge, a surgeon's probe. . . . You go where the path leads. At the end of the path, you find a box canyon. You hammer out reports, dispatch bulletins. The writing has changed, in your hands, and in a twinkling, from an expression of your notions to an epistemological tool. You attend. . . . Courage utterly opposes the bold hope that this is such fine stuff the work needs it, or the world. (Dillard, 1989, pp. 3–4)

Often, what is sought after is completely forgotten and discarded because it is no longer relevant to the search. The search, really, is the discovery of the important questions to address. If writers do their job earnestly, the questions are rarely the same at the finish of the story. Future work, similar to a program of scientific inquiry, progresses from the beginning of a work that the writer pares away. A piece may be technically well-written, perhaps the best written, but often a writer will realize that it is peripheral to the meaning of the story. The meaning itself changes as the story evolves. The writer is open to unpredictable and, if the writer has integrity, uncontrollable change within the story.

> The part you must jettison is not only the best-written part; it is also, oddly, that part which was to have been the very point. It is the original key passage, the passage on which the rest was to hang, and from which you yourself drew the courage to begin. . . . The writer returns to these materials, these passionate subjects, as to unfinished business, for they are his life's work. (Dillard, 1989, pp. 4–5)

The same ambiguity, unclear of purpose, distinguishes caring in the best of nursing practice as well fictional narrative. It is unfolding in purpose and, hopefully, has a surprise in the outcome. Creative fiction is appropriate to explore the caring situation in the clinical setting because the answer is not predetermined and because it can retain what is most human—the self, the other, the shared and unique context, feelings as well as thoughts, the smells, and the elusive.

CONCLUSION

Aesthetic inquiry through narrative is contrary to much of the current research trends in nursing. Nursing is justifying its existence as a scientific profession and is intent on highlighting and supporting those efforts in concert with that aim. But researchers are struggling to find methods to explore our shared world with patients that reflect the dance of intimacy and distance that is the heart of nursing. Few methods in nursing research are as elastic and contextual as the caring encounter in clinical practice.

Admittedly, aesthetic inquiry cannot lead to the clear answers suitable for a profession that is only scientific. If nursing values the privileged ontological stance we have with our patients, though, we must also value the ambiguous, the slippery knowledge of particular patients and individual contexts.

REFERENCES

Bartol, G. (1986). Using the humanities in nursing education. *Nurse Educator, 11*(1), 21–22.

Bartol, G. (1989a). Creative literature: An aid to nursing practice. *Nursing and Health Care, 10*(8), 453–457.

Bartol, G. (1989b). Story in nursing practice. *Nursing and Health Care, 10*(10), 564–565.

Benner, P., & Wrubel, J. (1989). *The primacy of caring: Stress and coping in health and illness.* Menlo Park, CA: Addison-Wesley.

Boykin, A., & Schoenhofer, S. (1991). Story as link between nursing practice, ontology, and epistemology. *Image: The Journal of Nursing Scholarship, 23*(4), 245–248.

Carper, B. (1978). Fundamental patterns of knowing in nursing. *Advances in Nursing Science, 1*(1), 13–23.

Charon, R. (1986). To the lives of patients. *Literature and Medicine, 5,* 58–74.

Churchill, L., & Churchill, S. (1987). Storytelling in medical arenas: The art of self-determination. *Literature and Medicine, 6,* 73–79.

Dillard, A. (1989). *The writing life.* New York: Harper & Row.

Hillman, J. (1983). *Healing fiction.* Barrytown, NY: Station Hill.

Le Guin, U. (1989). *Dancing at the edge of the world: Thoughts on words, women, and places.* New York: Harper & Row.

Lincoln, Y., & Guba, E. (1985). *Naturalistic inquiry.* Beverly Hills: Sage.

Long, T. (1986). Narrative unity and clinical judgment. *Theoretical Medicine, 7,* 75–92.

Lopez, B. (1980). *Crossing open ground.* New York: Vintage Books.

Parker, R. (1990). Nurses' stories: The search for a relational ethic of care. *Advances in Nursing Science, 13*(1), 31–40.

Preston, J. (1987). Necessary fictions: Healing encounters with a North American saint. *Literature and Medicine, 6,* 42–62.

Ricoeur, P. (1985). *Time and narrative, Volume 2.* Chicago: University of Chicago Press.

Robinson, I. (1990). Personal narratives, social careers, and medical courses: Analysing life trajectories in autobiographies of people with multiple sclerosis. *Social Science Medicine, 30*(11), 1173–1186.

Spence, D. (1982). *Narrative truth and historical truth: Meaning and interpretation in psychoanalysis.* New York: Norton.

Tisdale, S. (1986). *The sorcerer's apprentice: Medical miracles and other disasters.* New York: Holt, Rinehart & Winston.

Watson, J. (1985). *Nursing: Human science and human care.* Norwalk, CT: Appleton-Century-Crofts.

Watson, J. (1988). New dimensions of human caring theory. *Nursing Science Quarterly, 4*(1), 175–181.

Webster, G. (1990). Nursing and the philosophy of science. In J. McCloskey & H. Grace (Eds.), *Current issues in nursing* (3rd ed.). St. Louis: Mosby.

Younger, J. (1990). Literary works as a mode of knowing. *Image: The Journal of Nursing Scholarship, 22*(1), 39–43.

15

Nursing Intuition: The Deep Connection

Debra Woodard Leners

*T*he art of nursing must not be confused with the science of nursing"
(Abdellah, 1969, p. 393). As one ponders what the essence of nursing art is,
perhaps it is helpful to remember that art is intimately connected with skill
and expertise. The skill and expertise of nursing art seem to be intimately
connected with human experience.

Since the time of the classical Greeks and Romans, intuition has been
acknowledged as a significant human experience. Historically, intuition has
been identified as a natural mental faculty, a key aspect in discovery, a
problem-solving process, a source of creative ideas, and a way to reveal
"truth from God" (Goldberg, 1983; Noddings & Shore, 1984). The word
intuition is derived from the Latin *intueri,* meaning "to look upon" or "to see
within." A dictionary definition of intuition provides a more concrete explanation. Intuition has been defined as an immediate and direct knowing
without the use of conscious reasoning (Webster-Merriam, 1992).

Intuition has been scientifically studied from the traditional, quantitative research perspective. This type of research has produced interesting
self-report scales and numerically based personality surveys that reflect the

degree to which an individual is intuitive (Loomis, 1982; Myers & Myers, 1980; Myers & Myers, 1985). The basic sense of the experience of intuition has to do with spontaneity and immediacy of knowing something. Intuitive knowing is not mediated by deliberate rational process (Fuller, 1973; Goldberg, 1983; Noddings & Shore, 1984). I chose to research intuition from a qualitative perspective because the goal of the study was to seek an *understanding* of the phenomenon of intuition in the culture of nursing care practice.

The qualitative research design chosen to study intuition was ethnography. Ethnography is an approach to discovering knowledge and understanding culture from the informants' point of view (Spradley, 1979). Utilizing the design of ethnography signifies that the researcher views nursing practice as a culture. Nursing as a culture has received little in the way of description or formulation. There is also a dearth of literature on the cultural process of epistemology, or ways of knowing, in nursing practice (Conway, 1983). According to Leininger (1970), nursing as a culture has simultaneously refuted yet covertly valued and utilized intuition in nursing practice throughout history.

Within this ethnographic study, metaphorical analysis was used to gain a richer understanding of the way the cultural informants (nurses) perceived intuition in nursing practice. The use of metaphor implies a way of thinking or seeing that pervades how one understands the world (Morgan, 1986). Metaphors of intuition from the data were hermeneutically examined for language and content. One of the informants was an amateur artist. After the completion of the study, this informant asked permission to capture the metaphors of intuition on canvas. The illustrations provided are the result of the work of this nurse artist (Becker, 1990).

AIMS AND DESIGN OF THE STUDY

The aims of the study covered in this chapter were:

1. Describe examples of intuition experiences.
2. Describe actions taken on intuition.
3. Describe feelings associated with the experience of intuition.
4. Compare and contrast patterns and processes of intuition in the culture of nursing care practice.

The study took place in a Colorado medical center that employs approximately 350 nurses. Procedures for data collection included informant interview and participant observation within the ethnographic format. The study was designed to include data collection from nurses in administrative, hospital clinical, and home care nursing arenas. In keeping with ethnographic research format, the data uncovered the. experiences and understanding of intuition from the nurses' perspective.

THE STUDY SAMPLE

Participant observation took place over a period of 6 months. Time was spent on all shifts, in each hospital unit, observing at the main desk areas, patient care areas, report/lounge areas, and charting centers. All unit manuals, orientation and education materials, nursing care paperwork, and patient charts were examined for intuitive statements. When intuition-related statements or behaviors were observed or noted, the individual was approached for an interview. The sample size was 40.

Informants were largely female (92.5 percent) and about half of the sample held a baccalaureate degree. Twenty-five percent were educated in a diploma school, and 22.5 percent in an associate degree program. Only 5 percent of the sample held a master's degree. Slightly more than half (57.5 percent) of the sample had between 1 and 10 years of nursing experience. The remainder had between 11 and 34 years of nursing practice experience.

Approximately half (42.5 percent) of the sample were between the ages of 30 and 38 years. Thirty percent were 23 to 29 years, and 27.5 percent were 42 to 56 years of age. Most of the informants worked an 8-hour day or night shift in the hospital. Seventeen and one-half percent were graded "RN I," relatively new to the hospital. Half of the nurses were "RN II," meaning they had been in practice at least 2 years and were considered by the hospital to be "above average" in their job performance. Twenty-five percent of the sample were "RN III," the highest level of the hospital clinical promotion system. Fifteen percent of the nurses were in some type of management role.

Ethnographic interviews were conducted and audio tape-recorded with the consent of the informants. All interviews were transcribed verbatim and entered on the Ethnograph computer program (Seidel, Kjolseth, & Seymour, 1988) for analysis. Seven themes within 3 domains, and 1 pervasive cultural theme were discovered in the data. The language of ethnographic data is

Table 15–1
Themes and Domains of Nursing Intuition: The Deep Connection

Domains	Themes
I. The Process of Intuition	The Look: An Elusive Pattern Putting Yourself on the Line
II. Intuition Mediation Variables	It Just Gets Better and Better Environment- and Person-Related Variables
III. The Significance of Intuition	Enhancing the Tuning-In Process You Can't Nurse Without It The Hidden Reward

kept as close to the words of the informant as possible. Each of the themes is explained within the corresponding ethnographic domain (Table 15–1).

RESULTS OF THE STUDY

Domain I: The Process of Intuition

The first theme within this domain is "The Look: An Elusive Pattern." Informants were heard to say, "You can tell a lot about patients just by looking at them." This type of data dominated the description of the process of intuition. A patient's eyes were used frequently to describe where it was that "the look" came from. Beyond this "look," informants described a pattern in their clients that they "tuned into," "picked up on," or "cued in on" in the process of intuition. This "look" or "pattern" was described as unseen and elusive—something that had to be understood by "listening to the inner self" (Figure 15–1).

The patterns described by the informants were more obvious if there were *no* clinical *objective* data supporting the intuition. An intuition would be experienced, then the nurse would look for objective clinical data to support the intuition. If the objective data were *not* found, the intuition was fully explored and accepted as reliable knowledge. The knowledge that became apparent to the informants through intuition was deemed highly reliable and trustworthy: "I just *know* and I'm always right"; "It [intuition] will generally prove to be true."

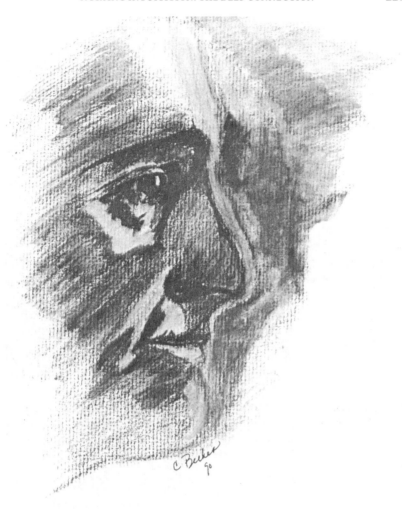

Figure 15–1
The Look: An Elusive Pattern of Intuition

The "look" or "pattern" of intuition also reflected some sort of energy activity, and was noted to be highly connected to nursing as an art of caring. Energy and the association of intuition with caring are typified by these three statements:

> Intuition is an energy exchange and very spiritual and very strong.
> If caring is the priority of nursing, then intuition is the process.
> I really think intuition is a hidden dimension to caring.

"Putting Yourself on the Line" is the second theme of the process domain. Taking action on intuition is a risk-taking behavior in nursing practice. The nurse risks losing credibility as a "good" nurse with peers and physicians. One informant stated:

> Now when you're seasoned like I am it's not as risky, but it's very risky for those that haven't got a lot of grey hair. You have to put yourself on the line with a statement that may make a fool out of you.

Three different types of nursing action were described by the informants in the process of the intuition experience. The first action was to "keep a closer eye on the patient." This might involve anything from rechecking charts to being more physically present or setting up equipment in anticipation of a particular change in the patient's condition. The second action was to share intuitions with other nurses to see what the peer group thought. This was only done if the peers were considered "safe" in terms of interpersonal interaction. The last action informants discussed was communicating the intuition to the physician. This action was clearly the most intimidating one:

> Some docs will listen to you and some just don't think you know anything. It depends on the doc . . . but it takes a lot of courage to tell them you "just know something" and can't explain it.

Domain II: Intuition Mediation Variables

The first theme explains the variable of experience: "It Just Gets Better and Better." The informants spoke of a relationship between nursing experience and intuition. The amount of experience had nothing to do with having intuition but had everything to do with recognizing, sensing, identifying, and listening to intuition. Experience was described as providing increased confidence in the use of intuition.

In the process of analysis, informants' data were compared across years of experience. There is a notable similarity to Benner's (1984) work on expertise in nursing practice. In the "novice" level of experience (1 to 2 years), informants commented on their inability to trust their intuitions. These same informants also expressed hope for increased confidence in their intuitions. In the "standard" level of experience (3 to 8 years), informants were noted to comment on their increasing sense of self-confidence in relying on intuition in nursing practice. Informants in the "veteran" level of experience (8 or more years), did not have to stop to think about recognizing or trusting their intuitions. Intuition appears to be an innate skill for the veteran nurse: "Intuition is simply part of my practice."

The second theme of the mediation domain delineates two categories of intuition variables: "Environment- and Person-Related Variables." The first environmental variable was patient status. Patients who are more critically ill elicit more intuition experiences in the nurses studied. Another environmental variable was technical support. Nurses felt their intuitions were more important to them in the event of less available technical and ancillary support.

External stimuli was a third factor associated with the environment. Fewer distractions, less noise, less activity, and fewer team members to rely on—all of these variables promoted the use of intuition in nursing practice. Organizational philosophy was the last environmental mediator discovered. Hospital or unit philosophy supportive of independence, autonomy, and assertiveness (on the part of the nurse) positively influenced the use of intuition by the informants. Nurses who are allowed to be assertive and independent are identified as being frequent users of intuition:

The ones that have intuition and use it a lot are also the ones that tackle things and don't sit back. So they are also the ones that are more assertive. I don't think nursing can function independently without intuition.

Personological (person-related) mediators are variables that relate to personal, psychosocial factors. The first person-related mediator is the quality of the nurse–client relationship. The deeper the relationship, the greater the intuitive ability of the nurse. Another person mediator was psychosocial–physical status. Fatigue, stress, illness, and low self-esteem were all noted by the informants to play a part in whether one "tuned into" intuitions in a quality way. Many of the informants spoke of their intuitions as a sixth sense that gets overloaded just like other senses:

There is a point of overload and just like your eyesight or your dexterity, your intuition fades too.

Self-perception is the third person-related variable. If an informant perceived himself or herself as trusted by peers and physicians, or if the informant was comfortable on the job (in terms of peer relationships), the informant was more apt to listen to and trust intuition.

The last person mediator was professional image. Informants identified a professional image as being important to the use of intuition. Intuition was frequently noted to make the difference between a good nurse and an excellent nurse:

Intuition is important to a nurse that excels in nursing. The more you have, the more potential you have to be a better nurse.

Domain III: The Significance of Intuition

The first theme of this domain is "Enhancing the Tuning-in Process." Informants consistently spoke of the need to develop and encourage intuition in nursing practice. The primary enhancement technique suggested was sharing or role modeling the use of intuition with student nurses and new staff nurses. Specifics of how to enhance intuition were also provided:

Enhancing intuition is certainly possible, by asking questions like "What are your feelings about this?", or "Listen to your inner self and tell me what you think."

You just have to be quiet and reflect on your feelings, then you can really empathize with the patients and begin to use your intuitions to help them.

A second theme that uncovers the significance of intuition to nursing practice is: "You Can't Nurse Without It." Informants provided very emphatic statements about the importance of intuition to their practice:

I just think nurses can't nurse without it.

We need to use it as much as we can.

It's really there for a reason even though it's not scientifically proven or whatever, but it's very important.

As the informants described the importance of intuition, they began to describe what nursing practice would be like if their intuition was taken away from them. Nursing without intuition was referred to by one informant as an "intuectomy." This metaphor was one that thoroughly reflected how the informants felt about a possible loss of their intuition. Table 15–2 provides informant quotes about an "intuectomy," or nursing practice *without* intuition. The summary analysis on the right side of the table indicates that nursing care without intuition was viewed as mechanistic, dependent, monotonous, nonrelational, ineffective, and substandard.

The final theme discovered in the significance domain was "The Hidden Reward." The primary reward for the use of intuition in nursing practice was that "the patient got better." Informants related that neither patients or physicians were aware of nursing's use of intuition, therefore any rewards were described as hidden. The informants were very articulate: "You aren't ever going to get a merit raise based on the use of your intuition." Informants perceived that nursing and hospital management were not aware of nursing's reliance on intuition or the significance of intuition to practice.

Table 15–2
Descriptions of an Intuectomy

Informant Statements	Summary Analysis
Mechanical, robot-like. Like machines taking care of people. Like a computer nursing patients—just the facts.	Mechanistic
Ball-and-chain-like. No autonomy or independence. Would need to be told what to do. Nursing by policy and procedure only.	Dependent
Stiff, rigid, inflexible. Boring, no fun. Task-oriented only.	Monotonous/lack of creativity
Empty. No sensitivity or feeling. Ineffective. No relationship with client. Couldn't build deep relationships with clients.	Nonrelational
Like having a lobotomy. No individuality. Like being led by the hand. I couldn't function.	Ineffective
No anticipation. Patients would suffer. Terrible handicap to caring. No caring. Lack of caring. Poor quality of patient care. The real stuff of nursing just wouldn't happen.	Substandard nursing care/lack of care

METAPHORICAL ANALYSIS

Within the ethnographic research format, the researcher looks for the data to manifest a cultural theme that embodies a cognitive map of informant experience. Informants provided synonyms for the experience of intuition by consistently referring to "an intense connection," "a true understanding," and "a deep recognition." In order to better understand these explanations of intuition, I examined all metaphorical statements in the data describing intuition in nursing practice.

Hermeneutical analysis was utilized to analyze the intuition metaphors. This type of analysis involves looking at the words, sentence structure, and context of the informant language to uncover meaning (Packer & Addison, 1989). The metaphors provided insight into the experiential meaning of intuition in nursing practice. Four categories of information surfaced:

1. Cues of intuition awareness.
2. Activity responses generated by the intuition.
3. Outcomes of the intuition experience.
4. Intuition as a nursing art form.

A sampling of the metaphorical analysis is provided in Table 15–3.

Cues of Awareness

Initial cues that brought intuition to the nurses' awareness were often described in metaphorical language. Examples of initial cues included: "the look in a patient's eye"; the patient's projection of an aura; "a light bulb going on overhead." These cues to intuition were found to be contextual and relational by nature, reflecting the necessary quality of interpersonal interaction. Sensory feelings associated with intuition experience were also described as initial cues that brought the intuition experience into awareness. These cues were spontaneous, sensory episodes described as: "the voice in the back of my mind," "the alarm clock going off in my head," "nebulous, uneasy feelings," "cold, hollow, empty feelings," and "goose bumps."

Table 15–3
Analysis of Intuition Metaphors

Metaphor	Initial Cue	Action	Outcome
It's like a pattern of dots coming together as one point.	Sensing a pattern	Dots come together	One point is identified
You are underneath the surface and it tells you something deeper is going on.	Nurse is underneath the surface	Being under the surface tells you something	A knowing that is deep
It's just a look in their eyes; green-grey, and you know. That look is all it takes to know something's going to happen.	The green-grey look in the eyes	Recognizing the look is all it takes	You know something is going to happen

Activity Response

The intuition metaphors provided rich information about activity generated by the intuition experience. Many of the activities reflected an anticipation or preparatory organizing on the part of the nurse. "Fine tuning," "getting on the right station," "antennae going up," "putting the bullet in the gun," "filtering information," "energy," "listening," "watching," and "waiting"—all seemed to connote a sense of anticipation or preparatory organizing for something to come. Other activities reflected a connection or coalescence of the nurse–client relationship; "building a bridge," "an understanding link," "thoughts of the nurse and client as one," "awareness of the other," "dots coming together," and "coming to a conclusive point."

Outcomes

Outcomes of the intuition experience consistently communicated a level of understanding or a sense of knowing reached by the nurse. Examples are "true knowing," "knowing that something deeper is going on," "knowing what is going to happen," "the bullet hits dead center," "understanding and connection," "true empathy," and "focused communication with the client."

Nursing Intuition as Art

The metaphors also provided a description of intuition as a professional nursing skill or tool that enhanced practice. The word skill implies the ability to use knowledge effectively or the execution of a learned physical task. Tool defines an instrument or apparatus to use for a purpose (Webster-Merriam, 1992). Skill seems to be internal to the nurse, where tool is external to the nurse. Some metaphors indicate that intuition allows for the use of the nursing self as the tool of practice. Table 15–4 summarizes some of the metaphors used to describe nursing intuition as an art of practice.

In order to provide a greater sense of the richness of the metaphorical language shared by the informants, four illustrated metaphors are presented in Figures 15–2 through 15–5 (Becker, 1990). The associated metaphorical analysis is provided for each figure.

Table 15–4
Intuition as an Art of Practice

Skill: Internal to the Nurse	Tool: External to the Nurse
Intuition is really another clinical skill.	It's the biggest tool you have as a nurse.
Intuition is a very active source of knowledge that takes a lot of energy.	Intuition is like a blind man with the sight-seeing dog.
Intuition is not a mystical force, it is like another sense you have to use.	Intuition allows you to use yourself to build a connection with others.

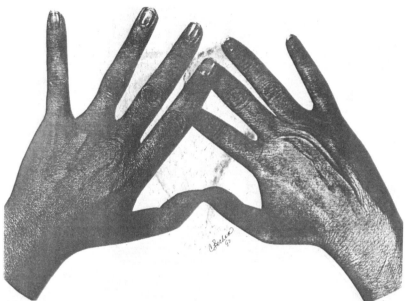

Metaphor: Intuition is two people with a bridge between them. I think intuition is like building a bridge to understanding and connection with people.

Initial Cue: Sensing the building of a connection between two people.

Action: The building of the bridge.

Outcome: Understanding and connection.

Figure 15–2
Intuition Is Like Building a Bridge

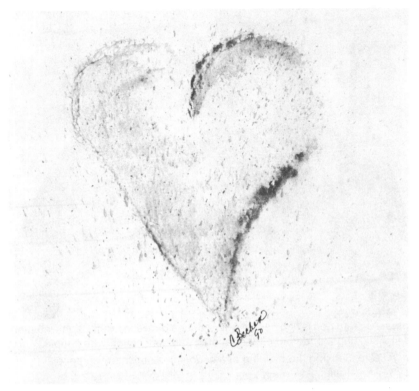

Metaphor: Intuition is the heart that's allowing itself to come out in order to connect with the patient.

Initial Cue: Recognizing the heart.

Action: Allowing the heart to come out.

Outcome: Connection with patients.

Figure 15–3
Intuition Is the Heart

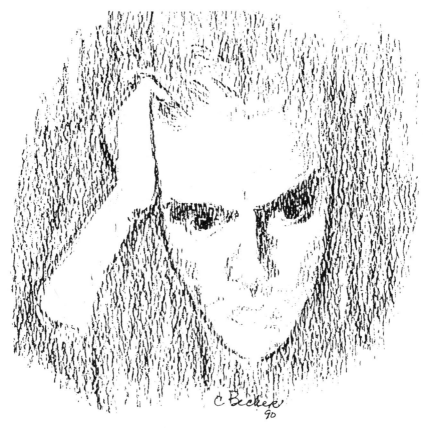

Metaphor: Intuition is an understanding link, a true empathy and coming together, or true communication with a focus—sort of a coming together in-depth.

Initial Cue: Recognizing an understanding link.

Action: True empathy, true communicating with a focus.

Outcome: True coming together in-depth.

Figure 15–4
Intuition Is an Understanding Link

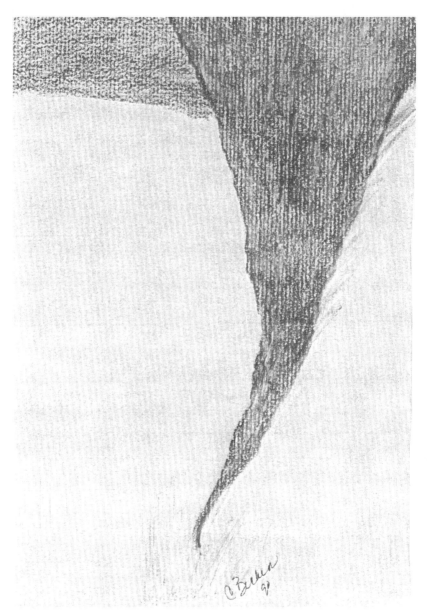

Metaphor: It's like a tornado funnel: these feelings are very nebulous but they come to a conclusive point where you know something.

Initial Cue: Nebulous feelings are recognized.

Action: Coming to a conclusive point.

Outcome: Something is known.

Figure 15–5
Intuition Is Like a Tornado Funnel

THE DEEP CONNECTION

Intuition experience was consistently described as involving a relationship between nurse and client that was "deep," not superficial. The ethnographic and metaphorical data reinforced nursing intuition experience as something that involves a deep connection of self to others. Therefore, the cultural theme of intuition as the "deep connection" was generated. One informant articulately explained the deep connection of intuition experience:

Intuition is my ability to connect at a soul level with another person. And in that connection, there is a deeper ability to understand and to heal. Intuition is a deep connection, that I feel.

The discovery of nursing intuition as a "deep connection" in nursing care practice may be an innovative way to view the transpersonal caring process described theoretically by Watson (1985). In transpersonal caring, the nurse enters into the experience of the one cared for. Transpersonal caring begins when the nurse experiences the patterns and spirit of the one cared for. In the process of the "deep connection," intuitive knowing facilitated the ability of the nurse to "tune into" the patterns of the client and experience a significant, deep knowledge about the one cared for. The "deep connection" theme may signify the experience of transpersonal caring in nursing.

Further research to study ways to enhance the use of intuition in nursing practice is imperative. Gender differences in the experience of intuition in nursing practice is an area yet to be explored. The fact that intuition is a cultural way of knowing in nursing makes rewarding the use of intuition a recruitment and retention factor. It would be expedient to research the specifics of how autonomy, independent decision making, and assertiveness reinforce the use of intuition in nursing practice.

CONCLUSION

Intuition in nursing practice was discovered to be a deep connection that is elusive, risky, promoted by autonomy and independence, and essential to nursing as an art of human caring. The tremendous significance of intuition to nursing care practice is appreciated when one realizes nurses have continued to rely on intuition even when the professional risk is great, the benefits are unrecognized, and the rewards are covert. A word of caution, however: The intuitive way of knowing is a valuable caring technique for nursing, but intuition cannot be itemized as a *duty* of the nurse. Intuition in nursing practice cannot be forced, tallied, or quantified. Rather, intuitive knowing may be a benchmark that nurse and client have achieved a deep, connected, caring relationship.

REFERENCES

Abdellah, F. (1969). The nature of nursing science. *Nursing Research, 18,* 393.

Becker, C. (1990, August). Personal communication. [Clinical Specialist, North Colorado Medical Center, Greeley, CO 80631.]

Benner, P. (1984). *From novice to expert. Excellence and power in clinical nursing practice.* Menlo Park, CA: Addison-Wesley.

Conway, M. E. (1983). Socialization and roles in nursing. In H. H. Werley & J. J. Fitzpatrick (Eds.), *Annual review of nursing research, Vol. 1.* (pp. 183–207). New York: Springer.

Fuller, R. B. (1973). *Intuition.* New York: Anchor Books.

Goldberg, P. (1983). *The intuitive edge.* Los Angeles: Tarcher.

Leininger, M. (1970). *Nursing and anthropology: Two worlds to blend.* New York: Wiley.

Loomis, M. (1982). A new perspective for Jung's typology. *Annals of Psychology, 27,* 59–69.

Morgan, G. (1986). *Images of organizations.* Beverly Hills, CA: Sage.

Myers, P., & Myers, K. (1980). *Gifts differing.* Palo Alto, CA: Consulting Psychologists Press.

Myers, P., & Myers, K. (1985). *Manual: A guide to the development and use of the Myers–Briggs Type Indicator.* Palo Alto, CA: Consulting Psychologists Press.

Noddings, N., & Shore, P. (1984). *Awakening the inner eye: Intuition in education.* New York: Teachers' College Press.

Packer, M. J., & Addison, R. B. (1989). *Entering the circle.* New York: SUNY Press.

Seidel, J., Kjolseth, R., & Seymour, E. (1988). *The Ethnograph.* Littleton, CO: Qualis Research Associates.

Spradley, J. (1979). *The ethnographic interview.* New York: Holt, Rinehart & Winston.

Watson, J. (1985). *Nursing: Human science and human care.* Norwalk, CT: Appleton-Century-Crofts.

Webster-Merriam. (1992). *Webster's new collegiate dictionary.* Springfield, MA: Webster-Merriam.

PART IV

NURSING PRACTICE AND NURSING EXPERIENCES

16

A Qualitative Analysis of Patient Responses to Caring: A Moral and Economic Imperative

Gwen Sherwood

*T*he Fourteenth Annual Human Research Conference brought together nurses from around the world to examine and honor a common, universal, and historical nursing ideal. The conference centered on exploring caring from a global perspective within frameworks representing multicultural (Leininger, 1978, 1981, 1986, 1988), philosophical (Watson, 1979, 1985, 1988), and feminist (Noddings, 1988) points of view. The universality of caring, as manifested in all cultures of the world, is permeated throughout nursing's history. Yet, the very broadness and global nature of caring leave both its meaning and its impact difficult to define, explain, or predict. As a concept and as a process, caring still lacks universal consensus of explication.

The search for common denominators in the theoretical and operational viewpoints of caring in nursing may never cease. Caring is not simple; its broad scope and diverse applications will supply material for debate and exchange for future generations of nurses. The increasing presence of caring in the nursing literature and the constant appeal by practicing nurses to

help determine the essentials of a caring practice are indicative of the perva-
siveness and importance, the *essentialness*, of caring in nursing.

Numerous studies have identified and described caring from a patient's
point of view (Brown, 1986; Cronin & Harrison, 1988; Greiner & Harris,
1992; Henry, 1975; Larson, 1984; Miers et al., 1991; Riemen, 1986; Sherwood, 1991; Swanson-Kaufmann, 1988) as well as from the nurse's perspective (Barr, 1986; Ford, 1981; Forrest, 1989; Kahn & Steeves, 1988; Knowlden,
1986). The limited examination of how patients react or respond leaves unde-
fined the outcomes of a caring nursing practice. As nursing pushes forward in
its professional development, it is imperative to continue the search for common denominators in the theoretical and operational viewpoints while beginning to establish a data base of patient responses to a caring nursing
practice.

PATIENT OUTCOMES AMID
MARKETPLACE REALITIES

Historically, rewards and incentives for efficiency and cost reduction
have dominated the health care arena in contrast to the person-centered
practice world valued by nurses. From observing the shifting paradigm in
health care delivery, it is evident that nursing is experiencing an opportune
time to promote nursing care delivery styles that embody caring as a human
mode of being and acting (Roach, 1987). The limited scope of directly applicable knowledge for constructing a caring practice constrains nursing administrators at the bargaining table in their efforts to ensure the necessary
policies and resources. Current conceptualizations of caring require expansion beyond the descriptive and topological level to higher levels of theory
where the nuances of a caring practice can be explained, predicted, and prescribed. In time, nurses will be able to demonstrate the expected economic
benefits, particularly as nurses' caring is believed to enhance recovery, thus
shortening hospital stays.

Identifying yet another trend, the current orientation of health care public policy strongly emphasizes patient outcomes. Indeed, the entire marketplace has shifted toward total quality improvement where quality and
effectiveness are determined by product outcomes. Given the entrenched belief that caring forms the basis and is the very essence of nursing (Leininger,
1981), explication and description of patient responses to nurses' caring set
the stage for extended study of patient outcomes, nursing's "product line."
Competition in the health care environment makes the impact of nurses'

caring on patient satisfaction an important issue. Within the policy guidelines of the Joint Commission on Accreditation of Hospitals Organization (JCAHO), quality improvement related to patient outcomes could be directly impacted by identification of patient responses to nurses' caring.

Motivated by a moral and professional concern for the patient's overall welfare, nurses seek an operational model to guide and direct a personalized plan of care. A nursing practice based on the interactive nature of caring empowers both nurse and patient through the freedom of reciprocal being and doing. To develop such systems, it is necessary to expand the current knowledge base, through systematic study, to substantiate claims of the benefits, outcomes, and power of a caring practice and demonstrate its effectiveness, efficiency, and economics.

CARING WITHIN MORAL AND ECONOMIC CONTEXTS

In the belief that the invisibility of caring reflects its virtue, many caring actions are hidden (Roberts, 1990). Protection of a person's integrity and dignity during the stresses of caregiving exemplifies what Roberts means by the hidden dimension of caring. "We will be more able to provide that kind of care if we know what it is, how it looks in practice, and how it is transacted interpersonally" (p. 69). Moving into openness, its value in nursing settings can then be described, demonstrated, and embraced so that it can be recognized, rewarded, and taught to both students and nurses.

Moral conflicts in nursing result from the clash of health care economics and human caring (Ray, 1987). Concurring, Watson (1985) referred to caring as the moral ideal of nursing, which, in order to be translated into an economic context, must be defined as nursing services to be rendered and outcomes documented. Ray stated:

> For society, nurses must be not only loyal to caring as a moral ideal in health care, but also responsible to society by involvement in the search to formulate the means to preserve human caring in an increasingly economic health care delivery system. (p. 36)

The study of caring in nursing can thus be given a moral context even within cost–benefit analysis. For a thorough composite of a caring practice, potential outcomes for the patient must be examined not only from a moral context but also in light of the resulting economic picture. Continued examination of the polarities of economics and the preservation of the human person through caring is necessary if health care economics is to become a human science, resulting in the capability to transform nursing practice.

In a comprehensive review article of nursing theories of caring, Morse, Bottorff, Neander, and Solberg (1991) found a dearth of theoretical foundations useful for solving real-world nursing problems with specified outcomes. Examining twenty-three theoretical formulations for definitions of outcomes, only nineteen identified *any* expected outcomes. Of the nineteen, five related outcomes were from the nurses' perspective, eight were from the patients' perspective, and six were from the perspective of both patient and nurse.

Nurses at the forefront of care delivery need the reassurance of well-defined and tested models. Lundh, Soder, and Waerness (1988) criticized caring theories as tending to lack sufficient empirical validation, failing to develop past a subjective approach. To confirm the legitimacy of caring as the essence of nursing, its uniqueness must be explored beyond an internalized feeling; the relevance of caring to practice must be demonstrated through observation of patient response and outcomes. Watson (1988) saw caring as the mutual, reciprocal, and interactive experiences between caregiver and care receiver, and the outcome as positive changes in the welfare of others. For Gendron (1988), caring is a part of the art of nursing wherein the nurse enhances skills used in creating and expressing caring, predicting identifiable patient outcomes will result.

A CARING CONCEPTUAL FRAMEWORK

To advance knowledge about nurses' caring by exploring its impact in the patient's world, research was undertaken to identify and describe the themes of patient responses to caring. A qualitative philosophy and method, phenomenology, was chosen to preserve the richness of the experience as it existed among those living it. A summary description or overall view of caring from the patient's perspective formed the conceptual basis for the study.

Based on an attitude of interaction, caring is marked by an overall concern and commitment communicated through nursing actions. Encompassing awareness of need and knowledgeable assessment, a personalized plan of care is established; appropriate interventions that will lead the patient toward positive well-being are chosen. Actions are validated and confirmed through evaluative assessment. As a conceptual model, caring encompasses patient assessment, personalized care planning, intervening for the good of the patient, and validating effectiveness of actions, all with an overall attitude of interaction (Sherwood, 1991).

METHODOLOGY FOR STUDYING PATIENT RESPONSES

With the above summary description providing the framework, ten adult patients were asked: "What is your response to demonstrations of nurses' caring?" The central purpose of the study, therefore, was to look at patient responses in order to examine the impact of caring. The open-ended interviews conducted privately with each participant in a large hospital in the southwestern United States during postoperative recovery were tape-recorded and transcribed. Steps were taken to safeguard patient confidentiality, assured by appropriate Human Subjects Review.

Analysis was completed using Spiegelberg's steps of phenomenology (1976). The basic steps involved reading and rereading the interview transcripts to capture the overall meaning while highlighting descriptive expressions of patient responses to nurses' caring. Reflecting upon the data, patterns emerged from the descriptive expressions. These patterns were coded and collapsed into increasingly specific themes describing patient reactions to nurses' caring. Themes were given clearer description and meaning from elements listed with each theme.

PATIENT RESPONSES TO NURSES' CARING

Overall, patients described responses to demonstrations of caring in physical and mental realms, in both physiological and affective domains. Moments between nurse and patient characterized by the conceptualization of caring forming the basis for this research uniformly led to a sense of positive well-being for the patient. In brief, the eight themes emerging from the data analysis describing patient responses to nurses' caring were: (1) a positive mental attitude; (2) movement toward recovery and healing or rehabilitation; (3) physical comfort; (4) gratitude; (5) reassurance; (6) dignity and acceptance; (7) trust; and (8) satisfaction. Table 16–1 provides an overview of the themes and descriptive elements of patient responses to nurses' caring.

Table 16–1
Major Themes and Elements: Patient Responses to Nurses' Caring

1. Positive mental attitude
   —improved coping
   —enhanced physical well-being

2. Movement toward recovery and healing or rehabilitation
   —satisfied mental and emotional needs
   —alleviated anxiety and worry
   —freed energy for physical recovery
   —feelings of elation/excitement
   —enabled by personalized plan of care

3. Physical comfort
   —relieved of pain by skillful intervention
   —knowledgeable assessment of needs
   —alleviated worry and anxiety

4. Gratitude
   —felt protected
   —experienced safety and protection
   —recognized and praised skillful nursing actions
   —freed for recovery as a result of feeling safe

5. Reassurance
   —offered "release and freedom"
   —felt existential presence

6. Dignity and acceptance
   —experienced wholeness
   —treated like a person, not a patient
   —felt respected as a competent individual
   —experienced positive, existential growth and development

7. Trust
   —experienced trusting relationship
   —responded to personalized nursing intervention with physical and mental comfort
   —felt unique, positive environment

8. Satisfaction
   —communicated feeling of quality care
   —noted caring as "being and doing"
   —felt attitude of interaction from nurse

The following discussion of each major theme encompasses descriptive elements along with patient statements.

1. *A positive mental attitude, increasing the ability to cope while enhancing physical well-being.* When patients felt better mentally, they felt better physically and recovered more quickly, indicating a perceived relationship of the physical and mental. Feeling good mentally, then, was related to getting well faster. "It really helps a lot—my mental attitude, as well as physically, because I know when I feel better mentally I actually feel better physically."

2. *Movement toward recovery and healing as a result of a personalized, coordinated care plan.* Patients felt better after a caring interaction, a feeling that built each day in exponential fashion. The satisfaction of mental or emotional needs alleviated anxiety and worry, freeing the self for physical recovery. "[Caring] helps me mentally to do it on my own and I start moving and sure enough it does work and I start feeling better."

3. *Physical comfort brought about by competent, personalized interventions.* Feelings of elation, excitement, and amazement were identified with having received personalized, coordinated attention. Relief from pain as a result of skilled intervention by the nurse was a frequent experience among patients. The nurse's knowledge of how to assess the pain and intervene appropriately brought about relief more quickly when encompassed by an attitude of concern and commitment. Use of relaxation techniques offered relief from worry, induced calmness, and reduced pain. "[O]ne of the nurses, when I was feeling really bad, stroked me on the forehead and I was too out of it to remember who it was, but it felt good and relaxed me."

4. *Gratitude for safety, protection, and skillful actions.* Appreciation was variously described. The positive experience of one patient even led *almost* to regret at discharge: "I'm almost happy I had to stay longer, it's been such a worthwhile experience." Recognition and praise for the nurses' skillful actions further instilled an atmosphere of being safe and protected from harm—again, freeing the patient for recovery. "That's real important . . . to talk to you to keep you from getting nervous." A protecting connotation, much like a motherly love but unrelated to gender, brought forth feelings of affection and acceptance. To experience safety and protection in a crisis time was a source of comfort and brought gratitude and

reciprocal feelings toward the nurse. To be with someone at such a precious, intimate moment was truly to experience a reciprocity of caring benefit.

5. *Reassurance provided by constant monitoring and attentive presence.* The skillful observation and assessment activities of the nurse offered reassurance of caring. Knowing the nurse was constantly checking on their status and condition offered patients release and freedom, allowing physiological responses to proceed unhindered. The attentive presence of the nurse, existential and transcendent, was reassurance of being *seen*, being *heard*, and being *with*. "I had a good feeling. I think with experiences of that sort they help you mend a lot quicker than if you had adverse reactions to things."

6. *Dignity and acceptance from being treated like a person, "like I was whole."* Experiencing caring from the nurse brought forth a feeling of being whole, of being an individual, not "just another patient." Nurses' demonstrations of respect for patient privacy, for personal competence, and for individual rights in making decisions about care led patients to a feeling of wholeness, positive well-being, and growth unrelated to any remaining physical limitations. "It made me feel good. I felt like I was whole, that I was being treated like a person and not a patient." A synergy of nurse–patient mutual helpfulness was generated where both felt a positive, existential growth and development.

7. *Trust developed between nurse and patient.* The demonstrations of nurse caring brought forth physical and mental changes, positive outcomes that resulted in a trusting relationship. As the nurse combined a personalized, coordinated plan of care and skillful actions to help move patients toward their own level of recovery, a measure of mental and physical comfort was achieved. The nurse provided safety and protection through monitoring, and presence with recognition of personhood. Patients relinquished responsibility for care to the nurse until they were able to resume self-care. "It was a real neat experience. I knew that I was hurting bad and she was there with me until I felt better." A unique environment had been created for the journey toward wholeness.

8. *Satisfaction from receiving quality care.* Patients not only expressed gratitude for the caring received, but also communicated a feeling of having received quality care. In other words, caring, as both being and doing, was equated with quality care. Technical and skillful competence carried out interactionally and with a

person-centered orientation resulted in an outcome of satisfaction. "[B]ecause you are here to get well, I think if they treat you well, say mentally and physically, it helps you recuperate fast, and altogether your experience will be great."

VALIDATION OF CARING
THROUGH RESEARCH

The emphasis on total quality improvement in health care demands a focus on patient welfare and subsequent outcomes. Identification of patient responses could be the basis for evaluation research of specific nurses' caring and the effect on patient outcomes as documentation of quality. Shiber and Larson (1991) cited an evaluation model based on Donabedian's work and encompassing structure, process, and outcomes. Structure includes the setting and instruments available and used to provide care; process includes the activities of the nurse in delivering care to patients; and outcomes for patients, as befitting a caring model, include growth and development, ability to cope better with illness, and ability to meet personal needs with nursing assistance. Linkages between caring as process and clearly stated, anticipated outcomes would document the usefulness of caring practice. Backed by administrative policies and decisions, nursing incentives and rewards can be based on provision of humanistic, personalized care. The ability to describe, explain, and predict caring, from structure, process, and outcomes, would empower and propel nursing to the forefront of health care delivery.

Valentine (1991), a leader in evaluation studies related to caring, reported a comparative analysis of nurse–patient interactions and outcomes related to productivity and concluded that caring is missing from the current productivity system. Building on the identification of patient responses presented here, evaluation theories and models can form the basis for more definitive quantitative studies.

Duffy (1992) measured the relationships between nurse caring behaviors and the selected outcomes of patient satisfaction, health status, length of stay, and nursing care costs in hospitalized patients. Using a descriptive correlational design with five data collection instruments, Duffy tested eighty-six patients. Caring behaviors of nurses positively correlated to patient satisfaction, but no relationship was found between nurse caring behaviors and perception of health status. Although no definite determination could be made that nurse caring behaviors reduced hospital costs for patients, both length of stay and costs showed a decline, demonstrating a trend toward the positive outcomes of nurse caring. More advanced study methods are needed to continue the important efforts begun by Duffy.

IMPLICATIONS FOR A CARING PRACTICE

Miller-Baden (1988) discussed predictors of patient satisfaction within a caring conceptual framework. Satisfaction with nursing care appears to be based in large part on perception of the nurse's affective behavior toward the patient. Patients were less satisfied with the way nurses met emotional and psychological needs of patients than with physical care, marking the importance of research defining nursing care that satisfies affective needs of patients. Nursing interventions meeting affective needs must be identified and systematically tested to establish the relationship with patient outcomes.

Changes occurring in the health care industry in this decade are of paramount importance to the future of nursing. Now is the time to validate the importance of caring in nursing. Buerhaus (1986) highlighted the economic impact of establishing the cost factor for nurse caring interactions with patients. Qualitative study was encouraged to identify patients' perceptions of nurse caring interactions and to determine the worth to the patient of the interaction. The quality of nursing care, with the main attribute "simple human caring," is a hospital's most important asset. The nurse is most intensely and constantly focused on the whole patient. It is essential that nurses take command of this indispensable commodity not only for moral integrity related to patient welfare but also to safeguard the economic future of nursing.

With increased emphasis on accountability in nursing and the move to project costs for nursing services, there is difficulty in measuring the nurse's full role. Activities involving technical skills and procedures are more easily measured; the interhuman dimension of nursing and its resultant outcomes are not easily quantified (Bottorff & D'Cruz, 1984).

CONCLUSION

Daily commitment to constructing and maintaining a caring nursing practice can affect patient outcomes in a positive way. Dedication to caring, with a connection and mutuality to one another, can make a difference in the lives and well-being of others by creating a positive response. Through construction of an operationally defined caring practice, the global nature and universality of nursing can be demonstrated.

REFERENCES

Barr, W. J. (1986). Critical care nurses' perceptions of caring: A phenomenological study. *Dissertation Abstracts International, 47,* 567B.

Bottorff, J., & D'Cruz, J. (1984). Towards inclusive notions of "patient" and "nurse." *Journal of Advanced Nursing, 9,* 549–553.

Brown, L. (1986). The experience of care: Patient perspectives. *Topics in Clinical Nursing, 8*(2), 56–62.

Buerhaus, P. I. (1986). The economics of caring: Challenges and new opportunities for nursing. *Topics in Clinical Nursing, 8*(2), 13–21.

Cronin, S., & Harrison, B. (1988). Importance of nursing caring behaviors as perceived by patients after myocardial infarction. *Heart and Lung, 27,* 374–380.

Duffy, J. (1992). The impact of nurse caring on patient outcomes. In D. Gaut (Ed.), *The presence of caring in nursing.* New York: National League for Nursing.

Ford, M. (1981). Nurse professionals and the caring process. *Dissertation Abstracts International, 43,* 967–968B. (University Microfilms No. 7516229)

Forrest, D. (1989). The experience of caring. *Journal of Advanced Nursing, 14,* 815–823.

Gendron, D. (1988). *The expressive form of caring.* Toronto, Canada: University of Toronto.

Greiner, D. S., & Harris, D. (1992). *Professional nursing caring as perceived by critically ill psychiatric patients: A phenomenologic study.* Unpublished abstract, University of Alabama School of Nursing, Birmingham.

Henry, O. M. (1975). Nurse behaviors perceived by patients as indicators of caring. *Dissertation Abstracts International, 36*(2), 652B. (University Microfilms No. AAC7516229)

Kahn, D. L., & Steeves, R. H. (1988). Caring and practice: Construction of the nurse's world. *Scholarly Inquiry for Nursing Practice, 2,* 201–216.

Knowlden, V. (1986). The meaning of caring in the nursing role. *Dissertation Abstracts International, 46,* 2574A.

Larson, P. J. (1984). Important nurse caring behaviors perceived by patients with cancer. *Oncology Nursing Forum, 11*(6), 46–50.

Leininger, M. (1978). *Transcultural nursing: Concepts, theories, and practices.* New York: Wiley.

Leininger, M. (Ed.). (1981). The phenomena of caring: Importance, research questions, and theoretical considerations. In M. Leininger (Ed.), *Caring: An essential human need* (pp. 5–20). Thorofare, NJ: Slack.

Leininger, M. (1986). Care facilitation and resistance factors in the culture of nursing. *Topics in Clinical Nursing, 8*(2), 1–12.

Leininger, M. (1988). Leininger's theory of nursing: Cultural care diversity and universality. *Nursing Science Quarterly, 1,* 152–160.

Lundh, U., Soder, M., & Waerness, K. (1988). Nursing theories: A critical view. *Image: The Journal of Nursing Scholarship, 20,* 36–40.

Miers, L. J., Kinney, M., Burfitts, S., Greiner, D., Branyon, M., Packa, D. P., & Connell, J. (1991). Professional nurse caring as perceived by critically ill patients: A phenomenological study. *Heart and Lung, 20,* 25A. (Abstract)

Miller-Baden, M. (1988). Nursing care behaviors that predict patient satisfaction. *Journal of Nursing Quality Assurance, 2*(3), 11–17.

Morse, J. M., Bottorff, J., Neander, W., & Solberg, S. (1991). Comparative analysis of conceptualizations and theories of caring. *Image: The Journal of Nursing Scholarship, 23,* 119–126.

Noddings, N. (1988). An ethic of caring and its implications for instructional arrangements. *American Journal of Education, 96*(2), 215–230.

Ray, M. (1987). Health care economics and human caring in nursing: Why the moral conflict must be resolved. *Family and Community Health, 10*(1), 35–43.

Riemen, D. (1986). The essential structure of a caring relationship: Doing phenomenology. In P. Munhall & C. Oiler (Eds.), *Nursing research: A qualitative approach* (pp. 85–108). Norwalk, CT: Appleton-Century-Crofts.

Roach, M. S. (1987). *The human act of caring: A blueprint for health professions.* Toronto: Canadian Hospital Association.

Roberts, J. (1990). Uncovering hidden caring. *Nursing Outlook, 38*(2), 67–69.

Sherwood, G. (1991). Patient descriptions of nurses' caring: The role of the compassionate healer. In D. Gaut & J. Watson (Eds.), *Caring: The compassionate healer.* New York: National League for Nursing.

Shiber, S., & Larson, E. (1991). Evaluating the quality of caring: The structure, process and outcome. *Journal of Holistic Nursing Practice, 5*(3), 57–66.

Spiegelberg, H. (1976). *The phenomenological movement: Vols. 1 & 2* (2nd ed.). The Hague: Martinus Nijoff.

Swanson-Kaufmann, K. M. (1988). Caring in the instance of unexpected early pregnancy loss. *Topics in Clinical Nursing, 8*(2), 37–46.

Valentine, K. (1991). Comprehensive assessment of caring and its relationship to outcome measures. *Journal of Nursing Quality Assurance, 5*(2), 59–68.

Watson, J. (1979). *The philosophy and science of caring.* Boston: Little, Brown.

Watson, J. (1985). *Nursing: Human science and human care.* Norwalk, CT: Appleton-Century-Crofts.

Watson, J. (1988). New dimensions of human caring theory. *Nursing Science Quarterly, 1*, 175–181.

17

"She Dares":
An Essential Characteristic of the
Excellent Swedish Nurse

Siv R. Bäck-Pettersson
Kirsten Pryds Jensen

"Good-bye," said the fox, "and now I am going to entrust you with my secret. It is quite simple: only with the heart you can see properly. The essential thing is invisible to the eye."

"The essential thing is invisible to the eye," repeated the little prince for better to remember it.

"It is the time you have spent on the rose that makes it so meaningful."

"It is the time I have spent on my rose . . . ," said the little prince for better to remember it.

"Mankind has forgotten that truth," said the fox. "But you must not forget it. You are for ever responsible for what you have tamed. You are responsible for your rose. . . ."

"I am responsible for my rose," repeated the little prince for better to remember it.

Antoine de Saint-Exupéry (1987)

257

Nurses are aware of the secret that caring is fundamental to human life; they take their responsibility to really care for their rose. Nurses know that the most important part of caring—the part that deals with pain, suffering, and human misery—is invisible. Most people have forgotten that truth, therefore that truth must be recaptured. Nursing and nurses are very important to their patients, but nurses' knowledge, skills, and efforts are more or less invisible to health care authorities. To preserve human caring in the health care system, nurses' experience must be regarded as a valued source of knowledge (Watson, 1990).

In an attempt to visualize the invisible caring, we regarded stories from caring situations to be very useful. Who could tell stories that expressed caring in all its nuances? Who could bridge the gap of understanding between the caring reality and the health care authorities? Who could give caring a voice? We believed that nurses recognized as excellent in clinical practice could do that. This was confirmed in a large research project tentatively entitled "The Green-Thumb Phenomenon in Nursing." The metaphor "green thumb" was used in the Swedish context: a synonym for excellent.

This research identified and described (1) the characteristics of Swedish nurses considered to have a green thumb for nursing and (2) caring moments in which these nurses were involved. From the data, a profile of the green-thumb nurse emerged. The green-thumb nurse was a woman. Her mean age was 42.6 years (range 24 to 60 years). She was a family woman with an extroverted personality. Apart from nursing, her main interests were her family, her garden, and her house pet. She was a lover of open-air life. She had an average working experience in nursing practice of 17.6 years (range 3 to 39 years). Her level of education was equivalent to a bachelor of science in nursing.

Three main concepts were identified as characteristics of the green-thumb nurse: competence, compassion, and courage. In the theme clusters, the nurse was characterized as "she can," "she wants," and "she dares." The green-thumb nurse knew when a caring moment was possible, she was able to act on the spur of the moment, and she created the caring moment by using her competence, compassion, and courage (Pryds Jensen, Bäck-Pettersson, & Segesten, 1992).

This chapter is focused on the concept of courage because courage appeared to be the salient feature in most of the statements and stories told by the green-thumb nurses.

PERSPECTIVES ON CARING AND COURAGE IN CARING

Courage in caring seems to be an important characteristic of a professional nurse and is described both explicitly and implicitly in various concepts. Caring was described by Watson (1985, 1988) as the ethical and moral ideal of nursing. Caring consists of transpersonal intersubjective attempts to protect, enhance, and preserve humanity and human dignity by helping people find some meaning in their illness, suffering, pain, and existence. Preservation of human dignity calls for love and courage from the nurse (Lanara, 1990). Roach (1984) stated that caring behavior in nursing is manifested through the attributes of compassion, competence, confidence, conscience, and commitment. Confidence is the integration of trust, hope, and courage. A trusting relationship is fostered by confidence (Boykin & Schoenhofer, 1990).

Watson (1985) proposed that caring is effectively demonstrated and practiced interpersonally only in the actual caring occasion, when the nurse is a co-participant in a process in which the ideal of caring is the human-to-human, subject-to-subject transaction. Through the richness of knowing—personal, empirical, ethical, and esthetical—the nurse as an artist creates the caring moment (Boykin & Schoenhofer, 1990). In the caring moment, the importance of authentic presence and connectedness with the other is stressed (Mayeroff, 1971; Parse, 1981; Roach, 1984; Watson, 1985). It requires courage to be authentic in a situation: to be a caring nurse who attends to the dignity of the person, who demonstrates respect for human life, and who expresses nonpaternalistic values related to human autonomy and freedom of choice (Watson, 1985). Joseph (1991) stated that "courage and devotion are necessary for nurses to consciously make a choice to be fully present and energetically open in a compassionate way that facilitates wholeness for clients" (p. 57).

POPULATION AND METHOD

Thirty-two nurses participated in the green-thumb study. The nurses were identified by their superiors as excellent nurses, as having that special gift—a green thumb for nursing. They were head nurses or staff nurses in inpatient units, working with adult patients with somatic diseases.

The method used was descriptive exploratory (Bogdan & Taylor, 1975; Parse, Coyne, & Smith, 1985). The descriptive exploratory method is an investigation of the meaning of a particular life event for a group of subjects who have shared the event (Parse et al., 1985). The nurses were subject to a semistructured interview that was tape-recorded and transcribed verbatim. The interview contained the following questions:

1. Please identify and describe the characteristics of the green-thumb nurse.
2. Please describe a situation (a caring moment) where your actions were of great positive importance to the patient.

The data were analyzed according to the method.
The procedure for the data analysis included the following steps:

1. Transcripts were read to achieve a sense of the whole.
2. Transcripts were analyzed and the essential points were summarized in paraphrases.
3. Major themes were extracted.
4. The import of the themes was formulated and organized into theme clusters.
5. The theme clusters were formed as concepts.
6. The essence of the phenomenon studied was described.

The descriptive method includes an elaboration of the context of the situation as well as the retrospective plans surrounding the event (Parse et al., 1985).

FINDINGS

The concept of courage appeared to be an essential characteristic to the green-thumb nurse and a prerequisite for her ability to create caring moments. Three major themes constructed the theme cluster "she dares." The first major theme was that the green-thumb nurse was expected to be courageous when connecting with people in crisis:

> *Even in troublesome situations she must dare to stay and contribute to solve the problem.*

In the first story narrated, the green-thumb nurse created the caring moment when being together with the isolated patient in chaos. She caught the moment and took the risk of being rejected. She stayed authentic, confirmed the patient, and was willing to go beyond conventional limits to alleviate suffering. The green-thumb nurse was able to maintain a close human-to-human relationship when caring for her dying patient.

This corresponds with the work of Parse, Eriksson, and Lanara. According to Parse (1981), "the beingness is risking, which includes having the courage to be authentic in a situation" (p. 130). Eriksson (1987) stated that "it takes courage to confirm another. . . . Every time the other is confirmed it results in courage and power to go on living" (p. 65). Lanara (1990) expressed the nurse's need for "heroism to face dying patients. . . . It requires heroism for the nurse to provide truly humane care for the dying patient" (p. 38).

The green-thumb nurse is courageous when practicing advocacy. To be an advocate means to be in opposition and to speak up for someone who is unable to speak for himself or herself.

In the second story, the green-thumb nurse demonstrated courage when trusting her own decisions, defending the patient's choice to go home, and opposing the physician's decision in an attempt to alleviate suffering. Practicing advocacy corresponds to Lanara's (1990) implication of courage in the concept of heroism. Lanara stated that "providing humanistic and personalized care in the midst of specialized care, mechanized, and depersonalized health delivery services requires strength, courage, motivation and strong will" (p. 38).

The green-thumb nurse must be courageous when coping with stressful situations in the working environment. In the third story, the green-thumb nurse showed courage when opposing the staff opinions and routines at the ward. Her acting seemed to be derived from an internalized caring value system based on solidarity with the patient; she was true to the caring philosophy of the ward in her attempt to alleviate suffering. This response corresponds to Lanara's (1990) description of "the heroic act of the nurse when transcending the fatigue and exhaustion the nurse often experiences after a feverish and laborious series of emergencies and unpredictable events, and yet provides 'caring' nursing" (p. 39).

The alleviation of suffering was viewed by Eriksson (1992) as the cornerstone of caring and a starting point within the profession. It takes courage to face pain, suffering, and human misery. It seemed that the green-thumb nurses were quite aware of the importance of alleviating suffering and, through competence, compassion, and courage, were able to seize the moment and act accordingly. It takes courage to be an independent professional nurse; as Watson (1990) proposed, "if caring is to be sustained, those who care must be strong, courageous, and capable of inner love, peace and joy—both in relation to themselves and others" (p. 64). The findings indicated that the green-thumb nurses are courageous, independent, and professional.

Still there are questions to be answered. Are green-thumb nurses more courageous than other nurses? Is it from lived experience that nurses are developing courage? Who taught them courage? Would patients have regarded the green-thumb nurses as courageous?

CONCLUSION

This chapter has attempted to visualize courage—the "dare" aspect of the invisible caring—by communicating statements and stories from caring situations in clinical practice, told by nurses recognized as having a green thumb for nursing. We believe that green-thumb nurses could give caring a voice that could bridge the gap of understanding between the caring reality and the health care authorities. We hope that courage as a force, once recognized among nurses, can be an important tool in our common mission to preserve human caring.

To help society recapture the truth that caring is fundamental to human life, and to identify caring as a global agenda, a united effort from courageous nurses all over the world—researchers, theorists, administrators, and nurses in clinical practice—is needed. We have a common responsibility to really care for our rose.

REFERENCES

Bogdan, R., & Taylor, S. J. (1975). *Introduction to qualitative research methods*. New York: Wiley.

Boykin, R., & Schoenhofer, S. (1990). Caring in nursing: Analysis of extant theory. *Nursing Science Quarterly, 3*, 149–155.

Eriksson, K. (1987). *Pausen*. Stockholm: Almqvist & Wiksell.

Eriksson, K. (1992). The alleviation of suffering—the idea of caring. *Scandinavian Journal of Caring Sciences, 6*(2), 119–123.

Joseph, L. (1991). The energetics of conscious caring for the compassionate healer. In D. Gaut & M. Leininger (Eds.), *Caring: The compassionate healer* (p. 57). New York: National League for Nursing.

Lanara, V. A. (1990). Heroism in nursing implications for nursing research. *Proceedings of the International Caring Conference.*

Mayeroff, M. (1971). *On caring.* New York: Harper & Row.

Parse, R. R. (1981). Caring from a human science perspective. In M. Leininger (Ed.), *Caring: An essential human need* (pp. 129–132). Thorofare, NJ: Slack.

Parse, R. R., Coyne, A. B., & Smith, M. J. (1985). *Nursing research: Qualitative methods.* Bowie, MD: Brady.

Pryds Jensen, K., Bäck-Pettersson, S., & Segesten, K. (1992). The caring moment and the green-thumb phenomenon among Swedish nurses. *Nursing Science Quarterly.*

Roach, M. S. (1984). *Caring: The human mode of being, Implications for nursing.* Perspectives in Caring, Monograph 1. Toronto, Canada: University of Toronto Press.

Saint-Exupéry, A. (1987). *Den lille prins.* Vyborg, Sweden: Lindhardt & Ringhof.

Watson, J. (1985). *The philosophy and science of caring.* Boulder: Colorado University Press.

Watson, J. (1988). *Nursing: Human science and human care.* New York: National League for Nursing.

Watson, J. (1990). The moral failure of the patriarchy. *Nursing Outlook, 38*(2), 62–66.

18

Humanistic Care and Nurses' Experiences

Joan Donoghue

Nursing is consistently described as a highly expressive and humanistic process that focuses on caring functions (Fenton, 1987). Caring makes curing possible—"though there can be caring without curing, there can be no curing without caring" (Leininger, 1986, p. 10). Kelly (1988, p. 17) stated that impersonal caring interventions may repair the patient's body but crush the soul. Issues related to caring now pervade current nursing literature; however, published research in Australia is limited in relation to the care concept. This chapter is based on a study that measured the degree to which nurses incorporate caring values into their practice and identified the characteristics, views, and experiences that influence nurses' care behaviors.

The author thanks Mary V. Fenton for the use of her Scale of Humanistic Behaviors, and the registered nurses who participated in this study.

REVIEW OF LITERATURE

Although no universal definition of nursing exists, there is agreement among nurses that the essence of nursing lies in its individualized, personalized care of patients. However, the caring aspects of nursing practice are often viewed as too complex and ill-defined to be measured in a meaningful way. For the purpose of this study, humanistic care was defined as "care that enhances the dignity and autonomy of patients and health professionals alike" (Howard, David, Pope, & Ruzek, 1977, p. 12).

Only a few studies have identified nursing behaviors that convey caring. Most of these reported studies have asked individuals, both patients and nurses, to identify specific actions and/or attributes of nurses that indicate care.

Henry (1975) and Brown (1981, 1986) examined patients' views of nurses' caring behaviors. The data supported the concept that caring is based on the attributes of the caregiver, as well as on expressive and instrumental behaviors. When Larson (1981) and Mayer (1986) examined the congruence of patients' and nurses' views of caring behaviors, both found that, although there was congruence overall, patients appear to value the instrumental technical skills more than nurses, and nurses ranked the expressive behaviors higher.

Several studies have examined nurses' views of caring behaviors. Ford's (1981) survey of 192 nurses identified two major categories of caring: genuine concern for the well-being of another and giving of oneself. From a list of seventy-five behaviors, Wolf (1986) identified the five highest ranked caring behaviors as attentive listening, comforting, honesty, patience, and responsibility.

Despite the increased emphasis on caring in nursing research and education, there are signs that nursing has lost its ethic of caring. In a qualitative study by Riemen (1986) on caring and noncaring nurse–patient interactions, the results revealed that noncaring interactions were consistently described first by patients and that a great majority of perceptions of noncaring interactions fall into two categories: being rough/belittling patients and treating patients as objects. Newburn (1987) studied 272 consenting participants from six caregiver disciplines working in acute-care and long-term facilities. The results revealed that patient abuse occurs in most health care settings and that females, the elderly, and those suffering from a chronic condition were perceived to be most at risk.

Other studies on care have narrowed the focus to specific behaviors or interventions that accomplish care ideals. The most widely studied variable of care is empathy. The most common measures of empathy employed in these studies are based on scales developed by Carkhuff, Hogan, and Barrett-Lennard. Studies conducted by Kalisch (1971), La Monica, Caren, Winder, Hasse, and Blanchard (1976), Hills and Knowles (1983), Brunt (1985), and Alverson (1987) concluded that nurses have low to moderate empathy. Forsyth (1979), however, found that nurses' empathy scores were average to above average. Based on these findings, it remains questionable as to whether empathy occurs routinely in hospital settings.

In relation to demographic factors and care, Forsyth (1979) tested the difference in empathic ability in relation to nurses' characteristics and found there was no significant relationship between empathic ability and the age, marital status, parental status, and length and level of practice of nurses. Sparling and Jones (1977) found that 28 medical-surgical nurses scored lower on empathy than did 29 psychiatric nurses. Brunt (1985) found no significant difference in empathy scores of nurses working in four specialty units—two intensive care and two nonintensive care.

The gender of nurses in relation to caring behaviors has also been explored. MacDonald (1977), in a study of 60 students, found that males in nursing scored slightly higher than females on the Hogan Empathy Scale. In contrast, Taylor, Pickens, and Geden (1989), in their study of interactional styles of female and male nurses and physicians, concluded that gender was not a significant factor in the approach used to influence patient decision making. The results of these studies suggest that the significance of demograhic variables on the care behaviors of nurses requires further exploration.

Fenton (1987) developed a Scale of Humanistic Behaviors to measure the concept of humanistic care in hospital settings as perceived by nursing staff. The scale was based on four dimensions from Howard's (1975) theoretical model of humanistic health care: status equality, empathy, shared decision making, and responsibility and holistic selves. The results of Fenton's study (conducted in the United States) indicated humanistic behavior scores of nurses to be lower in public hospitals in contrast to a university-affiliated hospital and a small private community hospital. The effect of the relationship among social desirability, the scale, and the differences in hospital means raised the issue of whether the main effect of humanistic care depended more on the characteristics of individuals who staff a unit than on the overall type of hospital (Fenton, 1987).

PURPOSE OF THE STUDY

The aims of the study were threefold:

- To measure the degree to which humanistic care behaviors are enacted by nurses in clinical nursing practice in hospitals.
- To explore the relationship between humanistic care behaviors and nurses' characteristics.
- To describe the attributes and experiences that affect nurses' care behaviors.

METHODOLOGY

Sample

The subjects in the study included 107 registered nurses working in ten adult acute-care public hospitals with an average of 150 to 350 beds available. These hospitals were selected for their similarity in size, complexity of care levels, and skill mix of nursing staff. Registered nurses working full-time or part-time on three shifts (day, evening, and night), and rostered on a permanent or rotational basis to units or departments that provided continuous twenty-four-hour direct patient care services, were included in the sample.

Instrument

The instrument was a semistructured four-part questionnaire. Part I was an adaptation of Fenton's Scale of Humanistic Behavior (Fenton, 1981), which was developed and tested based on four dimensions of Howard's (1975) theoretical model of humanistic health care: status equality, empathy, shared decision making, and responsibility and holistic selves.

The questionnaire was comprised of 70 items. For the purposes of this study, the subject noun of each question was a personal view ("I") rather than an objective assessment of behaviors on a particular ward. For example, some of the statements were "I refer to patients by the name they prefer to be called," "I tell patients their vital signs when they ask about them," and "I consider that the patient has a right to refuse treatment." Although Fenton used a 5-point scale, to increase the sensitivity of the instrument, respondents in this study were given a choice of 7 categories along a bipolar dimension of *never* to *always*.

Part II of the questionnaire was developed to explore the views of nurses in relation to caring dimensions. Information was sought on:

1. The words or phrases that nurses consider to be attributes of a caring nurse.
2. How nurses perceive nursing overall in relation to the caring dimension.
3. How nurses rate themselves as carers.
4. Nurses' level of expertise in the area in which they are working.
5. The care experienced if they had been hospitalized at any time.

Part III of the questionnaire was unstructured and asked nurses to be reflective and give an account, in order of importance, of what has influenced them to be caring persons.

Part IV sought background information. Respondents were asked to indicate their sex, age, marital status, parental status, length of nursing experience since graduation, educational preparation, level of appointment, caregiver status, area of clinical practice, length of time in present practice area, and employment status.

Procedure

A pilot study was conducted with eleven nurses working in a hospital that had characteristics similar to those included in the study. A cover letter and abstract of the proposed study were sent to the Director of Nursing in each of the selected hospitals, seeking approval to conduct the study in each facility.

A systematic, stratified, random sampling of every fifth person on individual unit/department rosters was employed to select participants. A cover letter, questionnaire booklet, and stamped self-addressed envelope were then mailed to prospective participants. A code number was assigned to each questionnaire as part of the process of ensuring confidentiality. Respondents and hospitals were informed that results would be reported in aggregate form, hence no individuals or hospitals would be identified in any report of the findings of the study. Ninety-one nurses completed the questionnaire for a response rate of 85 percent.

RESULTS

Demographic Data

Nurses' demographic data are presented in Table 18–1.

Nurses also rated how they personally saw both the nursing profession and themselves in relation to the caring dimension on a 1-to-5-point (low-to-high) graphic rating scale of noncaring to caring (Table 18–2).

Responses to expertise level, rated from 1 (low) to 5 (high), were more varied (Table 18–3).

Analysis of variance (ANOVA) and two-way t-test were utilized to compare nurses' demographic characteristics and humanistic behavior scores. The study revealed that nurses' demographic characteristics were not significantly related to nurses' care behaviors. There was a significant relationship ($f = 4.56$, $p = 0.002$, $df = 4$) between the care behaviors and level of expertise of nurses. Overall, younger nurses (21 to 30 years) who had had less than one year's experience as a registered nurse and self-reported a low expertise level had mean scores lower than all other nurses.

Humanistic Behavior Scores

Analysis of the data on humanistic care behaviors of nurses revealed a mean score of 5.0 for the 91 participants, from a possible score of 7.0. Standard deviation was 1.8. This result indicated that nurses self-reported average to high caring behaviors. The mean scores of each dimension of the scale are listed in Table 18–4.

Words That Describe Attributes of a Caring Nurse

Eighty words or phrases were documented by nurses as being attributes of a caring nurse. The five highest ranked attributes were: empathy, listening skills, understanding, sympathy/concern, and being knowledgeable (Table 18–5).

Table 18–1
Demographic Characteristics of Nurses

Variable	Groups	Number	Percent	Mean	Standard Deviation
Sex	Female	80	88	20.1	1.7
	Male	11	12	20.7	2.3
Age (years)	21–30	47	·52	19.9	1.7
	31–40	26	28	20.3	1.9
	41–50	10	11	20.5	1.4
	>50	8	9	21.0	1.9
Marital status	Single	42	46	19.9	1.7
	Married	42	46	20.0	1.7
	Other	7	8	22.2	2.1
Inpatient status	Previous hospitalization	63	70	20.4	1.8
	No previous hospitalization	27	30	19.7	1.5
Nurse experience (years)	0–1	16	18	19.1	1.4
	>1–3	12	13	21.0	1.2
	>3–5	13	14	20.1	2.5
	>5–10	16	18	20.0	1.9
	>10–15	13	14	20.4	1.6
	>15	20	22	20.4	1.6
Education level	*Certificate	77	85	20.2	2.7
	Diploma	8	9	19.9	2.6
	Degree	6	6	19.6	1.0
Employment status	Full-time	79	87	20.1	1.7
	Part-time	12	13	20.5	2.0
Practice area	Medical	30	33	20.0	1.8
	Surgical	27	30	20.2	1.5
	Critical care	15	17	20.1	1.8
	Psychiatry	2	2	17.2	1.2
	Midwifery	13	14	21.0	1.6
	Pediatrics	4	4	19.8	2.6

* Hospital-based training.

Table 18–2
Caring Dimensions—Respondents

	Rating Scale	Profession		Self	
Noncaring	1	0		0	
	2	2	(2%)	0	
	3	13	(15%)	8	(9%)
	4	44	(49%)	39	(43%)
Caring	5	30	(34%)	43	(48%)

Table 18–3
Expertise Level

Level	Percent	Number	Mean	Standard Deviation
1 (low)	2	2	19.1	0.4
2	7	2	18.8	2.6
3	17	19	19.0	1.2
4	37	41	20.6	1.8
5 (high)	27	30	20.7	1.4

Table 18–4
Total Mean Scores of Care Dimensions

Care Dimensions	Number	Mean	Standard Deviation
Shared decision making	91	5.6	0.5
Holistic selves	91	5.6	0.6
Status equality	91	5.2	0.8
Empathy	91	4.0	0.5

Table 18–5
Five Highest Ranked Attributes of a Caring Nurse

Attribute	Number of Respondents	Frequency
Empathy	37	40%
Listening skills	33	36
Understanding	31	34
Sympathy/concern	28	31
Knowledgeable	20	22

Anecdotes of Caring Incidents

Eighty-two nurses gave an account of what has influenced them to be caring persons. Individual accounts of personal experiences totaled 320. These were organized according to major themes (Table 18–6). The experience documented as the *most important* by nurses (N = 33) was the caring family upbringing. There was great variability in the order of importance of other personal experiences. The experience rated the *most often* by nurses (N = 35) was the personal satisfaction received from caring.

DISCUSSION

The overall humanistic behavior score suggests that nurses self-reported average to high caring behaviors. The study also revealed that nurses' personal characteristics are not significantly related to nurses' care behaviors. These findings are similar to those of Forsyth (1979), Brunt (1985), and Taylor et al. (1989).

In relation to level of education, it was hypothesized that there would be a significant positive relationship between humanistic scores and higher education levels, because of the increased number of humanities and social sciences courses offered in tertiary-level nursing programs. However, this relationship was not supported. A possible reason is the high percentage of nurses (85 percent) in this study who had trained in a general hospital. As more nurses are educated in the tertiary sector and at higher levels, it will be possible to examine the relationship between education and the humanistic care behaviors of nurses.

Their expertise level did have a significant effect on nurses' care behaviors. This result was not unexpected because novice nurses have limited experience with the situations they face and are therefore unable to use discretionary judgment in the care of patients. In contrast, more experienced nurses have the ability to interpret situations and implement care based on specific patient needs. This finding is consistent with the work of Benner (1982), who evaluated the practicality of applying the Dreyfus Model of Skill Acquisition to nursing and concluded that ongoing experience and education are essential to the development of expertise.

In relation to hospitalization status, although the majority of nurses (70 percent) had been hospitalized, the findings indicated that this variable is not a predictor of higher levels of caring behaviors. Eighty-three percent of

Table 18–6
Anecdotes of Nurses' Personal Experiences in Relation to Caring

1. *Personal satisfaction from caring (N = 35)*
   Patients' appreciation of my caring attitude.
   Receive satisfaction by caring for others.
   Feeling of contentment when you have helped someone else.

2. *Caring family upbringing (N = 33)*
   My upbringing—parents instilled caring values, especially with pets and visiting elderly neighbors.
   Loving, warm family—shared the ups and downs.
   Happy childhood—felt cared for and very much loved.

3. *Intrinsic factors influencing self as a carer (N = 30)*
   Don't like hurting people.
   Interest in well-being of others.
   Personality—innate desire to help people.

4. *Personal abilities in caring for sick people (N = 21)*
   Understanding love and comfort required by the sick.
   Ability to recognize patients' needs.

5. *Education and experience (N = 21)*
   Years of experience in identifying people's needs.
   Education helps to be caring by broadening your outlook on life.

6. *Positive and negative role modeling of other people (N = 10 + 10)*
   From modeling myself on positive role models.
   Role model of another nurse.
   Seeing how poorly some patients were treated.
   Anger at examples of uncaring people.

7. *Nursing as a job (N = 19)*
   Being a nurse promotes the care mode.
   Being in a position to help sick people.

8. *Putting myself in another person's position (N = 17)*
   Putting myself in the patient's position; imagine if it is Mum and Gran and want them to be treated well.
   To be treated with respect and kindness that I would personally expect.

9. *Personal experiences of death/sickness (N = 15)*
   Death of brother in tragic circumstances with subsequent emotional stress to myself and family.
   Death of two Grans; "life is short."
   Death of family members—easier to talk with patients.

10. *Positive/negative experiences as an inpatient (N = 15)*
    Personal experience as a patient being brushed off with inadequate replies to questions.
    Being a patient made me realize how much caring influences recovery.

nurses rated nursing as a high caring profession. This suggests that nurses see the profession of nursing as meeting its commitment to society in the delivery of humanistic health care.

Ninety-one percent of nurses rated themselves in the two highest categories in relation to their own view of themselves as caring nurses. Although the social desirability factor may have contributed to these high ratings, the responses are consistent with the overall humanistic behavior scores of nurses. It is evident, therefore, that nurses perceive caring as a central feature of their role. These findings are consistent with the views of nurses expressed in the Study of Professional Issues in Nursing Report (Marles, 1988), which specifically addresses professional aspects related to the practice of nursing in Victoria, Australia.

The five highest ranked words or phrases documented by nurses as being attributes of a caring nurse include both actions and attitudes that nurses consider important to the caring process in nursing. It is acknowledged that different words may have been used by nurses to denote similar attributes. These findings are comparable to those in similar populations in the United States.

The findings in relation to nurses' experiences suggest that a number of "nature" and "nurture" elements contribute to each individual nurse's propensity to care. Nurses' descriptive accounts of their experiences indicate the multidimensional nature and complexity of the care concept.

CONCLUSION

The findings of this study point to the existence of caring nursing practice in a system that is increasingly being influenced by technological developments and cost-contained health services. Both of these factors have the propensity to devalue the humanistic element of nursing services. Fenton's Scale of Humanistic Behaviors (1981) is valuable as a diagnostic tool of care behaviors because of its high reliability, low cost, noninvasiveness, and content validity, and the ease with which it can be administered.

This study has concluded that nurses' personal characteristics do not significantly affect their care behaviors; however, this area should be further explored in other institutions and other target populations. The findings in relation to the expertise level of the nurse, length of nursing practice, and nursing educational preparation have potential for further hypothesis formulation and, ultimately, new knowledge in relation to the caring concept.

REFERENCES

Alverson, E. (1987). The preoperative interview—its effect on perioperative nurses' empathy. *AORN Journal, 4*(5), 1158–1164.

Benner, P. (1982). From novice to expert. *American Journal of Nursing, 2*(3), 402–407.

Brown, L. (1981). Behaviors of nurses perceived by hospitalized patients as indicators of care. *Dissertation Abstracts International, 43*, 4361B.

Brown, L. (1986). The experience of care: patient perspectives. *Topics in Clinical Nursing, 8*(2), 56–62.

Brunt, J. (1985). An exploration of the relationship between nurses' empathy and technology. *Nursing Administration Quarterly, 9*(4), 69–78.

Fenton, M. (1981). The measurement of humanistic and dehumanistic behaviors in hospital environments. *Dissertation Abstracts International, 41*, 4456B.

Fenton, M. (1987). Development of the scale of humanistic nursing behaviors. *Nursing Research, 36*(2).

Ford, M. (1981). Nurse professionals and the caring process. *Dissertation Abstracts International, 43*, 967B–968B.

Forsyth, G. (1979). Exploration of empathy in nurse–client interaction. *Advances in Nursing Science, 1*(2), 53–61.

Henry, O. (1975). Nurse behaviors perceived by patients as indicators of caring. *Dissertation Abstracts International, 36*, 2652B.

Hills, M., & Knowles, D. (1983). Nurses' levels of empathy and respect in simulated interactions with patients. *International Journal of Nursing Studies, 20*(2), 83–87.

Howard, J. (1975). Humanization and dehumanization of health care: a conceptual view. In J. Howard & E. Strauss (Eds.), *Humanizing health care*. New York: Wiley.

Howard, J., David, F., Pope, C., & Ruzek, S. (1977). Humanizing health care: The implications of technology, centralization and self-care. *Medical Care, 5* (Suppl. 15), 11–26.

Kalisch, B. (1971). An experiment in the development of empathy in nursing students. *Nursing Research, 20*, 202–211.

Kelly, L. (1988). The ethic of caring and has it been discarded? *Nursing Outlook, 36*(1), 17.

La Monica, E., Caren, D., Winder, A., Hasse, A., & Blanchard, K. (1976). Empathy training as the major thrust of a staff development programme. *Nursing Research, 25*, 447–451.

Larson, P. (1981). Important nurse-caring behaviors perceived by patients with cancer. *Oncology Nurse Forum, 11*, 46–50.

Leininger, M. (1986). Care facilitation and resistance factors in the culture of nursing. *Topics in Clinical Nursing, 8*(2), 1–12.

MacDonald, M. (1977). How do men and women students rate in empathy? *American Journal of Nursing, 77*(6), 998–1004.

Marles, F. (1988, February). *Report of the Study of Professional Issues in Nursing.* Victoria, Australia: Health Department.

Mayer, D. (1986). Cancer patients' and families' perceptions of nurse caring behaviors. *Topics in Clinical Nursing, 8*(2), 63–69.

Newburn, V. (1987). Caregiver perceptions of human abuse in health care settings. *Holistic Nurse Practitioner, 1*(2), 64–74.

Riemen, D. (1986). Non-caring and caring in the clinical setting: Patients' descriptions. *Topics in Clinical Nursing, 8*(2), 30–36.

Sparling, S., & Jones, S. (1977). Setting: A contextual variable associated with empathy. *Journal of Psychiatric Nursing and Mental Health Services, 15*(4), 9–12.

Taylor, S., Pickens, J., & Geden, E. (1989). Interactional styles of nurse practitioners and physicians regarding patient decision making. *Nursing Research, 38*(1), 50–55.

Wolf, Z. (1986). The caring concept and nurse-identified caring behaviors. *Topics in Clinical Nursing, 8*(2), 84–93.

19

Understanding the Meaning of Chronic Illness: A Prerequisite for Caring

Barbara E. Place

While working with undergraduate and graduate nursing students, I've often noted their comments regarding patients with chronic illness. The comments reflect the frustration the students experience when working with people who "keep coming back," who are not compliant, who do not do "what we tell them to do"—the frustration of chronicity, of not being able to cure. I've also noted that people with such illnesses are identified with the disease: "She's diabetic," "He's an asthmatic." In a sense, they are perceived as an embodiment of the disease; they are objectified.

I'm also aware that people living with chronic illness do most of that living in the community—in their homes, at work, in the everyday settings of their world and their lived experience—and these aspects are unknown to most nurses. Yet caring, as Fry so clearly argued, involves concern about how others experience their world. (See Chapter 11.) It links us to these persons and to the meaning their illness experience holds for them. Caring therefore also requires knowledge.

It seemed essential to learn how those who have such illnesses experience their world. What does it mean to live with chronic illness?

This examination of the meaning of chronic illness is an aspect of the resulting study. The discussion is based on data drawn from examination of the meaning of chronic, life-threatening illness for the adults with such illnesses and for the ways in which they live with their illness on a day-to-day basis. Ethnography, together with Kleinman's (1988) work on illness narratives, provided the methodology for the project. I drew particularly on the works of Aries (1981), Geertz (1973, 1983), Leininger (1978), Sontag (1989), and Turner (1984). The study focused on the use of narrative to give meaning to lived experience and the role of meaning in the construction of reality. Although the study used multiple data sources of the same phenomenon, such as participant/observation and published accounts of personal experiences with chronic illness (Goss, 1989; Register, 1987), the major source was a series of narratives provided by twenty-seven people with chronic illness. They spoke of their experience with illness, their knowledge of their illness, the meaning it holds for them, and its impact on their lives. Their ages ranged from early twenties to mid-sixties. Some had had their illness since childhood; for others, the onset occurred in adult life. The minimum time since diagnosis was 2 years. The illnesses were those such as asthma, diabetes, and epilepsy, which, while potentially life-threatening, are not necessarily visible to others and possibly can be concealed.

The incidence of chronic illness is known to be increasing, partly because of the aging of the population and the influence of medical technology, which often has the paradoxical effect of converting formerly terminal illnesses into debilitating chronic conditions (Bates & Linder-Pelz, 1990). Yet, little is known of the experience of living with such illness in a society that values appearance, physical prowess, vigor, and health. Against these background values, the individual's experience of chronic illness, especially an illness that is not necessarily visible to others, creates a great many tensions and conflicts. Even if illness leaves no visible marks, it is a constant presence in the consciousness of those who live with it, and it can have a profound impact on all aspects of life.

This impact is due not only to the effects of the specific illness, but also to the meaning it holds for the individual and others. The interaction of illness experience and the meanings of the illness shape the experience of living with chronic illness.

THE ILLNESS EXPERIENCE

In contrast to a narrow focus on the disease—that is, the alteration in physical structure or function, which is more characteristic of the medical perspective—the distress and practical concerns caused by the pathological processes constitute the effects and the problems of chronic illness in day-to-day living. These illness-related problems, described by Kleinman (1988, p. 4) as the "principal difficulties that symptoms and disabilities create in our lives," are a major aspect of the experience of chronic illness. Rather than the diagnosis of asthma, diabetes, or coronary artery disease, it is the breathlessness, the exhaustion, and the pain that interfere with work, study, recreation, and the achievement of patients' goals and ambitions.

Chronic illnesses tend to oscillate between periods of exacerbation and periods of improvement or quiescence. Living with this oscillation requires close scrutiny of bodily processes and vigilant attention to circumstances and events that could be potentially harmful. Frequent decisions must be made about when to commence or terminate an activity, when to modify medications, when to initiate emergency plans, and when to seek professional help (Kleinman, 1988).

Living with chronic illness is expensive, both financially and emotionally. It consumes great quantities of time—attending doctors' offices and clinics; waiting in doctors' rooms, hospitals, and pharmacies; lying in hospitals; resting at home; monitoring one's health status; and carrying out sometimes complex treatment regimes. It interferes with daily activities, special occasions, careers, relationships, and, perhaps most distressingly, self-esteem. Fear of consequences and feelings of vulnerability and loss of control may result in an exhausting and often futile attempt to maintain two separate worlds—one at work, which aims to appear free from sickness, and another at home, where sickness is legitimized (Kleinman, 1988). The presence of chronic illness results in a changed relationship with one's own body. The usual taken-for-granted relationship is altered as time and attention are directed toward observing, assessing, and modifying the functioning of the body. Behind the activity, the worry, and the uncertainty looms the threat of complications and untimely death.

THE MEANINGS OF ILLNESS

In addition to the effects of the illness itself, the meanings associated with it constitute a major aspect of the experience of living with chronic illness.

Illness has many meanings, and illness experiences and events usually radiate (or conceal) more than one meaning. The meanings of illness are not fixed. Some may change as cultural beliefs and values and dominant ideologies change; others may change over the long course of a chronic disorder.

Illness may have many specific meanings, but there are basically two types: *cultural* meanings of illness, which are imposed on illness by the culture and shape the illness experience of the individual, and *personal* meanings of illness, which are derived from the life experience of the sick person. Cultural meanings of illness carry significance *to* the sick person; personal meanings of illness transfer significance *from* the person's life to the illness experience (Kleinman, 1988).

Cultural meanings of illness may be attached to illness per se or to the specific symptoms and labels of disease. One pervasive meaning of illness is death and, in considering the specific meaning chronic illness holds for the sick person, it is important to do so in the context of the cultural meaning of death as reflected in the prevailing beliefs and attitudes. In contemporary Western society, the dominant attitudes are a widespread refusal to confront the reality of death, and a denial of death as a part of human existence. The socially sanctioned avoidance of death has been noted by many commentators (Axelrod, 1987; Feifel, 1977; Fulton & Owen, 1988; Rando, 1984; Shneidman, 1984; Steinfels & Veatch, 1974). Chronic illness, by its existence, challenges the belief that ultimately all illness is curable and confronts us with the reality of death. Not surprisingly, there are many common aspects in the experiences of the dying and the chronically ill in current Western societies. Both states are devalued, lack clear social roles, and are preferably invisible to the rest of society.

The cultural meanings associated with specific symptoms and illnesses also change over time. Perhaps the current Western disorders that carry the most powerful cultural meanings are cancer, heart disease, and acquired immune deficiency syndrome (AIDS). As Kleinman (1988, p. 22) noted, for each of these disorders "meaning arrives with a vengeance together with the diagnosis." Each diagnosis is a label, and the web of meanings it conveys to the sick person shapes his or her subsequent illness experience and life history. Such meanings include a lack of control over one's own life and death, an inability to control the effects of technology, a fear of contamination and invisible pollution, a threat of disfiguring treatment with the concomitant loss of body- and self-image, discrimination, and the stigma of self-earned illness. Culturally marked illness carries a significance that, once applied to a person, marks that person's identity and is not easily removed.

Such meaning is most often linked to diseases such as cancer and AIDS, but it is not limited to them. This was apparent in the popular beliefs encountered by study participants about such chronic diseases as asthma and epilepsy. One of the most common and most pervasive beliefs encountered about asthma is that it is a childhood disease and that the child will "grow out of it." One implication of this belief is that asthma is not a serious disease because "it's only a childhood disease." Another implication is that adults who have asthma are in some sense childish or immature. This also exemplifies the common belief that disease reflects character. One participant in the study, who is now in his thirties, has had severe, incapacitating asthma since childhood. He has been regarded as "lazy" by his father and workmates since his midteens because he has not been able to work as physically hard or as long as they could. Another person, also with severe asthma, is regarded as a "nerd" and unfortunately also regards himself as one because he cannot participate in the active sports regarded as normal by both himself and his peers. Despite these beliefs, however, and the meanings they convey, the realities are: only one-third of children with asthma become asymptomatic on reaching adulthood; asthma may recur later (Spykerboer, Donnelly, & Thong, 1986); and asthma is a serious and increasingly fatal disease of adults (Robertson, Rubinfeld, & Bowes, 1990).

Epilepsy is another disease that has been marked by many myths supporting the belief that those with epilepsy are inferior (Beran, 1983). Despite increased knowledge of the disease, ignorance and fear continue to affect the experience of living with epilepsy. The identification of the brain with mental functioning has given rise to the most commonly encountered myth about epilepsy—that it causes diminished mental capacity and functioning. Studies by Beran (1983) and Larkins (1986) found that these beliefs and misconceptions about epilepsy influenced not only employers, teachers, and others in the general community, but also people with epilepsy and their doctors. Such myths result in marked stigmatization of people with epilepsy and affect all aspects of their lives.

Beliefs and values relating to illness are frequently expressed in myths and metaphors, and these provide a potent means whereby cultural meanings of illness are transmitted and reinforced. Metaphors, in particular, convey powerful images; when used in relation to illness, they can facilitate understanding and insight. They can make the strange familiar and, when used by those experiencing illness, can help convey the nature of that experience to those who do not share it. At the same time, however, as Sontag (1989) noted, metaphoric thinking, when imposed on the experience of others, can cause increased suffering and pain by obscuring the reality of the illness and giving it a meaning never intended.

Illness-related metaphors and myths therefore affect the way people interpret and learn to live with illness. The experience of being ill is shaped in part by our perception and acceptance of these different levels of meaning of illness as an image of something to be feared or dreaded, a character statement, or a personal judgment. Perhaps, as Sontag (1989) claimed, the "healthiest" way to live with illness is that most purified of, and resistant to, such thinking. From Sontag's point of view, disease is disease, no more and no less.

However, meaning is inescapable; illness always has meaning. In addition to cultural meanings, illness has powerful personal meanings. In the course of a life lived with chronic illness, the illness and life history become interwoven, and illness soaks up personal significance from the world of the sick person. The specifics of each life, like those of every other, create a unique texture of meaning for each person's experience of chronic illness.

Participants in the study spoke of the many meanings their illnesses held for them. The meanings varied for each person and individual life history, but, for many, the central meaning of illness was loss. In some instances, the losses were real; in others, they were anticipated and expressed as fears. The losses most frequently identified were loss of control of their own life and body, loss of independence, and loss of desired goals and ambitions. For one person, loss of his pilot's license because of his illness meant loss of a longed-for career in aviation; for another, her illness meant loss of the possibility of a senior administrative position; for a third, her inability to get disability insurance because of illness meant loss of an independent consultancy practice. Another loss mentioned by many was a loss of spontaneity in their lives. For many, each activity, each outing, each trip had to be considered in terms of possible consequences and planned for in detail. For others, illness meant loneliness, limited social contacts, and guilt because of the impact of illness and the associated way of life on partners and families. Other personal meanings of chronic illness were expressed as fears—fear of dying, fear of death, fear of not being available while children were growing up.

For many participants, illness also meant a sense of altered, and often less acceptable, self and social image and identity, although this sense was not universal. Thus, illness for one young man meant an undesirable role reversal that greatly threatened his sense of self and self-identity. He washed the dishes and minded the children while his wife went to work and mowed the lawn. For many people in the study, the major challenge posed by chronic illness was the impact it had on their self-esteem and their self-image. For some, there was a sense of loss of self, of depersonalization associated with emphasis on and identification with the illness: "He's a diabetic."

A person identified as chronically ill commonly experiences a changed self-image and faces a twofold separation. This separation is manifest both in society's rejection of the chronically ill and in the individual's alienation from the former self. In the process of avoiding the chronically ill, or denying the reality of their experience because of what it represents, people frequently impose on the ill a loss of social acceptability and in its place offer them an ambiguous and stigmatized identity (Stephenson & Murphy, 1986). This further reinforces the ill person's loss of previous self-image, of the self the person once was or had hoped to be.

Therefore, to become chronically ill commonly means to take on a new status and a new self-image, both of which are likely to be of lesser value to the person than those held previously. Those living with chronic illness may seek to mask their differences in order to maintain their previous social status and roles. However, roles and tasks may be limited by others, for decisions about appropriate roles for the ill are often made by family members, friends, employers, and statutory authorities. The chronically ill must then contend with the limitations imposed by the illness and those imposed by their social milieu, which may result in diminished and more passive roles for them. The converse may also occur, particularly in relation to people who have no visible signs of illness. They may continue to have expectations placed on them that far exceed their capabilities. They may then be forced into a separation from their previous roles and into a state of social limbo. This is particularly relevant for younger and middle-aged chronically ill people who are unable to meet society's expectations for an active life-style. This was a common experience for many people in the study.

Given that chronic illness is generally regarded as a negative and devalued experience, it is not surprising that positive aspects are rarely identified or acknowledged. However, although most discussion and research has focused on the negative aspects, some references hint at the possibility of another dimension to chronic illness. Viney and Westbrook (1984, p. 171), in their study of reactions to chronic illness associated with death, commented that "positive feelings have unexpectedly proved common in reactions to chronic illness."

Some of the positive meanings identified by study participants as associated with the experience of chronic illness included illness as a challenge, or as an opportunity for testing one's strength, courage, and feelings of competence. Others spoke of the increased insight and understanding that they had achieved and of increased empathy and tolerance for others, gained through their own experiences of living with long-term illness. Confronting chronic illness therefore may lead to a re-experiencing of self and reality and may provide a chance to break through to a fuller way of being in the world and an awareness of how illness has contributed to who they are and to the person they have become. As Kleinman (1988) noted, the experience of being ill need not be self-defeating; it can be—even if it often isn't—an occasion for growth, a point of departure for something deeper and finer.

I've focused in this chapter on the meanings of chronic illness as they provide insight into the experience of living with such illness. I'd like to make just a brief mention of how people live with long-term illness. Participants in the study had developed a range of strategies for living with illness. However, regardless of their main way of coping with their illness, everyone in the study used, or had used, two other strategies, concealment and minimization, in different situations and at different times in the illness experience. Concealment involved hiding the existence of the illness from others by such means as not taking any medications in front of people, not talking about the illness, and using explanations other than illness to explain absences or changes in arrangements. Many went to considerable lengths to conceal their illness. When concealment was not possible, people tended to minimize the nature and effects of the illness in interaction with others. If asked specifically about their illness, they dealt with the query casually and briefly. This approach was usually employed with strangers and casual acquaintances, but some people also used it with family members and close friends, particularly when they were known to become anxious when confronted with the reality of the illness. This meant that some participants had few if any people with whom they could really discuss their illness and their fears and concerns.

I mention these aspects because they reflect a pervasive belief about illness in our society, that is, the belief that illness is not normal. As one woman said to me, "People get tired of you always being sick; *normal people aren't sick*" (italics added). Another, when I asked her how she lived with her illness, responded, "I work twice as hard to appear normal." She did not say "to be normal," but "to appear normal," a belief and a response echoed by many. This is significant when considering caring in the context of chronic illness.

CARING IN THE CONTEXT OF CHRONIC ILLNESS

As noted previously, caring requires knowledge; to care for another, it is necessary to have knowledge of that other. Several theorists have identified knowledge as an essential element or characteristic of caring. For Roach

(1987), it was an aspect of competence, one of the five attributes of caring she identified; for Gaut (1984), it was the first essential condition for caring for another. However, these authors also emphasized that knowledge of the other alone is insufficient; caring also requires knowledge of the self. Thus, Gaut argued that caring involves various kinds of knowing, including understanding the other's needs and knowing how to respond to those needs (Gaut, 1984, p. 35). Mayeroff spoke of the need "to know many things" in order to care for another. In addition to knowledge of the other and of what is conducive to his or her growth and well-being, he emphasized the need for self-knowledge, the need to know "what my own powers and limitations are" (Mayeroff, 1971, p. 13).

To care for another therefore requires knowledge of the other and knowledge of ourselves. In the context of caring for those who live with chronic illness, this includes knowledge of what their illness means to them and the impact it has on their lives, as well as their hopes and goals, their beliefs and values. We also need knowledge of our own beliefs and values, particularly as they relate to chronic illness, and of the expectations that we bring to the interaction. An essential aspect of this knowledge is, I believe, an awareness that chronic illness is not, as it is so often presented, an abnormal state, but rather a part of life—"a normative experience" (Kleinman, 1988).

CONCLUSION

Knowledge of ourselves enables us to be there for others, to be present. However, as Karl (1992) noted, "being there is difficult." Yet, it is essential because, as Street (1992) has highlighted, caring requires "authentic presence." Being there for another involves our whole self, including our cultural self—the beliefs, values, and worldview we have derived both from our primary culture and from our nursing culture. This can require courage; however, it certainly contributes to more authentic caring for and caring about those who live with chronic illness.

REFERENCES

Aries, P. (1981). *The hour of our death* (Helen Weaver, Trans.). New York: Knopf.

Axelrod, C. (1987). Reflections on the fear of death. *Omega, 17*(1), 51–64.

Bates, E., & Linder-Pelz, S. (1990). *Health care issues* (2nd ed.). North Sydney: Allen & Unwin.

Beran, R. (1983). *Epidemiological studies of epilepsy in Sydney, Australia.* Report prepared for the Federal Department of Health, Sydney.

Feifel, H. (Ed.). (1977). *New meanings of death.* New York: McGraw-Hill.

Fulton, R., & Owen, G. (1988). Death and society in twentieth century America. *Omega, 18*(4), 379–395.

Gaut, D. (1984). A theoretic description of caring as action. In M. Leininger (Ed.), *Caring: The essence of nursing and health* (pp. 27–44). Thorofare, NJ: Slack.

Geertz, C. (1973). *The interpretation of cultures.* New York: Basic Books.

Geertz, C. (1983). *Local knowledge: Further essays in interpretive anthropology.* New York: Basic Books.

Goss, S. (1989). *Ragged owlet.* Ferntree Gully: Houghton Mifflin Australia.

Karl, J. (1992). Being there: Who do you bring to practice? In D. Gaut (Ed.), *The presence of caring in nursing* (pp. 1–13). New York: National League for Nursing.

Kleinman, A. (1988). *The illness narratives: Suffering, healing, and the human condition.* New York: Basic Books.

Larkins, R. G. (1986). *Report of Committee on Uncontrolled Epilepsy.* Melbourne: Epilepsy Foundation of Victoria.

Leininger, M. (1978). *Transcultural nursing: Concepts, theories and practices.* New York: Wiley.

Mayeroff, M. (1971). *On caring.* New York: Harper & Row.

Rando, T. A. (1984). *Grief, dying, and death.* Champaign, IL: Research Press.

Register, C. (1987). *Living with chronic illness: Days of patience and passion.* New York: Free Press.

Roach, M. (1987). *The human act of caring.* Ottawa, Canada: Canadian Hospital Association.

Robertson, C. F., Rubinfeld, A. R., & Bowes, G. (1990). Deaths from asthma in Victoria: A 12-month survey. *Medical Journal of Australia, 152*(10), 511–517.

Shneidman, E. S. (1984). *Death: Current perspectives* (3rd ed.). Mountain View: Mayfield Publishing.

Sontag, S. (1989). *Illness as metaphor and AIDS and its metaphors.* New York: Anchor Books.

Spykerboer, J. E., Donnelly, W. J., & Thong, Y. H. (1986). Parental knowledge and misconceptions about asthma: A controlled study. *Social Science and Medicine, 22*(5), 553–558.

Steinfels, P., & Veatch, R. (Eds.). (1974). *Death inside out*. New York: Harper & Row.

Stephenson, J., & Murphy, D. (1986). Existential grief: The special case of the chronically ill and disabled. *Death Studies, 10*(2), 135–145.

Street, A. (1992, July). *Being caring: Getting beyond the tyranny of niceness in healthcare.* Paper presented at Fourteenth Annual Caring Research Conference, Melbourne, Australia.

Turner, B. S. (1984). *The body and society*. New York: Blackwell.

Viney, L., & Westbrook, M. (1984). Is there a pattern of psychological reactions to chronic illness which is associated with death? *Omega, 17*(2), 169–181.

20

Care, Caritas, and Ego Development

Sandie S. Soldwisch

Research and theories centering on caring abound. Caring has been identified as intrinsic, evoked, or acquired; existential or ontological; and contextual, transcultural, or universal. One dimension of caring that transcends theories and research is that caring is essential to human development and perpetuity.

In this study, the concept of caring is viewed through a different lens. I believe that the ability to care is inherent. Whether people manifest caring is dependent on many things—exposure to caring, being cared for and about, receiving permission to care, instruction regarding "appropriate" caring, and successful attempts to care, among others. I also hold that nursing is a profession with caring at its core, and that caring is demonstrated more often and more predictably as one grows older. Therefore, the research question guiding this study was: Is there a relationship between ego identity development and the presence of caring in nursing students? Within this study, the term caring is understood to contain the following elements: attention to personhood—being aware of the presence and needs of the cared for; responsibility for—engaging with the cared for (to the extent possible) and making a commitment to act on the needs of the cared for; and regard—accepting and dignifying the inherent value of the cared for.

REVIEW OF LITERATURE

Examination of caring as a predominant theme has revealed expanding volumes of literature and research. Various arenas are investigating caring and caring behaviors. Scientific and historical studies demonstrate that care is a vital force for human growth, maintenance, and survival. Philosophy and theology explore the notion of an unfolding of innate characteristics that exist in all humans. Anthropology and sociology are examining the concept of care and caring by addressing conditions that promote and augment or inhibit and prohibit associated caring behaviors. Psychoneuroimmunology is researching biological determinants of caring. Contemporary nurse researchers are directing attention toward the definition, description, and delineation of caring. These are only a few fields in which caring is a focal investigative concern.

Nursing research in caring is expanding in response to recognition of this essential element of practice. Members of the International Association for Human Caring (IAHC) account for a significant portion of this expansion. A recent literature search using the key words "caring" and "nursing" resulted in over 1,846 citations during the past five years. The majority of these citations focused on identification of caring attributes and behaviors. Caring occurrences between the nurse and patients and families have also received considerable attention. Although the existing literature describes caring behaviors and caring occurrences, the notion of caring as a structural feature of human growth and development is only beginning to be explored (Griffin, 1980; Soldwisch, 1990).

Investigation of more global caring is also in its infancy. The fields of anthropology, ecology, biology, and political science are beginning to explore, coordinate, and communicate research findings. Informational and educational programs abound at the local and state levels. Communities are initiating programs and legislation to promote a better local future, to be more caring and responsive to their constituents. Nursing has joined this exploration by creating a new paradigm of caring for the community-as-client (Geoppinger & Schuster, 1988; McCarthy et al., 1991; Schuster, 1990). More work in this area is indicated.

This chapter represents beginning exploration of the relatedness of care, caritas, and ego development. A framework that incorporates the nature of human beings with psychological, biological, and social components was necessary for this study. One framework that takes these components into consideration is Erikson's epigenetic theory. Therefore, the conjecture set forth in this study was: In terms of Erikson's epigenetic theory, individuals at specific ages·are working at specific crises. It is asserted here that the ego-stage crises, prior to the one that is phase-specific, must have been positively resolved if the person is to show a significant degree of caring.

THEORETIC AND
CONCEPTUAL FORMULATION

Erikson's epigenetic theory was used as the framework in this study for several reasons. It is a comprehensive psychosocial theory that emphasizes the relativity of three processes—the biological, the psychological, the social—to personality development (1968, p. 73). It discusses the concept of caring specific to human interactions through the life cycle. And, Erikson suggested that care is the ego strength of adulthood.

Epigenesis, somewhat generalized, states that anything that grows has a general plan, and out of this general plan the parts arise; each part has its time of special importance, until all parts have arisen to form a functioning whole. A classic example of epigenesis is fetal development. One by one, the various organs of the body have their central dominance, each organ commanding all the energy for a period of time. At various times, the fetus is preoccupied with the development of the nervous system, then the lungs, the heart, and so forth, with one organ or system invariably developing before another in a predictable sequence. The fetus grows in a progressive hierarchical fashion, each part being very much related to all other parts. In sum, for the fetus to be whole, each part must have been allowed its proper rate of growth. In addition, that rate of growth must have taken place in a desirable sequence, neither ahead of nor behind the general plan of human development. If this rate and/or sequence is altered, the development of the organ in prominence, as well as all other organs with which it interacts, is affected.

Erikson argued that this developmental process continues after birth. The infant continues to develop epigenetically in a prescribed sequence of biological, psychological, and social capacities. Beginning at birth and continuing through old age, Erikson formulated eight stages (I–VIII) through which an individual's ego identity develops (see Figure 20–1). The ascendance of each stage is associated with a life-span period that indicates the earliest and latest moments when a developmental quality can come to

Stage	Lifespan	Psychosocial Crisis	Strength	Virtue
I	Infancy	Basic trust vs. Basic mistrust	Drive	Hope
II	Early childhood	Autonomy vs. Shame and doubt	Self-control	Willpower
III	Play age	Initiative vs. Guilt	Direction	Purpose
IV	School age	Industry vs. Inferiority	Method	Competence
V	Adolescence	Identity vs. Role confusion	Devotion	Fidelity
VI	Young adulthood	Intimacy vs. Isolation	Affiliation	Love
VII	Adulthood	Generativity vs. Stagnation and self-absorption	Production	Care
VIII	Old age	Ego integrity vs. Despair	Renunciation	Wisdom

Figure 20–1
**Evolution of Psychosocial Development According to
Erikson's Epigenetic Theory**

relative dominance for normal progress to occur. The time periods are not fixed; they vary with the conventions and customs of the prevailing society. The sequence, however, remains consistent.

Erikson also described core conflicts that the individual strives to master during each stage of development. Each crisis has two components, or oppositional qualities (trust vs. mistrust, for example), that must be resolved in order to result in positive ego development and progression to the next stage. One stage always merges into another, and each stage is expected to continue development as subsequent stages become dominant. At each successive stage, earlier conflicts must be re-resolved in relation to the current level of development.

Emerging from the positive resolution of each crisis is a psychological strength. From each strength a related virtue emerges. Figure 20–1 provides a summary of Erikson's epigenetic theory.

Again, one of the strengths of the utility of Erikson's theory for this study is the specification of care as the virtue of Stage VII. All the strengths arising from the earlier epigenetic developments, from infancy through young adulthood, are essential for this virtue. Therefore, this study examined the resolution of all psychosocial stages and identified the stage in ascendance.

A part of the generative responsibility of Stage VII is that of caring for whatever is generated. Adult care thus must concentrate on the means of taking lifelong care of what one has chosen, "or been forced to choose by fate, so as to care for it within the technological demands of the historical moment" (Erikson, 1982, p. 79). In these relationships, the individual seeks to integrate outward-looking care for others with inward-looking concern for self.

To Erikson, care meant both provision and caution. Provision conveys the notion of providing support and stimulation, and caution conveys the idea of screening the quality and quantity of stimulation and support. He also indicated care is reciprocal: both giving and receiving care are involved (1959). Additionally, Erikson addressed a new generative ethos calling for universal care—caritas (concern for a qualitative improvement in the lives of all), which has been assigned to this stage.

Maintaining the principles of epigenesis, Erikson argued that each person grows simultaneously biologically, psychologically, and socially, and does so in such a way that what was once experienced is continually significant and influential. There is a general plan for continued development to reach the state of a functioning whole organism. If there is disruption of this plan, the developmental stage in ascendance is altered, which reciprocally alters all other stages in some manner.

RESEARCH DESIGN AND METHODOLOGY

To examine a possible correlate of caring as the virtue of adulthood, this study was conducted in 5 NLN-accredited baccalaureate schools of nursing located in the midwestern United States. A listing of NLN-accredited baccalaureate schools was reviewed. Invitations for participation were sent to 14 randomly selected schools within a 3-state region. Five schools responded affirmatively and facilitated student contact for the study. Thirty-three students who volunteered to participate and who had completed at least an introductory nursing course and one or more terms of clinical experience constituted the sample. Because of the nature of this study, no attempt was made to have equal age distributions. Only one person who met the criteria for the study failed to complete it, bringing the actual sample to thirty-two participants.

A case study design using both qualitative and quantitative methodologies was employed. Case studies are appropriate when examining a contemporary phenomenon with some real-life context. This approach was adopted to conduct an in-depth investigation of caring in nursing students. The focus of case studies is typically on determining the dynamics of *why* the participant of the investigation thinks, behaves, or develops in a particular manner, rather than *what* his or her status, progress, or actions are. Following the principle of methodological triangulation, multiple data sources were utilized to elicit data. These included standard instruments, investigator-developed tools, and an audiotaped interview. The reliability and validity of each instrument was evaluated and/or demonstrated as appropriate, prior to use in the study.

The Personal History Questionnaire established biographical information and eligibility for the study. Two items, year of completion and level of nursing education, validated eligibility. Four characteristics (age, gender, marital status, and parturition) situated the participant within the lifespan for comparison with the ego identity stage.

The major instrument for the measure of ego identity was the Self-Descriptive Questionnaire (SDQ) developed by Boyd (1961). Boyd reported Hoyt reliability correlation coefficients of 0.80. The test–retest reliability demonstrated reliability. Additional studies utilizing the instrument supported these figures. This instrument gives a profile of the individual's positive and negative ego stage development at a given point in time.

The second ego stage determinant was the Card Sort. This instrument was developed for this study to determine the participants' phase-specific ego stage. Employing a Q methodology, statements were grouped and categorized representing each ego development stage. Participants ranked the cards as reflecting their concerns and priorities at that time. Face and content validity were established through expert review and test–retest reliability with pilot test participants.

The Relationship Inventory (RI), developed by Barrett-Lennard (1978), was employed to determine whether the participants demonstrated adequacy in professional relationships. This instrument is concerned with the feelings of one person about another. Four factors measured by this sixty-four-item inventory are:

- Level of Regard, the affective aspect of one person's response to another.

- Empathic Understanding, a process of "feeling with" another.
- Unconditionality, the degree of constancy of regard felt.
- Congruence, the degree to which one person is functionally integrated with another.

Barrett-Lennard reported extensive reliability and validity testing. Test–retest reliabilities ranged from 0.78 to 0.95. Again, successive use of the RI resulted in substantiation of high reliability.

The second caring measure used in this study is the caring episode. The purpose of the caring episode was to gather data on the presence and prevalence of the three elements of caring as set forth in this study. The participants were asked to recount a patient-centered interaction that was of importance to them. Data were derived from the audiotaped caring episode interviews using content analysis methodology. A mechanism to quantify the analysis was investigator-developed. The Caring Episode Rating Scale is a 7-point Likert scale developed to rate the intensity of the response for each of the three elements of caring of this study. The validity of the Likert scale was established through expert review. The reliability of intercoder consistency in application of the scale was examined using the intraclass correlation coefficients, revealing coefficients ranging from 0.97 to 1.0.

Data were collected during two sessions. The first meeting, usually in a small group format, included an overview of the study, an explanation of the extent of participant involvement, and a secured consent to participate. The Personal History Questionnaire and the SDQ were completed. The session concluded with setting individual appointments for the second session. Each participant was given an appointment sheet, which also displayed a reminder of the task of identifying an important patient-centered experience.

The second session, which occurred 1 to 14 days later, began with informal conversation to facilitate comfort with the 1-to-1 situation. The caring episode interviews were conducted. Each participant was directed to tell about "an experience you had while working with a patient that had meaning for you." At no time were the words care, caring, and caring behaviors used by the interviewer. Following the interview, the Card Sort was administered. The session concluded with the completion of the RI.

Descriptive and statistical analyses of the data were performed to test the research question. The $p < 0.05$ level was used as the criterion for statistical significance. As previously stated, content analysis was used as the primary method of analysis of the interview data. The focus was on episodes of caring and, more specifically, the presence of caring in association with ego stage development.

SUMMARY OF THE FINDINGS

Combining the two ego stage development data sources, the Card Sort and the SDQ, allowed bipolar assignment of ego stage development. The SDQ provided eight categorical scores that indicated whether the ratio was more positively or negatively resolved. When each ego development stage, prior to the phase-specific stage (determined by the Card Sort), resulted in a profile containing ratios that were more positive than negative, the participant was assigned to the "positive ego stage development" group (+ESD). Conversely, when the ratio was more negative, the assignment was to the "negative ego stage development" group (−ESD). Table 20–1 shows a summary of the distribution of the participants. Analysis indicated that the biographical characteristics of the members of these two groups were not statistically or practically different.

The next task involved comparing these two groups to the outcomes from the caring data sources, the RI and the Caring Episode rating. The SDQ had generated two groups—overall positive or negative resolution of ego stage development. The RI scores also generated bipolar groups—adequate or less-than-adequate demonstration of caring. To determine the relationship between RI scores and the SDQ groups, a 2 × 2 contingency table was generated for each subscale.

The frequency count and percentages for each of the subscales are indicated on Table 20–2. For each of the four subscales, Fisher's exact test was calculated in order to determine the goodness of fit and association between the RI and the SDQ groups.

There is a difference in proportion between the two groups for all of the RI scales. Significant differences were found in both the Empathic Understanding subscale and the Congruence subscale. Congruence has been argued by Barrett-Lennard as a foundation variable on which the other three variables are dependent; therefore, it can be concluded that the relationship is significant in all four subscales (1986).

Table 20–1
Comparisons of the Participants According to
Ego Stage Development Resolution

Variable	−ESD	+ESD
Frequency	18	14
Age	20 to 42 years old	20 to 41 years old
Mean age	23.67 years	30.71 years

Table 20–2
Contingency Tables to Report Each Relationship Inventory Subscale
Compared Against Positive and Negative Ego Stage Resolution

| Subscale | RI Group | Ego Stage Resolution | | Total | p |
		−ESD	+ESD		
Empathic understanding	−RI				
	Frequency	15	6	21	
	Percentage	83.33	42.86		
					.027*
	+RI				
	Frequency	3	8	11	
	Percentage	16.67	57.14		
	Total	18	14	32	
Level of regard	−RI				
	Frequency	6	1	7	
	Percentage	33.33	7.14		
					.104
	+RI				
	Frequency	12	13	25	
	Percentage	66.67	92.86		
	Total	18	14	32	
Unconditionality	−RI				
	Frequency	16	10	26	
	Percentage	88.89	71.43		
					.365
	+RI				
	Frequency	2	4	6	
	Percentage	11.11	28.57		
	Total	18	14	32	
Congruence	−RI				
	Frequency	17	7	24	
	Percentage	94.44	50.00		
					.010*
	+RI				
	Frequency	1	7	8	
	Percentage	5.56	50.00		
	Total	18	14	32	

* $p < .05$

These findings strongly suggest that psychosocial development is related to whether caring occurs. The critical issue coming out of these data is: unless schools of nursing help the student to become psychologically mature, that is, to move toward positive resolution of ego stage development, working on any caring may be extremely questionable. This strongly suggests that, unless negatively resolved ego stages are reworked to become a positive ratio, it is very likely that nurses will not show aspects of caring. In view of these findings, the entire domain of psychosocial development must be incorporated if caring is to be furthered as the practice of nursing.

The second measure of participants' caring was the caring episode interview. The content analysis procedure and Caring Rating Scale were employed, observing for each element of caring as set forth in this study. The total average category was calculated by adding together the three previous categories and averaging the sums across the number of judges reviewing the episode. The four scores were then analyzed using the Wilcoxin rank sums procedure. Table 20–3 displays the results.

The data yielded significant differences between the positively and negatively resolved ego stage development groups on all of the caring episode scales. These results more sensitively confirmed the finding because they

Table 20–3
Comparison of Participants' Caring Scores Based on the Caring Episodes, According to Ego Stage Resolution Group

Scale	Group	Sum of Scores	Expected Sum of Scores	Standard Deviation	Mean Score	p
CEATTN	−ESD	197.00	297.00		10.94	
	+ESD	331.00	231.00	25.36	23.64	.0001*
CERESP	−ESD	202.50	297.00		11.25	
	+ESD	325.50	231.00	25.48	23.25	.0002*
CEREGARD	−ESD	205.50	297.00		11.42	
	+ESD	322.50	231.00	26.03	23.04	.0005*
CETAV	−ESD	193.00	297.00		10.72	
	+ESD	335.00	231.00	26.19	23.93	.0001*

*$p < .05$

were based on the words of each participant. Thus, the relationship between caring and positive resolution of ego stages was supported.

A second component of the study focused on the relationship between the degree of ego stage development and caring. This was tested using the total average score from the caring episode interview as a grouping variable. This analysis examined only those participants in the positive ESD group (N = 14). The results of a scatter diagram indicated a positive monotonicity between the positively resolved ESD group and caring. The correlation coefficient of 0.86 indicated a strong association. Because this pattern was present, a post hoc analysis for the negatively resolved ESD group was conducted. The scatter plot for this group revealed no trend.

These findings suggest that positive resolution of ego stages could be identified as the difference. Further, the findings suggest that psychosocial development and the development of caring occur simultaneously.

Several educational implications were indicated by this study. It has been shown that caring is associated with ego stage development. Therefore, faculty must direct attention toward and support students' movement toward positive resolution of ego stage psychosocial crises. One mechanism is curricular adaptation so that biopsychosocial needs of students are addressed. A second mechanism is to emphasize caring in the curriculum. When caring becomes emphasized, interactions are done "caringly," which allows for progressive expectations of predictable caring between and among faculty and students. Finally, nursing education must make caring central to the nursing curriculum. In this manner, caring transfers from education into practice.

CARITAS

As shown earlier, this study supports Erikson's position that the development of care is associated with the positive progression through the developmental stages and becomes the prominent virtue of adulthood. Erikson extended the concept of caring to a broader perspective. He indicated that it is in adulthood that the universal caring, caritas, occurs. Caritas was further described by Erikson as a widening concern for what has been generated, for attending to the needs of *all* that has been generated. Erikson effectively argued that "a new generative ethos may call for a more universal care concerned with a qualitative improvement in the lives of all. Such new caritas would make the developed populations offer the developing ones . . . some joint guarantee of a chance for the vital development as well as for survival . . ." (1982, p. 86). Although the nature of this involvement varies, caritas is displayed. For example, volunteering as a Big Sister/Big Brother demonstrates caritas for another member of society. An individual actively participating in recycling shows a concern for the environment. Concern for an improved nation is demonstrated by members of the Youth Conservation Corps, who attempt to support conservation. Another form of caritas may be political activism for local, national, or global concerns. These are only a few examples of observable caritas.

The power and significance of the virtues of care and caritas were eloquently expressed by one of the participants interviewed for this study. The participant's profile revealed him as having very significant caring, and as having positively resolved ego stages prior to his current stage, Stage VII. His words were powerful:

> For almost ten years I had wanted to enter nursing school so that I could help other people and make a difference in their lives. But an experience which has really made a difference in my life was this one patient, Mark. . . . He was in his thirties, attractive, a flight attendant. I was working as an aide and was floated to a different floor one night; it was a floor that had 9 or 10 AIDS patients. He was put on respiratory isolation inappropriately and the nurses—although a lot of nurses cared, a lot of the nurses didn't care to learn about AIDS—they just stigmatized conditions and people. But Mark was getting more and more despondent and at the end of the shift I could see that he was getting weaker and weaker. He confided that he was afraid he was dying and of dying alone. Since he was in isolation and nurses don't like to gown up and stuff he really was alone a lot. I sat on the bed—which wasn't the most appropriate thing to do infection-control-wise but I wasn't concerned—I knew he didn't have the kind of TB spread by droplet nuclei. I knew he needed someone to talk to him. I tried to comfort him by holding his hand and just listening. He did eventually die, but all these things came together to affect me. I felt that I had compassion, warmth, understanding—I cared for him as a patient and as a person.

Later conversation with the participant illustrated the extension of his caring to a broader perspective:

> I became concerned that so many people in this area, and in nursing, know so little about AIDS. I became angry that a whole community of people, people with AIDS, are receiving less than appropriate and less than holistic care. When I considered all of these feelings I knew that I had to care enough, be strong enough, to do something. I accepted a nursing position on an AIDS unit.

The concluding segment of the conversation then shifted to discussion of the extension of his personal impact on the world, his caritas:

I joined an organization of professionals working with AIDS. After a while I took on more active roles and now I am an officer in that organization. I try, every chance I can, to share information about AIDS and the care of AIDS patients. But even that wasn't enough. This disease is worldwide so my information, my actions, my knowledge, my work must be larger. I still work at the individual level by caring for AIDS patients, usually in their home or in hospice units. I still try to inform my peers and anyone else interested about AIDS. But I am also a member of an AIDS Research Team. We need to learn all we can about AIDS to appropriately care for millions of people, to spare millions of people from this disease, and to protect our future if possible.

The construct of caritas is also sensitively supported by the words of other participants in this study. These participants were located in the sixth and seventh ego development stages. Their expressions ranged from concern for inadequate health care for poor populations to concern for the community related to an epidemic of a transmittable disease and, more globally, to concern for the environment related to disposal of excreta from patients receiving chemotherapy in areas with wells and septic systems.

CONCLUSION

It is important to return caritas to the primacy of caring as the center of a generational cycle. An individual's existence is ensured with a universe that is believed to be meaningful and purposeful. A wholeness that fosters caritas appears to characterize the nature of the stages of adulthood and older adulthood. Erikson articulated this when he wrote:

The experience of caring, nurturing and maintaining—which are the essence of generativity—make of the stages of life a life cycle, recreating the beginning of the cycle in each newborn. These same experiences make of the sequences of life cycles a generational cycle, irrevocably binding each generation to those that gave it life and to those for whose life it is responsible. . . . We understand middle adulthood's generative responsibility for the "maintenance of the world" in terms of the interrelated realms of people, products, and ideals. It is, therefore, the responsibility of each generation of adults to bear, nurture and guide these people who will succeed them as adults, as well as to develop and maintain those societal institutions and natural resources without which successive generations will not be able to survive. . . . Matured adulthood, then, contains the capacity for grand-generativity incorporating care for the present with concern for the future—for today's younger generations in their futures, for generations not yet born, and for the survival of the world as a whole. . . . However, grand-generative concern for the future, in the abstract, must be integrated with the simple, direct caring for the specific individuals who are part of life today (1982, pp. 74–75).

Erikson posited that the human being is, from the first kick in the uterus to the last breath, an organism comprised of three processes: biologic, psychologic, and social. The physiology of living is governed by a relativity of each process, which is dependent on the others; together, these are the indispensable processes by which human existence becomes and remains continuous. Ego development must receive attention equal to other forms of development. Simultaneous with the emphasis on ego stage development, attention must be directed toward the development of caring. More importantly, the development of caring must become a central educational aim. The development of caritas, a global perspective of human caring, can and does emerge in Stage VII and must also be supported. The findings from this study imply that the constructs of care, caritas and ego development, also share a receptivity. The importance of continuing to describe, explain, understand, and support this relationship remains pivotal to humankind. It is through the virtue of care and the evolution of caritas that worldwide improvement can occur.

REFERENCES

Barrett-Lennard, G. T. (1978). The Relationship Inventory: Later development and applications. *JSAS: Catalog of Selected Documents in Psychology, 8,* 55.

Barrett-Lennard, G. T. (1986). The Relationship Inventory now: Issues and advances in theory, method, and use. In L. S. Greenburg & W. M. Pinsof (Eds.), *The psychotherapeutic process: A research handbook* (pp. 439–476). New York: Guilford Press.

Boyd, R. D. (1961). *Self-Description Questionnaire: An instrument for the measurement of ego-stage development.* Madison: University of Wisconsin.

Erikson, E. H. (1959). Identity and life cycle: Selected papers. *Psychological Issues* [monograph], *1*(4).

Erikson, E. H. (1968). *Identity: Youth and crisis.* New York: Norton.

Erikson, E. H. (1982). *The life cycle completed: A review.* New York: Norton.

Goeppinger, J., & Schuster, G. (1988). Community as client: Using the nursing process to promote health. In M. Stanhope & J. Lancaster (Eds.), *Community health nursing.* St. Louis: Mosby.

Griffin, A. P. (1980). Philosophy and nursing. *Journal of Advanced Nursing, 5,* 261–272.

McCarthy, M. P., Craig, C., Bergstrom, L., Whitley, E. M., Stoner, M. H., & Magilvy, J. K. (1991). In P. L. Chinn (Ed.), *Anthology on caring.* New York: National League for Nursing.

Schuster, E. A. (1990). Earth caring. *Advances in Nursing Science, 13*(1), 25–30.

Soldwisch, S. S. (1990). *An examination of the association between caring in nursing and Erikson's epigenetic theory. Dissertation Abstracts International, 51,* 1748–1749B.

21

The Actualized Caring Moment: A Grounded Theory of Caring in Nursing Practice

Payom Euswas

A spirit of enquiry concerning "What nursing really is" began for me when I commenced nursing training in Thailand at the age of eighteen. It has remained with me ever since, over a seventeen-year journey in nursing. As a student and new graduate nurse-midwife, the experience of nursing consisted of procedures designed to assist the medical profession, for instance, administering oral medications, injections, giving and monitoring intravenous fluid, and attending to the admission and discharge of patients. The satisfaction came not only from the tasks themselves, but also from the opportunities they provided to help patients with relief of discomfort and pain. I learned that, while not all pain and suffering could be prevented, for

The author wishes to thank Professor Norma Chick, at Massey University, New Zealand, for her support and critical suggestions; and Professor Jean Watson, Center for Human Caring, University of Colorado Health Science Center, for her constructive suggestions.

these are part of the human experience, a nurse can often bring relief just by her presence and by providing a few words.

A desire for understanding nursing led me to undertake a study of nursing practice in Thailand, using a quantitative approach (Kanjanangkul & Euswas (Wiriya), 1985). It aimed at finding out "what nurses and other personnel do." The data revealed a picture of nurses mainly performing tasks directed by medical instructions. Examples of major activities performed by staff nurses were: documenting, administering medications and intravenous fluid, taking blood samples, and supervising nonprofessional nurses and student nurses. Practical nurses assisted patients to accomplish their personal daily activities and performed simple nursing procedures, such as recording vital signs. The findings provided some useful information about nursing practice, but they did little to further the understanding of nursing's essential nature.

Historically, nurses have affirmed that caring for people is their central focus (Henderson, 1966; Nightingale, 1964). However, because of the increasing use of technology in health care systems and the fact that nursing practice is dominated by a biomedical model, caring has been overshadowed in nursing practice and the investigation of the phenomenon of caring has been limited in the past. Recently, caring has been recognized by a number of nurse leaders and researchers as a topic of scholarly and practical importance (Benner, 1984; Gaut, 1984, 1986; Leininger, 1978, 1981, 1984; Reimen, 1986; Roach, 1984; Watson, 1979, 1985). Leininger (1984) asserted that "caring is the essence and the central, unifying, and dominant domain to characterize nursing" (p. 3). Watson (1985) stated that the core of nursing is caring. She defined caring as the moral ideal of nursing with "concern for preservation of humanity, dignity, and fullness of self" (p. 14).

In the past decade, a large number of studies have undertaken to uncover the phenomenon of caring in nursing, but this is still not well articulated. Although understanding has increased, an analysis of nursing literature on caring from thirty-five authors, by Morse, Solberg, Neander, Bottorff, and Johnson (1990), showed diversity in the conceptualization of caring. The five conceptual categories that emerged from the analysis are: "caring as a human trait; caring as a moral imperative or ideal; caring as an affect; caring as an interpersonal relationship; and caring as a therapeutic intervention" (p. 3). The authors identified two additional categories of the outcome of caring: caring as a subjective experience of the patient and caring as a physical response. They also made linkage relationships among all categories and suggested that further clarification was required regarding these relationships. The same authors also addressed the urgent need to develop a clearer conceptualization of caring by moving to include patient-centered theories as well as nurse-focused theories. "At this time, instead of enlightening the reader, examination of the literature only increases confusion. There is no consensus regarding the definitions of caring, the components of care, or the process of caring" (Morse et al., p. 2).

In the New Zealand context, the link between nursing and caring has been made explicit. The New Zealand Nurses' Association (1984) adopted the following definition of nursing:

Nursing is a specialized expression of caring concerned primarily with enhancing the abilities of individuals and groups to achieve their health potential within the realities of their life situation. (p. 3)

Despite the statement, no previous study focusing specifically on caring in nursing has been undertaken in New Zealand. The absence of significant studies in this context led me to undertake the present study, intending to clarify how caring is expressed in everyday nursing practice.

PURPOSE

The purpose of this study was to identify and authenticate those aspects of nursing practice that best typify caring. The aim of the study extends to theory generation.

THE RESEARCH QUESTIONS

What does caring mean for nurses in their professional practice?
How do patients perceive themselves as being cared for by nurses?

METHODOLOGY

This study concerned human experience: the nurses' experience of caring, and the patients' experience of being cared for. Therefore, a phenomenological perspective (Munhall & Oiler, 1986; Omery, 1983) was initially chosen as the most suitable approach. The study also intended to generate a grounded theory of caring nursing practice. Glaser and Strauss's (1967) grounded theory method provided strategies for the discovery of theory from data. The method finally chosen for this particular study, which aimed to uncover knowledge about caring in nursing practice, was a combination of the phenomenological approach and the grounded theory method.

SETTINGS AND PARTICIPANTS

Three nursing practice settings involving cancer patients—hospital, hospice, and community—were selected in two cities in New Zealand. Thirty-two registered nurses and thirty patients with cancer participated in the study.

DATA COLLECTION AND ANALYSIS

In line with the phenomenological perspective and the grounded theory strategies, data for the present study were obtained by three main methods: in-depth interview, participant observation, and audit of nursing and medical notes. The study aimed to uncover the human experience of caring and being cared for. In order to gain a naïve perspective of the participants' experience, I endeavored to set aside or suspend all my preconceptions on caring. The data were analyzed by the method of constant comparative analysis.

FINDINGS

A number of concepts and subconcepts were developed from the data, and the grounded theory of "the actualized caring moment" was formulated. The theory is a gestalt configuration of three main components: the preconditions, the situated context, and the ongoing interaction. This grounded theory provides a partial explanation of how the process of caring occurs in nursing practice.

The *preconditions* are the prerequisites for the caring process to occur. Nurse and patient are ready to be in contact, and each brings unique capacities and expectations into the situation. The nurse brings her personal and professional qualities of caring, benevolence, commitment, and clinical competency, and the patient brings his or her personal uniqueness with a specific life situation of health-related problems.

The *situated context* is the situation of the nurse–patient contact in a specific place and time in the environment of health care settings that promote the occurrence of caring processes.

The *ongoing interaction* is the actual caring process that evolves from the preconditions and the situated context. The actual caring process is composed of six caring elements: being there, being mindfully present, having a trusting relationship, participating in meeting needs, having empathetic communication, and balancing knowledge-energy-time. It is the process of the nurse–patient interaction in a continuously changing pattern. The nurse is fully aware of her commitment to give of herself to assist the patient in achieving personal health needs within the reality of the patient's situation. She is physically present with the patient and promptly responds to the patient in the immediate, present moment. She develops a trusting relationship with the patient and coparticipants with the patient to identify needs and to meet these needs.

Because the nurse and the patient are human beings, feelings are involved in the process. The nurse conveys empathetic understanding to the patient through verbal and nonverbal communication. In this process of caring, the nurse is aware of integrating all patterns of knowing—ethical, personal, esthetic, and empirical—in order to use an appropriate approach, and spends the amount of time that is appropriate for a particular patient in a particular situation. Ethical knowing motivates the nurse's state of moral awareness of helping the patient as a valued dignified person. Personal knowing facilitates the nurse's entry into the patient's personal world. Esthetic knowing allows a nurse "artist" to create a unique approach to the individual patient in a specific situation. Empirical knowing allows the nurse to reflect on scientific knowledge to understand the particular caring situation and make decisions that will help the patient. The nurse maintains her complementary position by working with the patient moment-by-moment, by imparting her compassionate intention and physical energy, and by spending time with the patient, always with the awareness of preventing overemotional involvement.

The process of caring is continually moving forward. At any moment of the interactions, both the nurse and the patient are realizing their intersubjective connectedness, "the actualized caring moment," which is dynamically changing and occurs within the wholeness of the three components converging together. The diagram representing the conceptual model is illustrated in Figure 21–1.

The moment of actualized caring represents the growth potential that allows the nurse and the patient to realize the fullest expression of their innate psychological, emotional, spiritual, and intellectual capacities, their best moment as human beings in this situation.

The actualized caring moment does not occur in a regular pattern of the nurse–patient interaction. It may occur once or more in an episode of a nurse–patient encounter, or it may occur only once in many episodes. However, once it occurs, there is a likelihood that it will recur. A diagram showing caring moments in an ongoing process is presented in Figure 21–2.

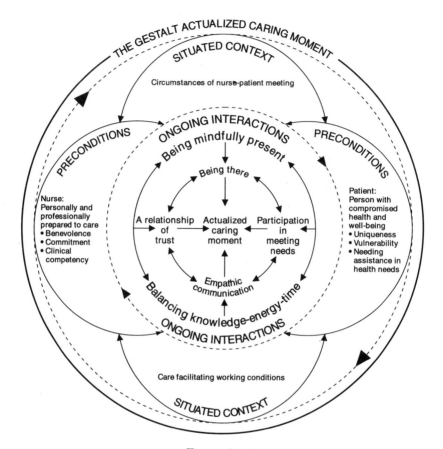

Figure 21-1
The Gestalt Actualized Caring Moment: A Conceptual Model of the
Nurse Caring Process (Euswas, 1991, p. 183)

In developing this grounded theory, two main existing theories—the
gestalt theory and the nursing theory of transpersonal human caring—and
a Buddhist concept of mindfulness were used to support the emerging theory of "the actualized caring moment." The moment of actualized caring is
relevant to the actual caring occasion of a transpersonal caring relationship
proposed by Watson (1985):

*In transpersonal human caring, the nurse can enter into the experience of
another person, and another person can enter into the nurse's experience.*

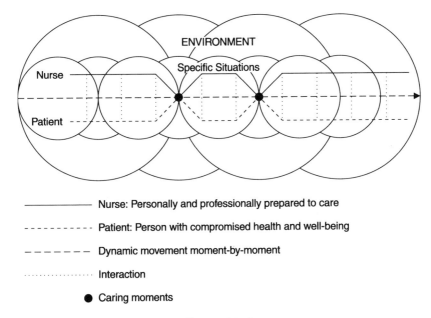

——————————— Nurse: Personally and professionally prepared to care

– – – – – – – – – Patient: Person with compromised health and well-being

– – – – – – – Dynamic movement moment-by-moment

. . . . Interaction

● Caring moments

Figure 21–2
Caring Moments Within Ongoing Process (Euswas, 1991, p. 182)

The ideal of transpersonal caring is an ideal of intersubjectivity in which both persons are involved. (p. 60)

Being mindfully present, a concept indicated by data, is an important element of the actualized caring moment. It describes the nurse's condition of being constantly present in the awareness of herself while she is involved in patient situations, and responding to the situations appropriately. As stated by three nurses:

. . . *you have to be aware of that moment being with them. You have to know yourself, what you are doing.*

. . . *you have to be mindful every second, every minute, dealing with the person, the drugs, and other things.*

I try to concentrate all my attention to them when I'm talking to them. They know that I'm concentrating on them and that I'm not thinking of a hundred other things at the same time. If I relax more, they think that you're competent and you are there to help them instead of quickly doing what you're doing and whiz away.

The state of being mindfully present is an activator for the nurse's readiness to act in her caring practice on a moment-to-moment basis; the nurse is fully aware of her thoughts, feelings, and actions in every moment in which she is dealing with the patient. In developing this concept, I have been sensitized by the concept of "right mindfulness" (*Sammasati*) from my Buddhist background. (*Sammasati* and *sati* (see below) are Thai words derived from Pali language.)

> Sati [Mindfulness] means to bear in mind or bring to mind. Sati is the state of recollecting, the state of remembering, the state of non-fading, the state of non-forgetting. Sati means the sati that is a spiritual Faculty, the sati that is a Spiritual power . . . . (Phra-Thepvatee, 1988, p. 2)

The actualized caring moment occurs when there is promptness of the caring preconditions and the caring situational context within the caring elements. It is a new characteristic, a gestalt configuration, as shown in Figure 21–1.

> A Gestalt is a whole whose characteristics are determined not by the characteristics of its individual elements, but by the internal nature of the whole. (Wertheimer, citing Katz & Tyson, 1951, p. 91)

This moment is a powerful and meaningful occasion for both the nurse and the patient. It potentiates the patient's self-caring and healing, and empowers the nurse in using herself as a therapeutic effect. The actualized caring and healing moment was described by a patient, his wife, and two nurses, as follows:

> . . . there's that personal contact as if it's circling you. It's very very close. It was a while ago a circle of pain, now they create a circle, a very comforting sort of circle. They've eliminated the pain and replaced the pain with themselves and made the circle that way. (Patient J, in a hospice)
> . . . when we walked in they were waiting for us and there was about three nurses and you could literally feel the love, possibly spiritual. You felt it radiating out and welcoming. (Patient J's wife)
> . . . the time I spent at helping and learning and what I gained is useful and a job that I'm doing isn't pointless. . . . I get quite a lot of satisfaction out of it, in this ward particularly; you spend a lot of time talking to them. And you get quite drained but you feel you achieved something maybe to put someone's mind at rest, especially if you can see a change in them. They tend to relax and you feel like you're being effective. (Nurse L)

If somebody like myself comes in and can help them over that problem which is an impediment to their quality of life, they are enriched in other ways, because they reprioritize their life, their relationships, and their whole view of the world. And so I see my job as being part of that. But in being a bit satisfied with the outcome, I get feedback so I'm re-energizing for the next. So it does help, but it also helps me as a person to grow in myself and I think that's important for us all and I think that if you can help somebody to grow, and also grow within yourself you are self-actualizing. (Nurse J)

CARING EPISODES

Following is a group of poems on episodes of caring in everyday nursing practice. I have transformed them from the data. My reflection on caring in nursing is portrayed in the analog diagram in Figure 21–3.

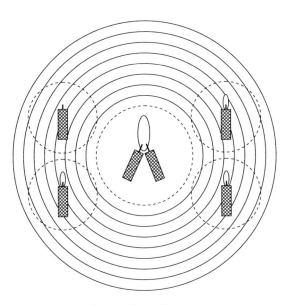

Candles = Caring Moments

Figure 21–3
An Analog Diagram of the Actualized Caring Moment
(Euswas, 1991, p. 238)

Taking Temperature

Having lymphoma, Mr. B
  Computer engineer is his career
    He needs explanation of things

Temperature high for two days
  Staying in a ward for investigation
    Moment of worrying, he experiences

A nurse comes for temperature taking
  Chatting away with him, his worries
    Telling him her finger hurt, she shares

Reading the scale 37.5 °C
  "I don't think it's long enough," he says
    "Could you put it in longer?," he asks

The nurse smiles, "Alright, we'll do it again"
  Three minutes thermometer is in his mouth
    Silence, eye touch, she waits

The scale shows 37.8 °C
  "Oh, it is not high as the other times," he says
    "Have you had a cold drink?," she asks
      "No." He smiles; she smiles

In the Hospice: Bedtime

Mr. K lies stretched in bed
  His wife sits close by
    Waiting for the nurse to come

Two come with a smile
  Close to him, his wife
    Eyes touch, soft speech, they listen

"I . . . . . . I . . . . . . feel . . . . al . . . . alright"
  Slow speech, stuttering, he speaks
    The nurses listen, talk, wait

Cleansing touch, soothing hand, they minister
   He talks about his garden, his wife shares
      The nurses share talking, and all laugh

Comforting him with pillows
   Puff the pillows...No, he says, Add a pillow...No, he says
      Tilt the pillow to the left...Yes...that...that's right

"I . . . I . . . heard . . . you . . . you . . . sing . . . this . . . this . . . morning
   Could . . . could . . . you . . . sing . . . sing . . . please," he asks one nurse
      She smiles, eyes touch . . . silence

Close to him, arms around his wife, they move
   "Edelweiss song" begins, they sing
      A circle of four in oneness
         He smiles . . . eyes close

When I Was First Told of Cancer

A lump was in my breast
   The biopsy was done
      I could not sleep well

Two forces pulling apart
   I might get it . . . my mother had it
      I hoped . . . I prayed . . . It would not happen to me

One morning I heard the word "cancer"
   It ran into my body, my mind
      Like a thundering storm . . . a shock

Nothing could I hear or see
   Cold and darkness
      My life was ending

Suddenly . . . a warm touch was creeping inside me
   Like a light spreading out
      A whispering of soft voice at my ears

She shared and guided me round
  When I went home
    I reflected on what she said to me
      "Try to think of one thing at a time"

She told my daughter
  "Your mother needs more love and caring"
    I gained the strength to have my breast off
      The caring from that nurse I remember

Having a Shower

A big operation, I had
  They helped me slowly down to the stool
    And gently let me down

They could feel what I felt
  "You are doing well," they reassured
    I felt good and tried harder

When I went into the shower
  I told them I could do by myself
    They listened to me and believed me

They let me do it
  They're always there
    "Are you alright? Are you alright?," kept checking

I felt really confident in myself
  I felt I'd achieved a really big milestone
    "I can do it"

PARTIAL THEORETICAL STATEMENTS DEFINING CARING IN NURSING PRACTICE

Caring in nursing practice is a situational-specific dynamic process that is actualized by the nurse and the patient, who engage in the helping relationship.

Caring in nursing practice is a series of the actualized caring moments occurring within a gestalt configuration of three main components:

- The *caring preconditions* are the prerequisite of the caring process. These are the nurse, who has capacities or qualities of caring, based on human care value and knowledge, and the patient with a specific health-related problem, who is in need of assistance.
- The *actual caring process* is the continuity of the interactive process between the nurse and the patient. The nurse translates caring into the action of helping the patient, and the patient participates in care. Both the nurse and the patient realize their intersubjective connectedness at a given point in time.
- The *situated context* is the set of circumstances in which the nurse and patient meet at a specific time and place in an environment that allows the nurse to practice caring.

The actual caring process in nursing practice consists of six caring elements: being there, being mindfully present, balancing knowledge-energy-time, having a relationship of trust, participating in meeting needs, and having empathetic communication.

The actualized caring moment occurs temporarily at a given point in time, at the place of the nurse–patient transpersonal lived experience. It brings a positive outcome for both the nurse and the patient—growth for both and potential healing for the patient. It may occur only once or at many points in the interactions. Sometimes, the circumstances may be such that it does not occur at all.

DISCUSSION AND IMPLICATIONS

The grounded theory of the actualized caring moment is developed from the nursing data. It includes both the highly visible and, particularly, the less visible aspects of caring nursing practice. It clearly captures what is actually happening when the nurse and the patient engage in the caring relationship because it explains how nurses care for the patients in everyday nursing practice. The essence of such caring has not been clearly demonstrated in the existing nursing literature. However, some of the findings of this study validate and are relevant to existing nursing literature (Brown, 1981; Gaut, 1984; Hernandez, 1987; Leininger, 1978, 1981, 1984; Riemen,

1983; Swanson-Kauffman, 1988; Watson, 1985; Weiss, 1988). The most closely related is the existing nursing theory of human caring (Watson, 1985). The actualized caring moment is relevant to an actual caring occasion of transpersonal human caring, as proposed by Watson. Watson's theory, developed from philosophical analysis, is highly abstract. It is a grand theory of human caring that prompts and stimulates further investigation and development. The grounded theory of the actualized caring moment is less abstract than Watson's theory because it is based on data. It is a midrange theory developed from practice (Bottorff, 1991) and it further clarifies how the actual caring occasion occurs in the real world of nursing practice. It clearly demonstrates that caring is actualized by the nurse and the patient, who engage in a helping relationship. This relationship occurs moment-by-moment in their interaction.

In their professional life, nurses experience special meaningful moments with their patients. There are very few detailed accounts of these moments because they are usually brief and invisible and because nurses, although they know these moments occur, find it difficult to relate them. As a result, this important aspect of nursing is not usually made explicit in efforts to communicate the essence of nursing both to nurses and to others. "I have experienced warm and generous relationships with patients, but . . . find them difficult to name. They are born, somehow, of a willingness of both to give and receive" (Fulton, 1987, p. 3).

The present study illuminated the details of this moment from actual nursing data and conceptualized it as a gestalt actualized caring moment. The theoretical framework of the gestalt actualized caring moment provides a basis for assisting nurses to understand their practice more fully and enabling them to articulate the essential nature of nursing. It is hoped that nurses who choose to use this theoretical framework will be helped to increase their therapeutic use of self to potentiate the patient's healing and growth and to gain satisfaction from their practice. Most importantly, it is intended to assist nurses in achieving personal and professional growth so that they can act as advocates to preserve humanity in a high-cost technology-driven health care system.

The framework contributes to the understanding of the actual caring process, which provides guidance and a means by which a nurse can transform the qualities of caring into a therapeutic effect for the patient. By increasing the intensity of the interaction with the patient, the nurse can provide a greater therapeutic effect. In order to do so, the nurse must increase her awareness so that she focuses on the patient at the immediate present moment; she must integrate within herself all patterns of knowing, in order to impart the appropriate energy and spend an appropriate amount of time. In this way, the nurse achieves a therapeutic harmony of verbal caring, nonverbal caring, and technically competent behaviours.

Although nursing has been recognized as a necessary human service for a long time, its image to the public is not clear and has not always been greatly valued. Quite often, patients say, "I never knew before what the nurses do. I thought they were just doing beds and pans, and what the doctors say." Nurses always say, "Most people don't understand what we actually do." In the public image, nursing is not far from subservience. The theoretical framework of the gestalt actualized caring moment provides a medium through which the public may gain more understanding of the nature of nursing as caring professional expertise in a partnership role with patients.

The actualized caring moment may not be limited to nursing. However, no other profession is equally predicated on achieving the preconditions to the caring moment.

LIMITATION OF THE STUDY

This study initiated the use of grounded theory strategy to develop a partial theoretical explanation of the phenomenon of caring nursing practice in the New Zealand context. Because time was limited, the study was terminated at this stage in order for a report to be written explaining the emerged theoretical framework. Development of propositions is the next step. Grounded theory is always in the process of development (Glaser & Strauss, 1967).

CONCLUSION

The theoretical framework of the gestalt actualized caring moment, which comes from the reality of nursing practice settings, has demonstrated the actual caring process in nursing. It has indicated clearly that not only is caring an essential component of nursing, but nursing in the full sense cannot be separated from caring.

The gestalt actualized caring moment gives a fresh perspective on the phenomenon of caring in nursing as a harmonious dynamic movement, moment-by-moment, of interhuman contact that transforms healing–growing so that suffering is transcended in a unique and whole situation. This framework challenges nurses to reflect on their practice and offers an aid to realizing the holistic nature of nursing.

EPILOGUE

A nurse searches for meanings
A journey has started
Years and years pass by

Questions still remain
After four years intensive searching
A little miracle is found

It is a beauty inside oneself
which all can see, feel, and know
What is it?

A hope is there
When the nursing circle comes together
with a pure heart, head, and hand

To search for our "spiritual bond"
Investigating "what really nursing is"
A journey continues

REFERENCES

Benner, P. (1984). *From novice to expert: Excellence and power in nursing practice,* Menlo Park, CA: Addison-Wesley.

Bottorff, J. L. (1991). Nursing: A practical science of caring. *Advances in Nursing Science, 14* (1), 26–39.

Brown, L. J. (1981). *Behaviors of nurses perceived by hospitalized patients as indicators of care.* Doctoral dissertation, University of Colorado.

Euswas, P. (1991). *The actualized caring moment: A grounded theory of caring in nursing practice.* Doctoral dissertation, Department of Nursing Studies, Massey University, New Zealand.

Fulton, J. S. (1987). Virginia Henderson: Theorist, prophet, poet. *Advances in Nursing Science, 10* (1), 1–9.

Gaut, D. A. (1984). A theoretical description of caring action. In M. M. Leininger (Ed.), *Care: The essence of nursing and health* (pp. 27–44). Thorofare, NJ: Slack.

Gaut, D. A. (1986). Evaluating caring competencies in nursing practice. *Topics in Clinical Nursing, 8* (2), 77–83.

Glaser, B. G., & Strauss, A. L. (1967). *The discovery of grounded theory.* Chicago: Aldine.

Henderson, V. (1966). *The nature of nursing.* New York: Macmillan.

Hernandez, C. M. (1987). *A phenomenologic investigation of the concept of the lived experience of caring in professional nurses.* Doctoral dissertation, Adelphi University, Marion A. Buckley School of Nursing, Garden City, NY.

Kanjanangkul, M., & Euswas (Wiriya), P. (1985). Nursing activities and categories of nursing personnel in Nakorn Chiag-Mai Hospital. *Journal of Nursing Education and Research (Thai), 7* (2), 7–13.

Katz, D., & Tyson, R. (1951). *Gestalt psychology, its nature and significance.* London: Methuen.

Leininger, M. M. (Ed.). (1984). *Care: The essence of nursing and health.* Thorofare, NJ: Slack.

Leininger, M. M. (1981). The phenomenon of caring: Importance, research questions and theoretical considerations. In M. M. Leininger (Ed.), *Caring: An essential human need* (pp. 3–15). Thorofare, NJ: Slack.

Leininger, M. M. (1984). *Care: The essence of nursing and health.* Thorofare, NJ: Slack.

Munhall, P. L., & Oiler, C. J. (1986). Philosophical foundations of qualitative research. In P. L. Munhall & C. J. Oiler (Eds.), *Nursing research: A qualitative perspective* (pp. 47–63). Norwalk, CT: Appleton-Century-Crofts.

New Zealand Nurses' Association. (1984). *Nursing education in New Zealand: A review and a statement of policy.*

Nightingale, F. (1964). *Notes on nursing: What it is and what it is not.* Philadelphia: Lippincott. (Original work published 1860)

Omery, A. (1983). Phenomenology: A method for nursing research. *Advances in Nursing Science, 5* (2), 49–64.

Phra-Thepvatee (Prayudh Payutto). (1988). *Sammasati: An exposition of right mindfulness.* Bangkok, Thailand: Komol Keem Tong Press.

Reimen, D. J. (1983). *The essence structure of a caring interaction: A phenomenological study.* Doctoral dissertation, Texas Woman's University, Denton.

Roach, S. (1984). *Caring: The human mode of being, implications for nursing.* Perspectives in Caring, Monograph No. 1. Toronto, Canada: University of Toronto.

Swanson-Kauffman, K. M. (1988). Caring needs of women who miscarried. In M. M. Leininger (Ed.), *Care discovery and uses in clinical and community nursing* (pp. 55–70). Detroit: Wayne State University Press.

Watson, J. (1979). *Nursing: The philosophy and science of caring.* Boston: Little, Brown.

Watson, J. (1985). *Nursing: Human science and human care.* Norwalk, CT: Appleton-Century-Crofts.

Weiss, C. J. (1988). Model to discover, validate, and use care in nursing. In M. M. Leininger (Ed.), *Care discovery and uses in clinical and community nursing* (pp. 139–140). Detroit: Wayne State University Press.

PART V

NURSING ADMINISTRATION AND ADMINISTRATIVE ROLES

22

Utilization of Research on Caring: Development of a Nurse Compensation System

Kathleen L. Valentine

Research on caring supports the concept that to be caring, one needs to demonstrate consistency among one's values, beliefs, and actions (Gaut, 1984; Leininger, 1988; Noddings, 1984; Ray, 1987; Valentine, 1991, 1992; Watson, 1985). This congruence is necessary on an individual basis and on an organizational level. Nurse administrators charged with the leadership of nursing within organizations must provide the necessary support and direction for caring to be evident within their practice environments. This caring organization must be provided for the benefit of staff as well as for the patients and families to whom they give care. Staff who perceive themselves to be working in a noncaring environment will find it more difficult to deliver care-based nursing.

This chapter describes how research on caring and participatory decision-making processes were used as the bases for the development of a nurse

The author gratefully acknowledges the willingness of the task force members to use these evaluation techniques in the completion of their project.

compensation system within one organization. Emphasis will be on the procedures used to develop this program rather than on the program itself. Any organization that uses caring as its theoretical base will need to develop its own context-specific program, rather than adopt a program from another organization. Therefore, the most transferable aspects of this program are the procedures used to develop it rather than the program itself.

BACKGROUND

The organization in which this program was developed is a multihospital system with 680 beds. After a period of "systematic downsizing," (Rozboril, 1987), the remaining staff were anxious to reactivate their reward system for clinical practice, which had been "frozen" during the downsizing. As the organization approached the reactivation of its clinical ladder system, dissatisfaction among the nursing staff was evident. Based on results from a survey of the registered nursing staff, it was found that the prior clinical ladder system was no longer acceptable: it had had limited positions for promotion and an unsatisfactory implementation of the performance review process once people were promoted. A task force composed of fourteen staff nurses and three representatives from nursing education, human resources, and nursing administration, respectively, was formed to examine the reward system for nurses. I was hired as a nursing administration consultant. My role was to integrate concepts of caring into the project, help facilitate the process, and provide technical assistance in evaluation and decision making.

ORGANIZATIONAL ASSESSMENT

Organizational diagnosis is one aspect of any major change process. The reward system is one of the interrelated components of any organization; others are purpose, structure, relationships, leadership, and coordinating technologies (Weisbord, 1983). In order to make a meaningful change in the reward system, one must examine other aspects of the organization and ensure that the various components are kept in balance. This is in keeping with a caring organization in which what one feels, thinks, and values is congruent with how one acts and interacts in relationship with the one cared for (Gaut, 1984; Valentine, 1989a, 1992). Congruence between purpose and rewards is also in keeping with concepts of total quality management and shared governance in nursing (Katz & Green, 1992). In order to focus its work primarily on the reward system, this task force also had to examine the mission of the division of nursing, the job descriptions, and the performance appraisal system for nurses. All of this examination was based on the foundation of caring.

CARING

Figure 22–1 depicts the integrated process used in the development of what came to be known as the Clinical Incentive Program. At the core of the process is research on caring. Prior to the establishment of the task force, this organization had participated in a research project that had defined caring from the patients', nurses', and administrators' viewpoints; measured its presence in specific nurse–patient encounters; and demonstrated care's relationship to available resources and patient outcomes (Valentine, 1991). The results from this research, as well as other literature

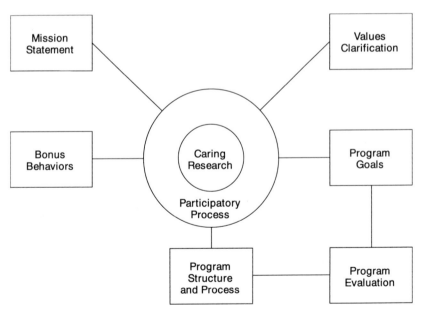

Figure 22–1
Clinical Incentive Program: Integrated Process

on caring, were shared with the task force and served as a theoretical foundation for the remainder of the task force's work.

VALUES CLARIFICATION/
PARTICIPATORY PROCESS

The task force had been charged by the new vice president for nursing to examine the mission, job description, review process, and reward system for the division of nursing. The task force would be participating in the process of transforming the nursing division from a bureaucracy to an organization in which the nursing professionals who practiced there were accountable for their practice and their subsequent rewards and recognition. The organization was moving toward a shared governance structure, but at the time the task force was formed, that structure was not yet operational. Many members who had experienced a bureaucratic organization with a history of autocratic leadership were distrustful of the process. Trust building was essential to the success of the task force's work. An exercise in values clarification was one of the first activities in which the task force engaged. Task force members were asked to draw some of their happiest and saddest moments in nursing; what would make them leave nursing; if they had a magic wand, what nursing would look like; as well as other representations related to their personal view of themselves as nurses. These drawings were then shared and discussed within the group. The exercise accomplished several goals:

1. All members had a chance to speak and be heard with understanding, not evaluation.
2. Common ground was established and many shared values emerged.
3. From the earliest moment, all members were role modeled as active contributors to the project.

Use of a participatory process and decision making was the key to the successful development of the project. Yet, some members were impatient with "process." They wished to quickly establish the revised reward system without "wasting time" on caring theory, values, or the mission of the department. They considered these to be "stalling" tactics employed by "administration" to avoid the real issue of rewards. Therefore, process activities had to move the project along, be inclusive, be data-supported, and produce concrete results quickly, in order to establish and maintain credibility and trust within the task force membership. Examples of these types of decision support aids will be described as they apply to each of the following topics.

MISSION

The mission of any nursing organization is essential to establish, because all other aspects of its operation flow from it. It helps to establish what nurses think and feel, and how they want to interact with the patients and families whom they care for. The mission establishes who and what the organization is, why it exists, and its constituency. The mission for this division of nursing was drafted based on a participatory approach called structured conceptualization (Trochim, 1989; Trochim & Linton, 1986; Valentine, 1989b). This approach uses a participatory process to help people take abstract ideas and make them concrete through a mathematical process called concept mapping. Concept mapping uses multidimensional scaling and cluster analyses to produce two-dimensional pictures of how concepts are related to one another. (For a thorough presentation of concept mapping

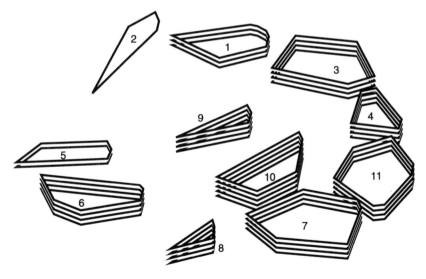

Figure 22–2
Ratings Mission

Support	(3.64)
Consumer advocacy	(3.55)
Value each person as a unique human being	(4.43)
Caring for individuals, families, and communities	(4.29)
Cluster Average	3.98

Figure 22–3
Cluster 10

methodology, see Trochim, 1989.) In concept mapping, participants follow six steps:

1. Choose a focus question.
2. Brainstorm.
3. Rate and sort the brainstormed items.
4. Compute the maps.
5. Interpret the maps.
6. Utilize the maps.

Figure 22–2 represents the concept map for this particular division of nursing's mission. Each cluster represents a grouping of ideas that are similar. The closer in space, the more similar the items are considered to be. The higher the border, the higher the rating for these items. Each cluster is then labeled by the participants. For example, Cluster 10 (Figure 22–3) had in it such items as support and consumer advocacy; it was labeled "why we exist." Cluster 8 (Figure 22–4) was labeled "outcomes." The numbers in parentheses represented the average rating given to that item on a 5-point scale. These numbers were then summed and averaged to determine the cluster rating.

Patient satisfaction	(4.21)
Maintenance of health	(4.00)
Cluster Average	4.11

Figure 22–4
Cluster 8

- Positive ideas.
- Cost-containment ideas.
- Positive attitudes.
- Risk taking.
- Problem resolution.
- Quality performance as a preceptor for new employees.
- Initiatives to improve patient care.
- Leadership.
- Demonstration of caring and empathy.
- Collegial support.

The goal was to create a system in which individual initiative, peer review, and commitment played an important part. Task force members identified certain criteria as essential to the success of the Clinical Incentive Program and the satisfaction of its participants. The system was founded on the belief that recruitment and retention of registered nurses would be positively affected by a program that met the following criteria:

- Elimination of any predetermined limits on the number of registered nurses able to become eligible.
- Renewable rewards.
- Recognition of expertise *and* longevity.
- Individualized rewards that vary according to the amount of effort exerted.
- Flexibility in the choice of behaviors to contract for and the amount of time to devote to the program on an annual basis.
- Use of objective criteria for meeting eligibility requirements and for evaluating performance.
- Unification of nursing colleagues through the creation of a system that provides equal opportunity for participation.
- Reward and accountability of participants in the system without punishment of people who choose not to participate.
- Recognition of education as one factor in achieving expertise.
- Inclusion of patient, peer, and supervisory input into evaluation of performance.

PROGRAM EVALUATION

Members of the task force rated each of the above criteria for their importance when they were deciding which program alternative to choose. This

---

Who and What We Are

The registered nurses   (4.
are professionals   (⁴
with specific knowledge,   (3.
skills, and standards of practice,   (
who value each person as a unique human being.   (4

Why We Exist and Our Constituency

The nursing professional exists to provide caring   (⁴
to the community's individuals (patients)   (⁴
families   (⁵
and groups   (community

Figure 22–5
Mission Statement: Excerpts

The mission statement was then drafted based on the insi
through this process. Excerpts from the mission statement are sh
ure 22–5. The numbers served to guide the areas of emphasis in
statement; in the final version, they were deleted.

From the mission statement, job description and performar
instruments were developed to be congruent with the mission o
division. Meeting biweekly, the task force took about four mo:
plete this work. Simultaneously, the group was conducting a
view of clinical ladders, bonus systems, and career ladders. T
then established program goals for the reward system.

PROGRA

The goals of the program were to provide a system in which
motivated registered nurses could be rewarded for initiatives 1
excellence as demonstrated through:

- Clinical skills.
- Education.
- Innovation.
- Expertise.
- Responsibility.
- Dependability.

generated much discussion; for example, how important was "patient review" of the nurses' performance in determining the rewards? The task force members decided to go back to their peers and solicit their opinion. The criteria were rated by registered nurses at large (RN) and the results were compared to the task force members' (TF) ratings of criteria (see Figure 22–6). Significant differences were found for some items. For example, task force members rated peer review higher than registered nurses at large did. The process of checking their perceptions with their peers and finding differences was a difficult issue for the task force members. They used a system of communication methods to ensure that they were representing the nurses at large. They met with nurses in small groups for unit meetings, they developed and distributed a newsletter, and they reported to and interacted with the nursing councils emerging through the development of the governance structure. In the end, they had to acknowledge that they were the representatives for nursing. They had to use their best judgment to produce a program that they could defend and one that would be acceptable to the majority.

To aid in the process of rational decision making, other heuristic decision aids were employed. Among them was multi-attribute utility analysis (Figure 22–7). In this process, each program was rated for the degree to which it met the program evaluation criteria (outline above). The weight represents the relative importance of each criterion as determined by the task force. The program that best met each criterion was then chosen. Based on this process and group discussion, the task force decided that a bonus system would best meet the goals of the reward project and the selection criteria. The task force then proceeded to develop a program structure and process based on the delineation of "bonus behaviors."

Criteria	Percent of Weight		Rating		Significant Difference
	TF	RN	TF	RN	
Peer review	7	6	4.71	3.35	*
Individual initiatives	7	6	4.71	3.92	*
Supervisor review	5	5	3.57	3.11	

* $p < .01$.

Figure 22–6
Testing Criteria with Peers

Criteria

	Patient Review	Open to All RNs	Objective	Points
Weight	37 (4)	64 (7)	67(7)	
Program 1				
Program 2				
Program 3				

Figure 22–7
Multi-Attribute Utility Analysis

PROGRAM STRUCTURE AND PROCESS

It was determined that a Clinical Incentive Program was to be developed that would recognize and reward the professional nurse who extended his or her work performance outside of the expected job requirements. The program was to be one part of a total compensation package that also included:

- Merit pay (for performance related to the job standards).
- Shift differentials.
- Market adjustments.
- Holiday and weekend differentials.
- Employee recognition programs.

The Clinical Incentive Program was intended to reward professional nurses who contributed to the improvement of quality patient care through contracting for "bonus points" in the following areas:

- Clinical.
- Educational.
- Administrative.
- Research.

Bonus points were to be assigned to specific individualized projects, tasks, behaviors, or processes that the nurses contracted to perform. A committee of peers would review and evaluate all contracts and recommend the award of bonus points and compensation upon completion of the contract.

BONUS BEHAVIORS

The challenge for the task force was to identify "bonus behaviors"—behaviors that were above and beyond the basic job description and were consistent with the mission of the division of nursing. It now became clear to the task force members why the mission and job descriptions had had to be addressed by this group. It made the identification of "bonus behaviors" easier, because the core activities had already been defined. The group proceeded to identify thirty-three "bonus behaviors." Each behavior was then rated, based on several criteria:

- Time or frequency of the behavior.
- Importance of contribution to the organization.
- Consequences of error.
- Difficulty.

After each behavior was rated, it was compared to all others and a weighted average was determined for each behavior (Figure 22–8). The task force determined that a minimum of 7 points must be achieved in order to receive bonus compensation. Each bonus point had an associated dollar amount, for example, $150. Each participant could earn up to 20 bonus points for any one contract year. Therefore, the amount of bonus compensation that an individual might earn could vary between a minimum of $1,050 and a maximum of $3,000. The task force predicted that approximately 30 percent of the registered nurses would choose to participate in the

Behavior	Relative Weight	Dollar Value
Preceptor—graduate nurse	5	1,100
Develop patient education tool	4	880
Journal (outside)	3	660
Resource consultant	3	660
Longevity	1	220

Figure 22–8
Bonus Behaviors: Partial List

program and would earn an average of 14 points. Based on a total of 475 eligible nurses, this would cost approximately $300,000. A range of 20 percent to 40 percent participation would cost the organization $200,000 to $400,000, respectively.

The task force went on to develop other aspects of the program. For example, it determined that each person who contracted to participate in the bonus program would need to have at least one behavior designated as direct patient care. The rationale was that the program was intended as a Clinical Incentive Program; therefore, the direct clinical application of a bonus behavior must be evident in at least one of the contracted behaviors. Figure 22–9 outlines one bonus behavior, showing its point value, dollar value, guidelines, evaluation criteria, need for peer adviser, and qualification as a direct patient care activity. These are discussed in the following sections.

Point Value

The assigned value ranges between 1 and 6 points. An applicant can accumulate up to 20 points per contract year by including several bonus behaviors in a contract. To enter the program, an applicant must contract for a minimum of 7 points. To contract for fewer points would not be worth the administrative effort needed to review the contract.

Dollar Value

The assigned dollar value is based on the total point value multiplied by $150. The dollar value may change from year to year, based on the amount assigned to each point.

Bonus Behavior	Value Point	Value Dollar	Guidelines	Evaluation Criteria	Peer Adviser?	Direct Patient Care?
Preceptor for graduate nurse or inexperienced RN	6	900	Designated by Head Nurse, actively serve one time	1 & 5	No	Yes

Figure 22–9
Sample Outline of a Bonus Behavior

Guidelines

The guidelines are intended to inform the applicant about the scope of activities that the Peer Board expects for each behavior, illustrated with some examples. It was not possible to include a description of all acceptable activities because the program was designed to be flexible and to respond to the creative ideas of the applicants. However, all behaviors awarded through the Clinical Incentive Program must fall within one of the thirty-three bonus behaviors.

Evaluation Criteria

Each applicant must submit evidence that the terms of the contract have been met. Necessary evaluation criteria are listed by their reference number. For individualized bonus behaviors, such as teaching projects, research, and consultant role, the evaluation criteria are to be thought of as guidelines for development of criteria specific to a particular project or program. Written documentation for evaluation may come from the following sources:

1. Input from Head Nurse about performance.
2. Input from Peers about performance.
3. Feedback from patients (e.g., comments after attendance at education program; change in clinical condition as documented in chart; number in attendance, etc.).
4. Feedback from family (e.g., comments after attendance at a support group or educational program; number of attendees).
5. Feedback from staff (e.g., comments about the contributions that a change, program, or policy has made to unit functioning; evaluation form completed by preceptee; inservice evaluation).
6. Evidence of outcome indicators (e.g., description of the degree to which clinical or learning objectives were met, as measured by posttests, change in patient condition, comments made by participants).
7. Review by expert in area (e.g., research project examined for its content or research procedure by a knowledgeable expert; cost savings for cost-effective changes, supported by review conducted by financial experts).
8. Evidence that the behavior occurred, as measured by a log of attendance, schedule of hours worked, transcript, certificate, minutes of

meetings, number of people precepted, or actual product (e.g., an article). For teaching programs, the number of people who attended a program and/or the number of hours of instruction or number of times an educational tool was used.

9. One- to two-page proposal (maximum) outlining the rationale for doing the project, the plan for implementation, and the means to evaluate the project for its effectiveness.

Need for Peer Adviser

This column designates those behaviors for which the applicant could benefit from input from a peer adviser. Because many behaviors are individualized, specific guidelines and evaluation criteria need to be individually determined.

Qualification as Direct Patient Care Activity

It is recognized that all the behaviors listed as bonus behaviors ultimately relate to patient care. Those that are designated as direct patient care activities are more directly linked to the patient as the recipient, and have an action component associated with them. In any one contract, the applicant must include at least one behavior designated as a direct patient care activity.

PROGRAM IMPLEMENTATION

Within one year, the task force had completed its task: it had developed a Clinical Incentive Program that met the goals of the organization and the criteria for an acceptable program.

The program was fully developed, with policies and procedures established for each of the following:

1. Eligibility criteria.
2. Application procedure, including:
   —Time frame for application submission,
   —Forms and procedures to complete,

    —Terms of the contract and how to submit it,

    —Procedures to withdraw,

    —Conflict resolution procèdures.

3. Review and approval of contracts by Peer Review Board.

4. Appeal process.

5. Compensation upon successful completion of the contract.

6. Composition, selection, and terms of the Peer Review Board.

In the compensation system that resulted from this process, individual initiative, peer review, and commitment were vital components. Task force members identified certain criteria as essential to the success of the Clinical Incentive Program and the satisfaction of its participants. The system was founded on the belief that recruitment and retention of registered nurses would be positively affected by a program that met the agreed-on criteria.

The task force proceeded with the Clinical Incentive Program on the premise that it met the criteria for a successful program and that it had the potential to meet the program goals. The extent to which the program would become a success would be determined by how well it resolved unanticipated as well as predicted problems. The intent was to provide an incentive program that met the current needs of the organization's registered nurses. Other issues that remained for consideration by the Peer Review Board included:

1. The reward system is not a promotion system appropriate for career planning. Career opportunities are important for the attraction and retention of nurses into the profession. Therefore, as the system was revised, these needs would have to be considered.

2. Absolute dollar amounts associated with bonus points need to be variable so that money earned through the bonus system provides adequate incentive and compensation.

3. Identified bonus behaviors need to be revised frequently enough to reflect changes in the role of the registered nurse.

4. The program requires ongoing evaluation in order to keep it responsive to staff and administrative needs.

Before the program could be implemented as designed, environmental changes occurred that caused the Peer Review Board to place the program on hold. There was an urgent need to remain competitive with salaries, in order to attract and retain nurses. The alternative plan was to give large market adjustments to salaries for registered nurses across the board. The money that would have been used to support the bonus program was needed for the market adjustments. The bonus program would have taken a year; the market adjustments were immediate. Therefore, the task force agreed to the immediate increase in salary rather than the year's wait.

CONCLUSION

The process of participating in this task force remained a positive experience because the nurses felt empowered to develop their own reward system and they had been significantly included in decision making. The work of the task force served as a model for how nurses would be involved in decision making in the future as the organization established its shared governance structure. The nurses on the task force developed a tolerance and appreciation for examining the "whole" of nursing. They recognized that, in caring organizations, rewards flow from the mission, and the two need to be congruent so that values, beliefs, and caring practices are reinforced.

REFERENCES

Gaut, D. A. (1984). A theoretic description of caring as action. In M. Leininger (Ed.), *Care: The essence of nursing and health* (pp. 27–44). Thorofare, NJ: Slack.

Katz, J., & Green, E. (1992). *Managing quality: A guide to monitoring and evaluating nursing services.* St. Louis: Mosby.

Leininger, M. (1988). History, issues and trends in the discovery and uses of care in nursing. In M. Leininger (Ed.), *Care: Discovery and uses in clinical and community nursing* (pp. 11–28). Detroit: Wayne State University Press.

Noddings, N. (1984). *Caring.* Berkeley: University of California Press.

Ray, M. A. (1987). Health care economics and human caring in nursing: Why the moral conflict must be resolved. *Family Community Health, 10* (1), 35–43.

Rozboril, A. (1987). Systematic downsizing: An experiment. *Journal of Nursing Administration, 17*(9), 19–22.

Trochim, W. M. K. (1989). An introduction to concept mapping for planning and evaluation. *Evaluation and Program Planning, 12* (1), 1–16.

Trochim, W. K., & Linton, R. (1986). Conceptualization for planning and evaluation. *Evaluation and Program Planning,* (9), 289–308.

Valentine, K. L. (1989a). Caring is more than kindness: Modeling its complexities. *Journal of Nursing Administration, 19* (11), 28–34.

Valentine, K. (1989b). Contributions to the theory of care. *Evaluation and Program Planning, 12* (1), 17–24.

Valentine, K. L. (1991). A comprehensive assessment of caring and its relationship to health outcomes. *Journal of Nursing Quality Assurance, 5* (2), 59–68.

Valentine, K. L. (1992). Strategic Planning for Professional Practice. *Journal of Nursing Care Quality, 6* (3), 1–12.

Watson, J. (1985). *Nursing: Human science and human care.* Norwalk, CT: Appleton-Century-Crofts.

Weisbord, M. (1978). *Organizational diagnosis: A workbook of theory and practice.* Reading, MA: Addison-Wesley.

23

Shared Governance: A Model of Caring in Practice

Alanna Wells

Caring is a phenomenon that affects all humanity. Each person has the natural inclination and desire to be "cared for" and "to care" (Leininger, 1988a; Noddings, 1984). The expression and practice of this caring ethic are defined within one's cultural boundaries (Leininger, 1988b). This definition includes nurses.

Nurses are a group of caregivers who have their own values, beliefs, opinions, and needs that define their cultural identity (Leininger, 1988a). As caregivers, they also need to be care receivers and to have their care needs attended to as they are defined by their culture. This renews their energies and maximizes their caring for patients (Keen, 1992). With caring described as the essence of nursing (Leininger, 1988a), this need for caring by nurses is the ideal opportunity for nursing administrators to embrace the caring ethic as the essence of their practice. Nursing administrators are the "leaders of a caring contingent" (Johnson, 1992, p. 11) and can care indirectly for patients by nurturing a caring relationship between themselves and staff nurses, that is, by responding to the need of staff nurses to be cared for as professionals and human beings. The approach that nursing administrators and leaders take in caring for and about staff nurses' relationships and the environment in which they take place can affect nurses in a most positive way. These caring actions shape the structure, character, and behavior of the nursing organization they guide (Johnson, 1992) and, thus, are responsible for much of the success of the organization.

The caring constructs that have been defined in caring literature regarding patient care can be applied within the nursing administrator–staff nurse relationship. They are similar to transformational leadership practices defined by Senge (1990), Covey (1989), and Porter-O'Grady (1992a). The caring constructs referred to include listening (Mayeroff, 1971), presence (Leininger, 1988a; Watson, 1988), and trust, facilitation, and compassion (Leininger, 1988a). If nursing administrators listen to the needs of the nurses, they will hear what nurses and studies on nurses' dissatisfaction have been saying for some years. Nurses, to practice and be accountable as professionals, need autonomy, authority, and control over their practice (Department of Health and Human Services, 1988; Moloney, 1992; National Commission on Nursing, 1982; Porter-O'Grady, 1992b).

Nurses state that these are primary needs for their continued growth, development, and self-actualization. Nursing administrators have felt and should recognize the natural conflicts that exist between a professional and the traditional hierarchical structures of hospitals:

1. A professional's primary commitment is to the public versus the organization (Stichler, 1992).

2. The nursing professional's view on life is holistic versus mechanistic, flexible versus rigid, and knowledge-based versus task-oriented (Porter-O'Grady & Finnegan, 1984).

Indeed, bureaucratic structures are very limiting to the full development of nursing and "fail to nurture a caring philosophy of administration" (Leininger, 1988b, p. 381).

Upon hearing the staff nurses' needs, it becomes part of the nursing executives' accountability to their profession to act by changing the stifling, rigid environments of bureaucracy. Caring requires action and attention to the care receiver's decisions, values, and claims (Gaut, 1983). Caring also implies the creation of an environment that fosters another's growth by meeting his or her stated needs (Mayeroff, 1971; Ray, 1988). It is here that shared governance becomes the natural outcome of a nursing leader's acting on the needs and requests of nurses. In the past 10 years, this management practice has been shown to be a valid and useful means of supporting the growth of nurses individually and as a profession within hospital practice settings (Porter-O'Grady, 1992b). This growth is defined as increasing self-confidence, maturation as leaders and followers, and fulfillment in being a nurse.

In this chapter, it is my intent to define shared governance, describe its principles, and identify the key components of its implementation process. It is my primary goal to show how the determinants of shared governance embody caring theory. Further goals include:

1. Showing how shared governance is a natural outcome of nursing leaders' caring for nurses.
2. Demonstrating how shared governance is a practical application of caring behaviors between administration and the patient care nurse.
3. Discussing the gestalt of caring behaviors and shared governance principles.

The fulfillment of nursing's need for growth and its progress toward self-actualization as the primary goal of caring is honored. This goal achievement is explicated by imparting outcomes of shared governance discussed in the literature and experienced by me at Santa Rosa Memorial Hospital, Santa Rosa, California, and Petaluma Valley Hospital, Petaluma, California.

SHARED GOVERNANCE: KEY COMPONENTS AND THEIR RELATIONSHIP TO CARING THEORY

Definition of Shared Governance

Shared governance is a management theory and practice requiring collaborative processes that balance power and provide for reciprocation through communications and interpersonal valuing (Stichler, 1992). The primary objective of shared governance is to transcend the frustrations and dependency experienced in bureaucracy by creating an environment in which nurses feel renewed and satisfied in their profession (Porter-O'Grady, 1986, 1992a).

Principles

The principles of shared governance are its core and substance (Porter-O'Grady, 1992b). Its structures can be designed and implemented, but there will be little commitment to those systems without acknowledging and practicing the principles that drive those systems. These principles, which are fairly straightforward, include:

1. *Decentralization.* Decisions and problem solving should occur at the lowest level of the organization (Porter-O'Grady & Finnegan, 1984). This requires respecting the authority and knowledge of staff nurses within departments, who are the experts in patient care.

2. *Democratic representation.* Full representation of all nurses is provided for in the decision-making process (Porter-O'Grady, 1992b), so each person's cultural care values can be expressed.

3. *Shared power.* Leaders must be willing to share their power with staff nurses (Porter-O'Grady, 1989, 1992b; Stichler, 1992) and thus balance power. There is no single locus of control in shared governance. Staff nurses and managers have their defined areas of autonomy.

4. *Empowerment.* When empowered, an individual grows in his or her sense of self-worth. Empowerment is provided through treating individuals with respect and dignity, providing recognition for their contributions, and continually finding ways for their power to grow within. A rewarding result of empowerment is that shame-based behaviors such as manipulation, anger, rage, passive aggressiveness, and perfection (Potter-Effron & Potter-Effron, 1989) are no longer necessary or useful. Instead, new level of self-fulfillment and participation in our destiny enrich our work experience and, concomitantly, our response to it (Shidler, Pencak, & McFolling, 1989; Stichler, 1992).

5. *Collegial and collective bonding.* Leininger (1981) stated that nursing is a culture with its own cultural care values that influence caregiving and care receiving behaviors. This culture of caring has been submerged or lost because of bureaucratic frustrations (Porter-O'Grady, 1986; Stichler, 1992), physicians' paternalism, society's de-emphasis on caring and emphasis on separation, and

nurses' drive to be high-tech and part of the medical model (Gordon, 1991). Competition among ourselves as nurses has also contributed significantly to separation among ourselves (Keen, 1992; Styles, 1982). Shared governance provides a means for reawakening our culture and finding our shared meanings so that we can be collegial with each other and collectively together as a whole profession.

6. *A basis of trust.* This principle is not immediate but is supported and allowed to grow by the practice of the previous principles, transformational leadership, and effective communication (Porter-O'Grady, 1992b).

Implementation: Initial Change Strategy

Leaders proposing a change to shared governance could be the chief nursing executive, managers, or staff nurse leaders. They must express their view of the environment and their perceptions regarding the kind of change needed to make a positive impact on those they serve in their environment.

It is, however, very important to broaden this assessment to the entire environment, which means listening to staff nurses' responses to their environment. Do they identify symptoms such as poor morale, frustration and apathy among nurses, poor productivity, or a desire to do things differently in the nursing organization? If so, then this is indeed an opportune time to initiate a shared governance process as a response to their environment.

Thoroughness in this assessment is essential to caring, because intentional caring implies that the caregiver is trying to reach a goal. For the care receiver to be receptive to this goal, the care receiver must also identify the need for change and want the proposed action (Gaut, 1983). For a change to a shared governance model to be successful, it must have the support of the nursing executive, key management staff, and key nursing staff leaders (union officers, charge nurses, and informal staff leaders) as caregivers and care receivers (Porter-O'Grady, 1992b).

In this process, if there is enough support to continue pursuing this management model, then there is a need to decide on its name, structure, and operational strategies. This begins the reawakening of collegiality and collectivity because there is a natural exploration of the shared meanings and values of the nurses within the organization, who have their own unique characteristics.

Structure

Names and Designs. Shared governance can have different names—collaborative governance, advocacy, professional practice model, and total quality management. It can be designed as a senate, a congress, an assembly, or a council.

The most popular structure within organizations and nursing divisions seems to be the council model (Porter-O'Grady, 1992b; Smith, 1992). Councils were first discussed within the scope of shared governance by Porter-O'Grady and Finnegan (1984) and subsequently by Porter-O'Grady (1992b). Councils typically grow out of committees that currently may be dealing with procedures, quality improvement, documentation, and professional practice.

What's different? Councils have more autonomy, authority, and control over final decisions related to their area of accountability. The councils and areas of professional accountability recommended by Porter-O'Grady (1992b) include nursing practice, education, quality assurance, research, and management of resources. An overseeing body such as Coordinating Council is used in congress and council models and generally includes council chairs (and/or union officers in a union setting), the chief nursing executive, and management staff. Each hospital and nursing department needs to decide on the correct number and type of councils that best fit their strategies and goals.

Authority Levels. The goal regarding authority levels is to allow councils to have control over their own decisions, once they have sought appropriate input into their work at hand. This is usually a developmental process, and mistakes must be allowed to engender growth. It is very important to give this autonomy to councils in order for them to accept the reciprocal accountability afforded to professionals (Stichler, 1992).

Veto power retained by the nursing executive defeats this goal (Porter-O'Grady, 1989) and does not allow trust to flourish. Veto power may need to be retained for fiscal decisions in union settings and in organizations that are struggling to maintain fiscal viability. However, efforts should be made to educate nurses of fiscal matters and to allow them to share in this decision making.

Bylaws. Each council must develop its own set of bylaws or structure standards that describe its purpose, scope of responsibility, membership, and authority level. Written bylaws that guide the conduct and business of each council give it direction and help to build trust by setting expectations within which the council can operate.

Membership Guidelines. Each department is represented on the council. Management representation is no more than fifty percent and preferably less. This helps to balance power. Members can be voted on by their departments, but frequently in the beginning stages they need to be solicited. The election of staff nurse chairpersons is encouraged. These membership guidelines naturally promote independence and growth within staff nurses.

Department Level Process. The structure design needs to include communication systems that allow for feedback from councils to individual departments and input from those departments back to councils via representatives. These systems preserve the democratic nature of shared governance. Perhaps one of the most difficult steps of implementing shared governance is finding the systems that work effectively in this feedback loop. It also takes patience (Mayeroff, 1971) to wait for staff nurses to be interested and trusting enough to participate fully in the loop (Smith, 1992). This trust is built by caring about, respecting, and acting on their thoughts and ideas.

Developmental Purpose of Councils. The most important function of councils and departmental collaboration is to capture the individual abilities of each nurse. Each nurse has a unique contribution to make to the success of the collective whole (Stichler, 1992). Leaders must probe ways to bring the strengths of each nurse to the forefront; each person's strengths complement another's weaknesses, and together we make a complementary whole. In doing this, the embodiment of caring is demonstrated in the governance model. We empower each other so that we can grow in our strengths, reverse our weaknesses, and create health for the organization.

Mission and Vision

A mission statement tells nurses and their constituencies about the present image of nursing within the organization. It helps to define and strengthen nurses' identity to themselves and others. A vision creates the image, goals, and hope for the future. It is the driving force behind present and future decision making. Frankl (1984, p. 94) reminded us of the basic need for our humanity; "It is a peculiarity of man that he can only live by looking into the future."

Establishing the mission and vision of a nursing organization is an integral component of shared governance and a key area in which cultural caring occurs. The mission and vision are generally written early in the development of shared governance. They are dynamic documents: they change as nurses evolve and have higher-level needs for self-development. These documents must be written collaboratively through the Coordinating Council or by a group that includes top nursing executives and key staff nurse leaders. Each person's thoughts, values, beliefs, and ideals need to be heard and, wherever possible, incorporated into the mission and vision.

The top nursing executive frequently initiates this process by planning a retreat of the key developmental team. The executive also ensures that the essence of nursing's mission and vision is compatible with that of the organization. When the mission and vision are drafted, they are shared in each nursing department. Input from all staff nurses is encouraged and added to the mission and vision statements after evaluation by the developing team.

At this time, it is also very effective to write behavior statements that are based on the core principles of shared governance, as they have been described. These statements will help to guide relationships among nurses, administration, peers, and other health care workers as shared governance progresses in the organization.

This exercise is a consensus-building event and an exciting team-building experience. It provides a strong mechanism for staff nurses and managers to align themselves by creating a common and shared purpose (Koerner & Bunkers, 1992). This work generates and helps sustain in a changing environment a synergism that those who are caring for nurses and those who are receiving that care can support. Figures 23–1 through 23–3 are examples of mission, vision, and principle statements.

Education and Publication

For the growth of shared governance, to provide to the staff at large many educational sessions and publications about the principles of shared governance and how it is being implemented within the organization. It takes at least 5 years to really capture and rejuvenate the majority of nurses who have mistrusted administration or who have had a general malaise regarding their profession. Changing their beliefs about what is actually possible with shared governance requires persistence and commitment to this caring process. Education at both division and department levels by the manager and council representatives is vital to changing beliefs and behaviors. Education

The mission of the nurses at Petaluma Valley Hospital is to provide patient/family-centered care and:

—Facilitate an optimal level of health by caring for the individual as a whole person throughout all stages of life.

—Be accountable health care professionals by utilizing appropriate technology and resources in our role as patient advocates.

—Expand our knowledge and expertise in response to the need for change.

—Exert a positive influence as compassionate health care professionals within our community.

—Share our knowledge as health educators, with patients, families, peers, and the community.

Figure 23–1
Mission Statement: Petaluma Valley Hospital, Petaluma, California

is part of "caring for" others because they need the tools necessary to be receptive to this caring and to reciprocate with anticipated changes (Noddings, 1984).

Publicizing the work of councils, particularly their successes, provides invaluable recognition of their members. This nurtures a continued desire to participate in their future and encourages other nurses to become interested in the process.

The vision of nurses at Petaluma Valley Hospital is to excel in our own development in order to:

—Participate and plan for effective, progressive nursing practice.

—Honor patient and family rights through consideration of each individual's dignity.

—Be politically active and respond to our community's health care needs.

—Create an environment that promotes trust, mutual respect, confidentiality, and collaboration.

—Share our experience, strength, and hope with our peers, colleagues, and other health care providers.

—Implement an effective shared governance model that meets the needs of the nurses at Petaluma Valley Hospital.

Figure 23–2
Vision Statement: Petaluma Valley Hospital, Petaluma, California

1. Knowledge is power.
2. Given adequate information, people will make appropriate decisions.
3. Risk taking with or without success is growth.
4. Effective communication requires attentive listening and a thoughtful response.
5. We recognize each individual's unique contribution to our organization.
6. All problems identified are mutually owned, and responsibility for resolution begins with problem identification.
7. We acknowledge that a commitment to collaborate among departments is necessary for success.
8. We are committed to provide educational and developmental opportunities in an atmosphere that shares knowledge and directs organizational energy toward common goals.
9. We accept the responsibility of providing a systemwide climate of learning which promotes the development of the nurse from novice to expert.
10. Our actions will comply with federal and state regulations and acknowledge reasonable economic constraints.

Figure 23–3
Principle Statements of Petaluma Valley Hospital, Petaluma, California

Behaviors

In addition to the principles previously described, shared governance provides facilitative systems that increase among nurses the sense of being cared for. If nurses and leaders are to really feel the joy of being cared for as Noddings (1984) described, the effort must be augmented by making a commitment to change the behaviors that supported bureaucratic management structures such as controlling, heroism, co-dependency, and authoritarian and manipulative coping mechanisms (Bradford & Cohen, 1984).

There is a calling in shared governance for transformational leaders who can demonstrate the courage, commitment, compassion, and competence described by Roach (1984) as caring phenomena. These personal behavior changes in leaders, and subsequently in nurses, are predictive of the success or failure of shared governance and measure the depth of nurses' caring. Substantive behavior changes such as these can be achieved through the learning and practice of new leadership styles and effective communication.

Leadership

Transformational nurse leaders are congruent with shared governance because their primary role is to facilitate, coordinate, and integrate the work and decisions of nurses' councils and ensure their correlation with the needs of other departments (Porter-O'Grady, 1992a). The characteristics of transformational leadership are not always innate; frequently, they must be learned by nursing executives, managers, and staff nurse leaders. These leaders in turn have a personal accountability to model these new learned behaviors to staff nurses, who can then make the choice of becoming leaders in their practice areas or effective followers.

Transformational leadership characteristics include:

1. Transformational consciousness—identifying change as a constant, valuing it, and incorporating this value into the culture of the workplace (Porter-O'Grady, 1992a).

2. Facilitator—assisting nurses in their adaptation to a constantly changing environment and removing barriers so that they can work to their full potential (Peters, 1987).

3. Focus on relationships—understanding that the quality of patient care is directly affected by staff nurses' satisfaction with their environment (Porter-O'Grady, 1992a). If leaders focus on building and adapting to mature relationships with nurses, the product of their efforts will be enhanced success for the organization.

4. System-oriented versus blaming—recognizing that failures in the organization are typically related to malfunctioning systems, not individuals. Leaders are able to guide nurses through systems changes that are responsive to the needs of the profession and organization as a whole (Senge, 1990).

5. Coach and mentor—educating oneself and others in the new leadership behaviors (Nyberg, 1989).

6. Risk taker—trying new ways of doing things without the fear of failure, and trusting others to do the same, when their intuition drives them (Peters, 1987). "It must be safe to risk and to stretch the boundaries of thinking and doing" (Porter-O'Grady, 1992a). Risk takers also:

   —Communicate directly and in a caring way the dysfunctional behaviors they observe in their colleagues, employees, and leaders (Covey, 1989).

—State their needs and, therefore, their vulnerability.

—Deal with conflicts in a timely way and strive for win–win resolutions (Bradford & Cohen, 1984).

—State their expectations that each person will work to his or her full potential, which is a strong caring message (Schaffer, 1991).

7. Expert management of resources—managing the resources of the environment well, with employees, so that there is security and, in turn, space for self-growth and actualization.

8. Self-care—"caring for" oneself and being receptive to one's own needs (Nyberg, 1989). Transformational leaders need to demonstrate self-care and assist others to gently care for themselves (Watson, 1985).

These leadership characteristics assist nursing executives in caring for and about nurses, because there are ways of being with nurses that respond to their needs and fulfill their goals. These characteristics are demonstrated through actions such as working with nurses in establishing the structure of shared governance, facilitating a retreat to write a mission and vision, providing resources for education, and working through conflicts. However, in facilitating and coordinating these changes, effective communications by all parties directly affect the enthusiasm and ease of moving through the change. Communications that engender a feeling of being cared for build trust and confidence between nurses and administration. It is my belief that effective communications reflect "care" and therefore are named caring communications for the purpose of this discussion.

Caring Communications

Caring is seeking out what matters to another (Benner & Wrubel, 1989). In order to do this, we must be willing to communicate through attentive listening, and openness to hear and understand what another has to say. This skill takes much effort, but its rewards are endless in building relationships between nurses and their cohorts on the health care team, including administrators. If we respect others enough to listen to them and be clear on our perceptions of the message they are trying to send, conflicts can usually be avoided or resolved and a healthy environment ensues.

Connection is another caring action that we usually reserve for our patients, but it is also necessary for the nurses providing this care. Connection is a transpersonal experience in which the energy of our spirits is shared. We all have experienced this with patients, but we need to offer this to each other when our associates are feeling angry, vulnerable, scared, or sad for any reason. This transpersonal caring accesses the higher human spirit and, therefore, has the capacity to expand human consciousness, transcend the moment, and potentiate healing and trust (Watson, 1985).

Other components of caring communications include the expression of:

1. Compassion—understanding and sharing the pain and joy of another's life experience (Roach, 1984).
2. Confidence—being confident in one's self-worth and self-understanding. Leaders' demonstration of this is required through words, actions, and care of self (Nyberg, 1989).
3. Humility—resisting the role of hero that leads to overcontrol; taking more blame and less credit (Heider, 1985).
4. Honesty—being rigorously truthful with ourselves and others by verbally owning our feelings, actions, and motivations.

The last major expression of caring communication is patience. Caring is not always fun. In fact, it is frequently frustrating and rarely easy (Mayeroff, 1971). We must remember, however, that everyone has his or her own process for growth and this evolution will come in its own time. We cannot force it; we can only teach and practice what we would like others to absorb. They may or may not grow in the direction and in the timeframe we desire. There is no right or wrong involved. We as leaders and nurses must allow for either outcome and have the patience to honor each individual regardless of this outcome.

These are rather rigorous behaviors to expect leaders and staff nurses to learn and adapt to. There can be a great deal of resistance to these changes. Those who take the step forward beyond their feelings of resistance must provide mechanisms of care for themselves so they can continue to evolve. To care for and love ourselves is a very rich expression of caring and a significant means of self-empowerment.

SHARED GOVERNANCE OUTCOMES

Shared governance meets the requirements of nurses for maturation in an evolving professional culture. I found empirical evidence of this in outcomes that are documented in shared governance literature and through my personal implementation of shared governance.

The identified developmental needs that have been satisfied include increased autonomy, improved communications, trust and a sense of pride and satisfaction in being a nurse.

These outcomes are demonstrated in the following ways:

1. Continued increase in staff nurses' interest level and in their involvement in councils and special projects. This energy begins with leaders and moves forward to energize all staff (Ludemann & Brown, 1989).

2. Staff nurses' sharing of information and opinions in councils (Porter-O'Grady, 1992b).

3. Increased risk taking in nurses' writing or stating their frustrations to nursing managers and executives.

4. Managers' taking risks in dealing effectively with conflict.

5. Staff nurses' and managers' working together to develop and maintain budgets. (Staff nurses delayed a salary increase at Petaluma Valley Hospital. This was so phenomenal that it was reported in *California Hospitals* in July 1992.)

6. Peers' becoming accountable for mitigating conflicts in councils and within departments.

7. Council members' learning how to delegate to their peers within departments (Ludemann & Brown, 1989).

8. Staff nurses' engaging in the study of nursing theory and finding an even higher level of professional identity through this activity. (Caring theory has been chosen by staff nurses as a theoretical base for their practice at Santa Rosa Memorial Hospital, Santa Rosa, California. This choice was made when staff nurses recognized the explicit relationship between caring and shared governance, and caring theory's natural application to patient care.)

Shared governance in the future can guide nurses to an ever increasing level of professionalism (Porter-O'Grady, 1992c). It should never remain static. If caring theory can be envisioned as the basis for shared governance, then nurses experienced in this caring should begin to extend its practice to other departments. If caring is the essence of nursing, then let us care for and about the entire organization. This can have amazing outcomes, as we have experienced at Petaluma Valley Hospital, where caring is also a base theory for the nursing division. The effects on the organization from applying caring theory through shared governance have been:

- Caring is identified as a core value of the organization.
- Shared Management Teams govern ancillary departments. These teams usually include nursing representatives, department staff, department managers, physicians, and an ancillary director.
- Innovative and creative ideas have increased productivity and decreased financial losses and there is a commitment to maintain these changes.
- Morale and communications have improved throughout the institution.
- Staff members feel "safe" visiting with the CEO and directors to express concerns and frustrations.
- Staff nurses attend board meetings.

CONCLUSION

This chapter has pointed to the linkages between caring for another and shared governance as a natural outcome of nursing administrators' caring for staff nurses. The practices as well as the principles of shared governance and the caring ethic are interwoven. There are practical applications of caring theory for the administration–staff nurse relationship.

Porter-O'Grady (1992a, p. 18) has said that "complementarity between practice and theory is the essential foundation of the emerging leadership role." Nursing leaders have an ideal opportunity to demonstrate to nurses the real value of theory by applying caring in this valuable management framework of shared governance.

Additionally, nursing leaders have the responsibility for setting the tone of caring in health care facilities (Miller, 1987). There could be no better way of establishing this ethic than by using caring theory as the theory base for their organization and, as a result, establishing shared governance as a means of caring for and about staff nurses.

REFERENCES

Benner, P., & Wrubel, J. (1989). *The primacy of caring.* New York: Addison-Wesley.

Bradford, D., & Cohen, A. (1984). *Managing for excellence.* New York: Wiley.

Covey, S. (1989). *Seven habits of highly effective people.* New York: Simon & Schuster.

Department of Health and Human Services. (1988). *Secretary's commission on nursing: Volume 1*. Washington, DC: U.S. Government Printing Office.

Frankl, V. (1984). *Man's search for meaning*. New York: Washington Square Press.

Gaut, D. (1983). Development of a theoretically adequate description of caring. *Western Journal of Nursing Research, 5* (4), 313–324.

Gordon, S. (1991). Fear of caring: the feminist paradox. *American Journal of Nursing, 91* (2), 45–49.

Heider, J. (1985). *Tao of leadership*. New York: Bantam Books.

Johnson, L. (1992). Structure, strategies and synthesis: The nursing executive as social architect. *Nursing Administration Quarterly, 17*(1), 10–16.

Keen, P. (1992). Caring for ourselves. In R. Neil & R. Watts (Eds.), *Caring and nursing: Explorations in feminist perspectives*. New York: National League for Nursing.

Koerner, J., & Bunkers, S. (1992). Transformational leadership: The power of symbol. *Nursing Administration Quarterly, 17*(1), 1–9.

Leininger, M. (1981). Cross-cultural hypothetical functions of caring and nursing care. In M. Leininger (Ed.), *Caring: An essential human need.* (pp. 95–102). Thorofare, NJ: Slack.

Leininger, M. (1988a). The phenomena of caring: Importance, research questions and theoretical considerations. In M. Leininger (Ed.), *Caring: An essential human need.* (pp. 3–16). Detroit: Wayne State University Press.

Leininger, M. (1988b). Some philosophical, historical and taxonomic aspects of nursing and caring in American culture. In M. Leininger (Ed.), *Caring: An essential human need*. Detroit: Wayne State University Press.

Ludemann, R., & Brown, C. (1989). Staff perceptions of shared governance. *Nursing Administration Quarterly, 13*(4), 49–56.

Mayeroff, M. (1971). *On caring*. New York: Harper & Row.

Miller, K. L. (1987). The human care perspective in nursing administration. *Journal of Nursing Administration, 17*(2), 10–12.

Moloney, M. (1992). *Professionalization of nursing*. Philadelphia: Lippincott.

National Commission on Nursing. (1982). *Nursing in transition: Models for successful organizational change*. Chicago: Hospital Research and Education Trust.

Noddings, N. (1984). *Caring*. Berkeley: University of California Press.

Nyberg, J. (1989). The element of caring in nursing administration. *Nursing Administration Quarterly, 13*(3), 9–16.

Peters, T. (1987). *Thriving on chaos*. New York: Harper & Row.

Porter-O'Grady, T. (1986). *Creative nursing administration*. Rockville, MD: Aspen Publications.

Porter-O'Grady, T. (1989). Shared governance: Reality or shame? *American Journal of Nursing, 89*(3), 350–351.

Porter-O'Grady, T. (1992a). Transformational leadership in an age of chaos. *Nursing Administration Quarterly, 17*(1), 17–24.

Porter-O'Grady, T. (1992b). A decade of organizational change. In T. Porter-O'Grady (Ed.), *Implementing shared governance.* St Louis: Mosby.

Porter-O'Grady, T. (1992c). Shared governance: Looking towards the future. In T. Porter-O'Grady (Ed.), *Implementing shared governance.* St. Louis: Mosby.

Porter-O'Grady, T., & Finnegan, S. (1984). *Shared governance for nursing.* Rockville, MD: Aspen Publications.

Potter-Effron, R., & Potter–Effron, P. (1989). *Letting go of shame.* New York: Harper & Row.

Ray, M. (1988). A philosophical analysis of caring within nursing. In M. Leininger (Ed.), *Caring: An essential human need.* (pp. 25–36). Detroit: Wayne State University Press.

Ray, M. (1989). The theory of bureaucratic caring for nursing practice in the organizational culture. *Nursing Administration Quarterly, 13*(2), 31–42.

Roach, M. S. (1984). *Caring: The human code of being, implications for nursing.* Toronto, Canada: University of Toronto Press.

Schaffer, R. (1991). Demand better results and get them. *Harvard Business Review, 69*(2), 142–149.

Senge, P. (1990). *The fifth discipline.* Garden City, NY: Doubleday.

Shidler, H., Pencak, M., & McFolling, S. (1989). Professional nursing staff: A model of self-governance for nurses. *Nursing Administration Quarterly, 13*(4), 1–10.

Smith, S. (1992). Nursing staff roles in unfolding shared governance. In T. Porter-O'Grady (Ed.), *Implementing shared governance.* St. Louis: Mosby.

Stichler, J. (1992). A conceptual basis for shared governance. In T. Porter-O'Grady (Ed.), *Implementing shared governance.* St. Louis: Mosby.

Styles, M. (1982). *On nursing.* St. Louis: Mosby.

Watson, J. (1985). *Nursing: Human science and human care.* Boston: Little, Brown.

Watson, J. (1988). New dimensions of human caring theory. *Nursing Science Quarterly, 1*(4), 175–181.

24

Caring Behaviors of Nurse Managers: Relationships to Staff Nurse Satisfaction and Retention

Joanne R. Duffy

*I*n the health care industry today, nurse managers are faced with numerous challenges: cost and quality concerns, environmental issues, and the retention of satisfied, competent staff. This last area is a chronic and poorly understood phenomenon and one of national concern. It has been studied under the guise of nursing turnover. The purpose of this chapter is to explore the impact of nurse managers' caring behaviors on staff nurse satisfaction and retention.

Traditionally, turnover has been defined as "the percentage of employed nurses who leave their jobs during a time period" (Davis & Bertram, 1991) and is usually expressed as a percentage. The national nursing turnover rate has recently been reported at 28 percent (Ambrose, 1990); however, in some regions of the United States, this figure may be higher or lower. Although some positives have been attributed to nursing turnover (Abelson, 1986; Miller, 1988), most of the literature on the subject suggests negative consequences. Most often reported is the cost of nursing turnover. In financial terms, turnover represents a major source of expense for hospitals. In one study of four acute-care hospitals in the southeastern United States, Jones (1988) reported a 28.8 percent turnover rate with costs averaging about 11 percent of the average annual RN salary budget. Jones further calculated the average cost of replacing one nurse to be greater than $10,000.

The cost of replacement is a serious issue; recruitment and hiring expenses, orientation, training (including the use of preceptors and decreased productivity), and termination costs are involved (Jones, 1988; Wise, 1990). According to Jones (1988), the two largest expenses associated with turnover are: covering the unfilled positions, and orientation and training costs. Jolma (1990) reported additional expenses such as lower employee morale, decreased quality of patient care, and fewer successes in new programs and services. Wall (1988) stated that these consequences may jeopardize the public image of the hospital and negatively influence medical-staff relationships. Several studies have indicated that an important reason for turnover among staff nurses is lack of job satisfaction (Kramer & Schmalenberg, 1991; Prescott, 1986; Price & Meuller, 1981; Seybolt, 1986; Sigardson, 1982).

Job satisfaction is a subjective perception from the employee's point of view and implies fulfillment of work expectations. Job satisfaction is composed of many factors (Kramer & Schmalenberg, 1991; Price & Meuller, 1982; Seybolt, 1986): organizational structure, professional practice, professional development, management style, and quality of leadership (Kramer & Schmalenberg, 1991). These last two factors, which concern the characteristics and behaviors of nurse managers, are crucial to our understanding, especially because the literature is beginning to support humanistic and/or caring administrators as predictors of staff nurse retention (Kramer & Schmalenberg, 1988, 1991).

Nurse managers play a critical role in the development and retention of staff. Through role modeling and human interaction, nurse managers ensure that caring remains central to nursing practice. Dunham (1989) noted that caring for staff must pervade the nursing profession and suggested several behaviors through which nursing administrators might display caring: leadership, communication, meaning/value, power, decision making, problem solving/conflict resolution, change, organizational behavior, futurology, planning/marketing, and re-education/continued learning. Nyberg (1989) described commitment, self-worth, ability to prioritize, openness, and the ability to bring out potential as necessary requisites for administrative caring. Through these behaviors, enhanced satisfaction of nursing staff may result. The nursing administration research literature, however, reflects few actual studies of caring. In fact, Brenner et al. (1986), in a major review of the administrative literature, found no use of caring as an independent variable.

A few qualitative studies have been completed. In the Magnet Hospital Study, McClure (1983) concluded that nursing administrators who communicate, acknowledge employee needs for recognition, and demonstrate genuine concern enhance staff participation and satisfaction. Ray (1989) examined the meaning of caring in an acute-care urban hospital and found many meanings that were contextually based. In other words, individuals' roles, actual work units, power, and position in the organization seemed to influence the meaning attached to caring. MacPherson's (1989) work also reminded us of the impact of corporate culture on the meaning of caring.

In an important study of 203 RNs, Bucchieri (1986) found higher satisfaction levels among staff nurses when perception of supervisor support was present. This study was consistent with others in which supervisors' interactions with staff were a key factor in satisfaction and retention. Finally, in a small nonexperimental study of staff nurse perceptions of important leadership characteristics, Meighan (1990) reported that 71 percent of the sample believed that "caring" was important.

These few studies of administrative caring are disheartening, especially in the face of reports that double standards presently exist in hospitals (Norris, 1989). Nursing administrators have been reported to "demand loyalty, blame instead of problem-solve, sanction excessively harsh punishments, fail to promote self-esteem, fail to allow time for feelings of grief, anger, or failure, and fail to make allowances for nurses' personal concerns" (p. 548). Consider the following remarks from a staff nurse in this study: "I find my nursing coordinator difficult to approach. She is frequently angry when asked questions and sometimes rude. Her main concern on the unit seems to be cleaning." These behaviors are counter to the human caring attitudes and actions that staff nurses are expected to implement and that have been reported to contribute to positive patient outcomes (Duffy, 1992). It is logical to consider that these feelings may provoke dissatisfaction and may negatively impact the work environment. Nurses who have negative experiences with their managers may even begin to look for work elsewhere, increasing the turnover burden on an organization. Watson's (1985) theory of human care supports this stance and is the theoretical basis for this study.

Rushton (1992) espoused nurses' being "enabled to care by being empowered to care. . . . Administrators . . . have a responsibility to create an environment where the burdens and suffering of caregivers can be appreciated and addressed in a supportive and constructive manner" (p. 305). Knowledge of nurse manager caring and its relationship to staff nurse satisfaction and turnover will contribute to nursing's knowledge base and provide guidelines for nursing administration. To control for the impact of unit type and number of employees on turnover, these variables were statistically controlled for in this study.

PURPOSES

The purposes of this study are:

1. To describe the caring behaviors of nurse managers.
2. To describe the relationship between nurse-manager caring behaviors and staff nurse satisfaction.
3. To describe the relationship between nurse manager caring behaviors and turnover rates among staff nurses.
4. To establish the reliability and validity of the Caring Assessment Tool-Administrative Version (CAT-A).

ASSUMPTIONS

1. Caring behaviors can be measured.
2. Staff nurses responded truthfully to all questionnaires.

RESEARCH HYPOTHESES

1. There will be a positive relationship between nurse manager caring behaviors and staff nurse job satisfaction.
2. There will be an inverse relationship between nurse manager caring behaviors and staff nurse turnover.

METHODS

A descriptive correlational research design was selected to investigate the study hypotheses. A voluntary, 535-bed, university teaching hospital comprised the setting.

SAMPLE

I chose a purposive, random sample of 100 subjects based on the following criteria: (1) full-time and part-time registered nurses (2) assigned to a

Department of Nursing designated cost center. The sample size was based on a medium effect, an alpha of .05, and a power of 80 percent (Cohen & Cohen, 1975). In total, 100 staff nurses were approached and 56 willingly completed the questionnaires within 48 hours; thus, the sample return rate was 56 percent. Of the 44 nurses who did not respond, there were no significant differences in age, educational preparation, years of experience, and employment status.

INSTRUMENTATION

Two instruments were used to collect data for this study. The CAT-A (Duffy, 1992) was amended to reflect the staff nurses' perceptions of their managers. Items such as "enjoy taking care of me" were changed to "enjoy working with me." Although the words were amended, the original idea behind the supporting item remained. Similar to the original instrument, this amended version is theoretically based on the Carative Factors (Watson, 1985) and consists of 94 items scored in Likert format (low caring to high caring). Internal consistency reliability of the new version was measured during this study.

I developed a Staff Nurse Information Form to collect sample demographics and to measure job satisfaction. Staff nurse job satisfaction was measured by a one-item question that allowed three possible responses: not satisfied, satisfied, and very satisfied. This form of measure was chosen for its ease and timeliness.

Finally, a qualitative question was posed to the subjects to expand and enrich the data. The following question was located at the end of the CAT-A: "If you were asked to advise head nurses/nurse administrators on what they need to do differently, what would you advise?"

Procedure

Following institutional review board approval, data collection was initiated. The study extended over 3 months. Subjects were randomly selected from the Department of Nursing Computerized Data System using a table of random numbers. I personally approached each selected participant and offered the chance to participate. After informed consent procedures were completed, the participants were asked to complete the questionnaires within 48 hours. To respect confidentiality, responses were coded and placed in sealed envelopes. Concurrently, turnover and unit-specific data were also collected.

RESULTS

Characteristics of the Study Sample

Of the 56 staff nurses who participated in the study, the distribution of males (7.1 percent) and females (92.9 percent) was representataive of the population. Most of the subjects were between 20 and 39 years of age (71.4 percent) and 57.1 percent were BSN graduates. Individuals who participated varied in race, religious affiliation, and marital status. The majority (85.7 percent) of the sample were employed full-time and 41.1 percent enjoyed over 10 years of nursing experience. Seventy one percent of the sample had been managed by the present nursing coordinator for at least one year.

Table 24–1 represents a description of the types of units in which the sample staff nurses were employed. A total of 24 (65 percent) of the nursing units were represented. By far, medical-surgical and critical care areas were more highly represented. These areas are consistent with the current patient populations in acute-care hospitals.

Table 24–1
Sample Units

Unit	Frequency	Percent
ER	1	4.2
DR	1	4.2
ICN	1	4.2
Pediatric stepdown	1	4.2
PICU	1	4.2
GYN	1	4.2
Postpartum	1	4.2
Intensive care	5	20.8
Surgical	5	20.8
Medical	7	29.2
Total	24	100.0

Sample units = 65 percent of total.

Table 24-2
Description of Study Variables

	Range	Mean	Standard Deviation	Number
Perception of nurse manager caring behaviors	196–470	339.84	66.98	56

Possible range: 94 (low caring) to 470 (high caring).

Description of Major Study Variables

The distribution of scores for the variable nurse manager caring behaviors is represented in Table 24–2. The overall mean score for nurse manager caring behaviors reflects that staff nurses' perceptions hovered toward the higher end of the scale. This breakdown of scores depicts a possible range of 94 to 470; however, most nurses rated their managers in the highest category. Cronbach's alpha, used to measure internal consistency of the CAT-A, was 0.9849, indicating excellent reliability of the instrument. The distribution of staff nurse job satisfaction scores (Table 24–3) revealed that 75 percent of the sample perceived themselves to be satisfied. The mean turnover rate for the sample was 10.6 percent.

Study Hypotheses

Hypothesis 1 suggested a positive relationship between nurse manager caring behaviors and staff nurse job satisfaction. A Pearson correlation

Table 24-3
Description of Study Variables

Satisfaction Level	Frequency	Percent
Not satisfied	6	10.7
Satisfied	42	75.0
Very satisfied	7	12.5
Missing	1	1.8
Total	56	100.0

Table 24–4
Pearson Correlation

	Nurse Job Satisfaction
CAT-A	$r = .35802*$

* p < .0067

yielded a significantly positive relationship fully supporting the hypothesis (Table 24–4). Thirteen percent of the variance in staff nurse job satisfaction was explained by the caring behaviors of the nurse manager.

Hypothesis 2, an inverse relationship between nurse manager caring behaviors and nursing turnover, was not supported. To control for the effects of unit type and number of employees on nursing turnover, a stepwise multiple regression analysis was performed. The variable, nurse manager caring behaviors, was entered last in this model. Unit type was the only variable that significantly explained any of the variance in nursing turnover. Medical units were significantly linked to higher turnover in this sample. The number of employees and nurse manager caring behaviors failed to meet the significance level for entry into the model.

Results of Content Analysis

Content analysis of the item "If you were asked to advise nursing coordinators on what they need to do differently, what would you advise?" yielded

Table 24–5
Content Category: Communication

Suggestions for Improvement	Frequency
Visibility	1
Available	2
Listen	2
Inform	2
Use staff meetings to problem-solve	2
Solicit staff feedback	1
Offer positive feedback/praise	5
Total	15

Table 24–6
Content Category: Open, Trusting Unit Culture

Suggestions for Improvement	Frequency
Open-minded	2
Nonjudmental	1
Approachable	2
Believe staff	1
Sincerity	1
Confidentiality	2
Total	9

Table 24–7
Content Category: Investment in Staff

Suggestions for Improvement	Frequency
Get to know us personally	2
Share responsibility in decision making	2
Understand outside demands	1
Respect staff's judgments	1
Total	6

Table 24–8
Content Category: Sharing Oneself

Suggestions for Improvement	Frequency
Laugh with staff	1
Don't be so detached	2
Relate more with staff vs. menial tasks	2
Total	5

four categories: communication; open, trusting unit culture; investment in staff; and sharing oneself. Tables 24–5 through 24–8 depict frequencies and specific suggestions for improvement from the respondents. Finally, relationships between staff nurse demographics and perceptions of nurse manager caring behaviors were analyzed. No significant relationships were found.

DISCUSSION

Using Watson's (1985) theory of human care as a framework, relationships between nurse manager caring behaviors and staff nurse satisfaction and turnover were examined. Perception of nurse manager caring behaviors yielded higher scores. Nurses in this sample perceived their managers to be more caring, supporting the inherent nature of nursing. The CAT-A version was found to be a valid and reliable instrument requiring only 18 minutes to complete on average. No demographic variables were found to influence staff nurses' perceptions of their managers.

Staff nurse satisfaction, however, was not as positive. The majority of the sample reported satisfying jobs, but only 12.5 percent reported being very satisfied. This may reflect the many factors comprising job satisfaction that could not be captured by this study's satisfaction measure and were not specifically addressed. The overall sample turnover rate was far below the national average, indicating a general trend at this hospital for staff to remain in their positions for many years.

Hypothesis 1 was supported as expected. This finding confirmed the work of others in which nurse manager behaviors were related to staff nurse satisfaction (Bucchieri, 1986; Kramer & Schmalenberg, 1991). However, this study specifically identified that the caring behaviors of nurse managers impacted staff nurse satisfaction, which is a new finding. This lends support for Watson's (1985) proposition that caring interactions promote satisfaction and growth. Caring nurse managers can now be linked to staff nurse satisfaction, an important predictor of nurse turnover (Cavanaugh, 1989). Hypothesis 2 was not supported. Many explanations are plausible, but the most credible is the low turnover rate in general for this sample. Tenure, in several studies, has been inversely correlated with turnover (Seybolt, 1986). The limited sample size may have also contributed. The only variable explaining turnover variance was the type of unit. Medical units (N = 7) were associated with higher turnover rates, which is consistent with local trends.

Analysis of the qualitative data was interesting. The four categories, reflective of staff nurse perceptions, indicated strong feelings about communication practices, interactions with staff, and the culture at this institution. The following quote from a respondent typifies other remarks about nurse managers:

> I sincerely hope that my coordinator is not the "norm" for coordinators. I feel very strongly that she lacks visibility and influence on the unit. I have worked here four years and know nothing about her—I don't even know where she went to school or what degrees (if any) she has! I can only recall two instances when she approached me directly and asked for my opinion . . . I don't recall her ever once speaking personally with me. The coordinator's role on my unit is very vague—you have no idea where she is—or what she does. When she is on the unit, it is only to do some housekeeping thing.

It is evident that staff nurses in this sample desire more meaningful interactions with nurse managers that reflect changes in old ways of behaving.

IMPLICATIONS FOR NURSING AND FUTURE RESEARCH

As the study suggested, nurse manager behaviors affect staff nurse job satisfaction. The nurse manager generally sets the tone and plays a pivotal role in a nursing unit. He or she is in a unique position to minimize barriers to nurse caring in an environment that continuously threatens it. Nurses who feel "cared for" by their manager are more satisfied workers who may be able to provide more caring experiences for patients and families.

The findings suggested implications for research, education, and administration. First, larger, multicentered replication studies would add to this beginning effort and help establish causative links. Second, quality educational preparation at the graduate level may help nurse managers examine their behaviors, study caring theories, and develop strategies for changing the environment to a more caring one. Nursing educators should examine their curricula and offer challenging programs that emphasize the humanistic aspects of leadership. The use of journaling that highlights interactions between individuals, role playing, and communication courses are a few creative methods. Some "unlearning" of old ways of doing things may be required. Because unlearning requires personal examination and continued relearning, educators' largest contribution may be in fostering a philosophy of continuous learning and self-study. Joint appointments between education and service may facilitate this philosophy.

CONCLUSION

Administrative practices in today's hospitals need immediate attention. Have we, as administrators, divorced ourselves too much from the clinical realities of everyday nursing practice? Are we connected with those we serve? As the nurses in this study attested, the creation of open, trusting work units in which nurse managers interact personally with staff is desired. Clinically present (Duffy, 1992) nurse managers facilitate communication and, ultimately, shared work values. As Burns (1978) stated, "the essence of the leader–follower relationship is the interaction of persons with different levels of motivations and of power potential, including skill, in pursuit of a common or at least joint purpose (p. 19)." How can the manager interact if he or she is not there? Leadership development programs, along with fellowships, good mentoring, and regular reflective brainstorming sessions may help the novice nurse manager become more intuitive to the needs and values of those he or she serves. Surrounding new nurse managers with caring role models and nurturing future leaders will ensure that caring permeates the work environment.

Finally, an accurate and reliable data base will add quality information concerning staff nurses' perceptions of their managers. Regular institutional assessment of nurse manager caring behaviors is now possible with CAT-A. These data may become the impetus for future leadership directions within an institution.

Little has been studied regarding caring for the staff nurse or the economic worth of caring. Yet, just as caring nurses influence patient outcomes (Duffy, 1992), caring nurse managers may, in fact, increase staff nurses' job satisfaction and enhance retention. At $10,000 per nurse, this is a serious cost savings. In this time of economic crisis in health care, human caring must remain an organizational priority.

REFERENCES

Abelson, M. A. (1986). Strategic management of turnover: a model for the health service administrators. *Health Care Management Review, 11* (2), 61–71.

Ambrose, U. (1990). Nursing in 2001: Are you ready? *Nursing Management, 21* (2), 45–48.

Brenner, P., Boyd, C., Thompson, T., Mary, M., Buerhaus, P., & Leininger, M. (1986). The Care Symposium. Considerations for nursing administrators. *Journal of Nursing Administration, 16* (1), 25–30.

Bucchieri, R. C. (1986). Nursing supervision: A new look at an old role. *Nursing Administrative Quarterly, 11* (1), 11–25.

Burns, J. (1978). *Leadership* (p. 19). New York: Harper & Row.

Cavanaugh, S. (1989). Turnover. *Journal of Advanced Nursing, 14*, 587–596.

Cohen, J., & Cohen, P. (1975). *Applied multiple regression analysis for the behavioral sciences.* New York: Wiley.

Davis, V., & Bertram, D. (1991). Staff methodologies. In D. Bertram & J. Wilson (Eds.), *Financial management in critical care nursing.* Baltimore: Williams & Wilkins.

Duffy, J. (1992). The impact of nurse caring on patient outcomes. In D. Gaut (Ed.), *The presence of caring in nursing.* New York: National League for Nursing.

Dunham, J. (1989). The art of humanistic nursing administration: Expanding the horizons. *Nursing Administration Quarterly, 13* (3), 55–66.

Jolma, D. J. (1990). Relationship between nursing workload and turnover. *Nursing Economics, 8* (2), 110–114.

Jones, C. B. (1988). Staff nurse turnover costs: Part II, Measurements and results. *Journal of Nursing Administration, 20* (5), 27–32.

Kramer, M., & Schmalenberg, C. (1988). Magnet hospitals: Part I, Institutions of excellence. *Journal of Nursing Administration, 18* (1), 13–24.

Kramer, M. & Schmalenberg, C. (1991). Job satisfaction and retention: Insights for the '90s. *Nursing 91, 3*, 50–55.

MacPherson, K. I. (1989). A new perspective on nursing and caring in a corporate context. *Advances in Nursing Science, 11* (4), 32–39.

McClure, M. L. (1983). Magnet hospitals: Attraction and retention of professional nurses. Kansas City: American Nurses Association.

Meighan, M. (1990). The most important characteristics of nursing leaders. *Nursing Administration Quarterly, 15* (1), 63–69.

Miller, J. J. (1988). Strategies: Calculating the cost of staff nurse turnover. In *Nurse executive management strategies,* Chicago: American Hospitals Association.

Norris, C. M. (1989). To care or not care—Question! Questions. *Nursing and Health Care, 10*, 545–550.

Nyberg, J. (1989). The element of caring in nursing administration. *Nursing Administration Quarterly, 133* (3), 9–16.

Prescott, P. (1986). Vacancy, stability, and turnover of RNs in hospital. *Research in Nursing and Health, 9*, 51–60.

Price, J. L., & Meuller, C. W. (1981). A causal model of turnover for nurses. *American Medical Journal, 24,* 543–565.

Ray, M. (1989). The theory of bureaucratic caring for nursing practice in the organization culture. *Nursing Administrative Quarterly, 13* (2), 31–42.

Rushton, C. (1992). Care-giver suffering in critical care nursing. *Heart and Lung, 21* (3), 303–306.

Seybolt, J. W. (1986). Dealing with premature employee turnover. *Journal of Nursing Administration, 16* (2), 26–32.

Sigardson, K. (1982). Why nurses leave nursing: Survey of former nurses. *Nursing Administration Quarterly, 7* (1), 20–24.

Wall, L. (1988). Plan development for a nurse recruitment–retention program. *Journal of Nursing Administration, 18* (2), 20–26.

Watson, J. (1985). *Nursing: Human science, human care.* Norwalk, CT: Appleton-Century-Crofts.

Wise, L. C. (1990). Tracking turnover. *Nursing Economics, 8* (1), 45–51.

25

Caring Nurse Managers: Have They a Future in Today's Health Care System?

Judy Lumby
Christine Duffield

*T*here can be little doubt that the face of health care provision has changed markedly since the late 1970s as a result of considerable transformations within the external environment, not the least of which is the significant downturn in the economy (Duffield, 1988, 1992b). As the largest employee group in the health care sector, nurses have both contributed to these changes and felt many of their effects. This chapter explores the apparent dissonance faced by nurse managers in a health care system in which the decisions made are increasingly controlled by business principles. The climate in which managers of health care are expected to function are analyzed and juxtaposed with the culture within which women and nurse managers have developed their skills in making decisions.

Presently, our health care institutions are highly competitive for scarce resources, and individuals become caught up in the game merely because they are part of the institution. Ray (1989) argued that health care has become a corporate enterprise that emphasizes competitive management and economic gain, which, in turn, challenge nursing's humanistic approach to clinical practice. She further argued that the bureaucratic structure in which health care is offered reinforces management strategies that are dominated by rational legal principles. A feature of this model is the equal treatment of all (Ray, 1989). Equity in health care provision within the society has always been a priority for nurses in their day-to-day practice, but they have individualized their care in order to best meet the needs of every person for whom they care. As a result, some individuals have received a greater slice of health care resources, based on their needs. The resulting problem for nurses is "the contradiction between their mission to care for people and the profit orientation of a health care system that systematically curtails their opportunities to deliver nursing care" (Moccia, in MacPherson, 1989, p. 37). As a consequence, nurses see economics as a threat to their caring practices (Nyberg, 1990).

The shift of health care in the United States from a charitable public service to one that is profit-oriented has changed the way that doctors and nurses do their work (MacPherson, 1989). The move to managing organizations through principles of economic rationalism has altered the way in which wards are managed and care is provided. Decentralization within the health care sector, while espousing greater accountability, nevertheless has the potential to increase competition. Units become fragmented and the goals of the total organization often become obscured by the goals of the individual units, which are busy developing strategic plans and coping with a budget that never seems to be realistic. The mission of the organization can thus be lost.

This situation is as true now in Australia as it is in the United States, where much of the writing has occurred. Management-centered funding and federal government guidelines, such as Care Aggregated Module (CAM), Standard Aggregated Module (SAM), and soon-to-be introduced diagnosis-related groups (DRGs), set the tone for decisions to be made largely on the basis of economic factors. For example, CAM is the funding provided to cover the nursing and personal care staffing required as determined by the Resident Classification Instrument (a measure of dependency). This tends to encourage the administrators of nursing homes to admit the highly dependent long-term resident, thus stabilizing their care hours and financial budget. DRGs have the potential for encouraging early discharge, thereby increasing community dependence. As a result of these requirements, members of the nursing profession now feel constrained by the system in which they find themselves working (Moccia, 1986).

This feeling of constraint is understandable if one examines the literature and the reality, which reflect the central focus of nurses and therefore the culture from which nurses emerge. This culture involves the relationship between the nurse and the one who is nursed, which is inherent in any nursing situation. Caring has been shown to be an essential component of this relationship (Leininger, 1990; Peplau, 1988; Noddings, 1984; Watson, 1988), and this has implications for the way in which nurses think and act when they make decisions. Noddings (1984) spoke of the way in which human caring requires a move toward the "cared for," and she identified this as the foundation of an ethical response as well as accountability in commitment. Watson (1990a,b) also argued for caring as a moral ideal and, in doing so, linked it with the healing relationship offered through transpersonal caring. This healing extends to not only the "cared for" but also to the "one who cares;" as a result of such caring experiences, Noddings (1984) believed, we are then able to care for and about ourselves.

The culture from which nurses emerge involves attributes and attitudes seen to be feminine rather than masculine. The work nurses do has historically been the work associated with women and has mainly been unpaid, dirty, and nurturant. As a result of the position of women in society, this work has been undervalued (Chodorow, 1974), as has the work that professional nurses do. Noddings (1984) argued that feminine approaches to moral action are through a "different door." Those with feminine values exist in the world "rooted in receptivity, relatedness and responsiveness" (p. 2), and managers who work from such roots make decisions differently from those who have masculine roots and work from principles such as the "detached" father.

Schultz (1990) argued for the "one cared for" to be extended to a "plurality of persons" in order to include those nurses who work within communities and those who work as educators or managers. Thus, the ethical ideal embedded in caring can be extended to public policy and to wider issues concerning health within society. Because nurses care for and about human beings who are often diseased as a result of the society in which they live, nurses have knowledge of and care about the issues surrounding such disease. It is vital that nurses are included in the wider arena in which decisions are made and that the way in which they make their decisions is valued for its roots.

The move to reclaim the caring nature of nurses' work through writing and research has been interesting and has even been pursued by nurses in management and education (Nyberg, 1990; Watson & Leininger, 1990). This positive response may be a reaction to the rapid movement by the health care delivery system toward an ethic based on competition and cost effectiveness. The economic rationalists' perspective dominates now and is reflected in the jargon used to describe health care. Terms such as efficiency, productivity, microeconomic reform, performance indicators, variance analysis, and outcomes are prominent (Finkler, 1991; Gardner, 1989; Hodges & Poteet, 1991; Keegan, 1990; Macintosh, 1991; Palmer & Short, 1989). The result, in the words of one Australian writer, is that Area Health Boards, which were introduced to meet the perceived health needs of the community they serve, are now more concerned with "technical efficiency" (Leeder, 1992).

The caring ethic in practice has no overt rewards in such a competitive system motivated by financial return. The group most likely to be compromised in this system are those nurses who have a management role; they are under the greatest pressure to increase productivity. Nurse managers carry the burden of concern for staff as well as for patients. Ray (1989) argued that the meaning of caring to individuals is influenced by their role and position. Non-nurse administrators see themselves as caring by maintaining the organization economically and politically. Nurse administrators, on the other hand, view their role more humanistically as one that supports the nurse and patient directly, as well as the organization politically and economically (Ray, 1989). In other words, nurse managers endeavor to provide holistic patient care while still understanding cost constraints (Nyberg, 1990).

Some Australian research supports the dissonance faced by nurse executives with a caring ethos who find they must work in an economic rationalists' environment. In his national study of chief executive officers, directors of nursing, and directors of medical administration, Rawson (1988) found that directors of nursing, more so than the other two groups, considered that interpersonal skills contributed most to their success. Rawson (1986) was critical of the reliance of nurse executives on their clinical background, arguing that this experience has exerted a disproportionate influence on their thinking and behavior. Their lack of managerial expertise increases their reliance on other staff for skills related to financial management, interpreting and understanding statistical data, and computer applications; these skills, he argued, are vital for health care managers. One wonders where the "other" staff go for the interpersonal skills that nurse managers demonstrate so successfully.

The consequence for nursing in this competitive environment includes a loss of self-identity, alienation, and confusion (Ray, 1989). However, it is not only the nursing profession that faces alienation. In the United States, the scrutiny under which both nurses and doctors have been placed by corporations endeavoring to measure and emphasize productivity has alienated both groups. The violation of confidentiality by financial reviewers and the use of patient classification systems are only two of several prominent causes (MacPherson, 1989). The latter in particular are unreliable in measuring the true worth and productivity of nursing because they fail to capture the essence of caring. Caring is fundamental to understanding a client's total needs, to be effective patient interaction, and to providing information and education. None of these activities is measured well, if at all, in current patient classification systems and certainly not in DRGs.

This emphasis on humanistic or caring functions is also reflected in the qualities now expected of managers in the Australian health care system. A recent Australian study found that there were seven clusters of competencies required of health managers, including directors of nursing (Harris & Bleakley, 1991). Interestingly, when the competencies in each of these seven clusters are examined, all but one (financial acumen) contain significant numbers of "people management" skills. The Australian study also highlighted differences between other management groups and the caring professions of medicine and nursing, which placed greater emphasis on participative consultation.

Important to this general discussion on management is the notion of the ideal manager, who in the past has been modeled on patriarchal values. Consequently, managers have reflected the attributes that men in Western society have been taught are valued and effective. Still (1988) described the model of management that occurs in most Australian organizations as being "rational, efficient and unemotional when performing daily tasks" (p. 25). In this statement, she echoed the beliefs of McGregor: managers are aggressive, competitive, firm, and just, and not feminine and emotional (Still, 1988).

One can see this notion of the ideal manager reflected in our history by the low number of women appointed to senior management positions. The employment of women, and therefore their potential to attain management positions, has been limited to a few specialist areas such as personnel, public relations, and training rather than areas that "drive" the organization managerially and financially (Still, 1990, p. 60). In Australia, recent statistics indicated that only 45 women held senior management positions compared to 1,873 men. More specifically, females represented only 2.4 percent of professorial positions, less than 5 percent of barristers, and 4 percent of chief executive officers in the public health sector (Cloher, 1991; Still, 1988). Women have not been accepted into management because of the myths and stereotypes that surround them (Still, 1988). These myths stem from the nurturing and mothering roles that women have played in society and the belief that they must leave these roles behind to enter the male world of management. Although there is much confusion in trying to understand why women would want to enter management, generally women are more supportive of women managers than men are (Cromie, 1981; Donnell & Hall, 1980; Stevens & DeNisi, 1980; Terborg, Peters, Ilgen, & Smith, 1977). Furthermore, nothing in the literature supports a view that men are more capable of managing than women are. The qualities women bring to these management positions include superior communication skills and a greater willingness to listen to others. They are also "more focused, less political and more democratic" (Jinman, 1992, p. 39). This augurs well for nurses, who are mainly female, to manage not only their own divisions but also those unrelated to nursing.

Helgersen (1990) studied four women who are leaders in their highly productive organizations yet use what she calls the "female advantage" to manage—management styles and philosophies based on female values. Helgersen (1990) found that these women worked differently from the five male leaders studied by Mintzberg. The main differences were the priority the women gave to caring, being involved, and helping their employees, and the women's willingness to give time to "live-action" encounters where they shared rather than withheld information. Helgersen (1990) believed that the warrior age is coming to an end, to be replaced with feminine principles that reduce aggression and alienation and increase nurturance and connectedness through focusing on the growth of individuals, individual responsibility, an ecological view, and the process rather than the outcome.

Such a view is evident in the values that are increasingly becoming highly regarded by today's employees. A study of Australian academic staff revealed significant differences between the values that the heads of departments (academic units) felt were important and those selected by their staff (Moses & Roe, 1990). Heads felt that the four most important functions they undertook were:

- Selecting staff members.
- Maintaining morale.
- Developing long-range plans.
- Implementing long-range plans.

Staff, on the other hand, emphasized administrative functions less and humanistic skills more:

- Serving as an advocate for the department.
- Considering staff's point of view.
- Developing long-range plans.
- Consulting staff and encouraging them to communicate ideas on departmental matters (Moses & Roe, 1990).

The authors concluded that staff are looking for leadership manifested as an identity with the department rather than values associated with productivity and efficiency (Moses & Roe, 1990). Staff need to feel that their opinion is valued and they are cared about.

It could therefore be argued that Rawson's (1986, 1988) contention that the clinical background of nurse executives had exerted too great an influence on the decisions they make was based on the male business perspective promulgated in the past.

More recent work indicates that employees now value a humanistic or caring approach to making decisions (Harris & Bleakley, 1991; Moses & Roe, 1990). Nurse managers will be ideally placed to offer the desired caring ethos within the health care sector as they continue to have a strong clinical background on which to base their decision making. Recent data indicate that 89 percent of first-line nurse managers in New South Wales are female and their average period of prior clinical experience is 10 years (Duffield, 1992a). Because the majority of those sampled intend to remain in nursing management, with many progressing to a director of nursing position within the next 10 years (Duffield, 1992a), this caring ethos will rebound throughout the various managerial levels. If nurse managers continue to have a long history of clinical practice, they should have the potential to incorporate the attributes shown by Helgersen (1990) to be advantageous for leadership.

Although it is important that nurses value their clinical experience and make decisions based on a caring ethos, organizations must in turn value these attributes that nurses are able to bring. Despite harsh economic times, decisions based purely on economic rationalism may, in the long run, cost more. The discharge of a patient to the community before he or she is able to manage independently, simply because the DRG funding code says the patient should be well enough to return home, is a case in point.

MacPherson (1989) argued that strategies to facilitate the maintenance of caring include: educational programs informing nurses of the dilemmas they face when introducing caring; values clarification for future nurse administrators; greater concern and involvement by nurses in developing health care policy; and increased social activism by nurses joining with other professions to ensure the provision of humane health care. Nyberg (1990) argued that nurse administrators must find ways to help nurses understand the interdependence of economics and human care so that cost-effective nursing can be provided without sacrificing the caring dimension. Ray (1987) believed that it is incumbent on nurses to be involved in developing new forms of economic evaluation that will capture the essence of caring. This will require an acknowledgment by policy makers that caring has a role in the promotion of consumer well-being or health.

However, the way in which one introduces a caring perspective to management and decision making in a bureaucratic structure must be thought through carefully. Nyberg (1990), in her empirical study of human care and economics, developed a model that attempts to integrate the humanistic perspective with both the economic perspective of nursing administrative practice and research. The attributes she described were: commitment involving interest and knowledge; self-worth, including self-confidence and self-understanding; the ability to prioritize; openness; and an ability to bring out potential. One needs to make a commitment that involves being interested in getting to know others, being open to sharing oneself, and encouraging growth in others. Nyberg (1990) urged nurse managers to understand the differences in philosophical theories and concepts of caring and economics that underlie the practice of nursing administration, in order to provide positive leadership.

Ray (1989) developed a theory of bureaucratic caring as a result of using a dialectical synthesis between the thesis of caring as humanistic, social, educational, ethical, and religious/spiritual, and the antithesis of caring as economic, political, legal, and ideological. She believed that through the application of this theory new organizational development was possible. This development facilitates a new look at the initial nature of the organizational culture, and shifts from a narrow to a much broader focus where management and caring can work together. Perhaps more importantly, Ray (1989) argued that nurses, who control quality by their caring activities, have a primary role to play in directing the health care system.

Nurse executives have a responsibility to develop an organizational culture in which caring dominates and is valued not only in the nursing division but throughout the organization. Nurses are the largest employee group in many health care settings; as a consequence, nurses can be very influential in determining the culture of an organization. The dominant values identified in the "magnet hospitals" follow-up in 1989—value, respect and care for each other, cost-effectiveness, and quality of care—are examples of nursing's influence (Kramer, 1989). First-line nurse managers form the interface between management/staff and patients and can therefore be significant in ensuring quality through caring. The ways in which they may do so revolve around creating and maintaining a favorable working environment and the means by which they subsequently link management with nursing care (Duffield, 1989). These values are not costed into current economic models. However, Ray (1989) has argued that existing models should be expanded to include interpersonal resources. Such a move would more accurately reflect the work of nurses and nurse managers. We must value caring, as society does, to ensure that all health care workers can continue to provide the quality of care expected by society.

The health care system of today may value decisions based on sound business principles, but to permit this emphasis to continue only serves to devalue the importance of caring in an industry that must always be "care-focused." There appears to be an emerging body of thought and text that reinforces the feminine values of responsibility, connection, and inclusion, which have been devalued in a society where individualism and competition have been the catch cry (Helgersen, 1990; Miller, 1976). This emergence has come about through many factors: an increased awareness of the environment, an increased alienation of individual from individual through social violence and technology, and an increase in the number of women brave enough to stand outside the patriarchal guidelines on management. Consequently, society is increasingly demanding that the machinelike bureaucracies listen to and endeavor to understand the needs of individuals. This is particularly important in the health care industry. The product is less clearly defined than in many industries, is based on an understanding of human needs, is costly, and, for most of us, is a product we will use at least once. In Australia, we still have the opportunity to ensure that caring is captured and reflected in activities associated with the costing of nursing services. Nurses with a strong clinical background are well-placed to ensure that the activities associated with managing a clinical service are identified and costed appropriately.

There would be little debate about the overt signs of increased loneliness and alienation expressed in our society. Nurses know all about this through their practice. In their special place within society, they are privy to the most intimate needs of individuals and of society. They come from a culture where the decisions they make are grounded in the reality of daily living and in the needs of others rather than being governed by objective principles. Nurses must now make the personal political and being to influence the decisions made at all levels of our health care system, knowing that their clinical background is perhaps their strongest ally in doing so. To do this, they will need the support of their colleagues so that they begin to value the very attributes that are now being recognized as essential to effective management.

CONCLUSION

To ensure this valuing, we must make the invisible visible, through action and text. We must continue to deconstruct the myths surrounding feminine values and feminine ways of acting in the world, and reconstruct alternative ways of viewing those things that have been constructed as reality but are found wanting. We need to take heed of the studies from the United States, where the system we are now emulating has been shown to be severely flawed. Perhaps more importantly, we need to influence the power brokers by using this evidence and arguing that the essence of quality care is the caring embedded in the practice of clinicians. These values must then be translated into the decisions made by managers. Future studies need to be based on the unknown rather than the known and focused on the real world of management practice and the real world of those who continue to need care within our rapidly changing health care system. The nursing profession is ideally placed to form a bridge between these two worlds.

REFERENCES

Chodorow, N. (1974). Family structure and feminine personality. In M. Z. Rosaldo & L. Lamphere (Eds.), *Women, culture and society.* Stanford, CA: Stanford University Press.

Cloher, T. P. (1991). Career progress: design or destiny. *Australian Health Review, 14* (2), 163–169.

Cromie, S. (1981). Women as managers in Northern Ireland. *Journal of Occupational Psychology, 54* (2), 87–91.

Donnell, S. M., & Hall, J. (1980). Men and women as managers: A significant case of no significant difference. *Organizational Dynamics, 8* (4), 60–77.

Duffield, C. (1988). Nursing in the 1980s and 1990s—A challenge for managers. *International Journal of Nursing Studies, 25* (2), 125–134.

Duffield, C. (1989). The competencies expected of first-line nursing managers—An Australian context. *Journal of Advanced Nursing, 14,* 997–1001.

Duffield, C. (1992a). Future responsibility and requirements for first-line nurse managers in New South Wales. *Image: The Journal of Nursing Scholarship, 24* (1), 39–43.

Duffield, C. (1992b). Role competencies of first-line managers. *Nursing Management, 23* (6), 49–52.

Finkler, S. A. (1991). Variance analysis: Part I. Extending flexible budget variance analysis to acuity. *Journal of Nursing Administration, 21* (7/8), 19–25.

Gardner, H. (1989). *The politics of health: The Australian experience.* Melbourne: Churchill Livingstone.

Harris, M. G., & Bleakley, M. (1991). Competencies required of health service managers in the 1990s. *Australian Health Review, 14* (4), 363–379.

Helgersen, S. (1990). *The female advantage: Women's ways of leadership*, Sydney: Double Bay.

Hodges, L. C., & Poteet, G. W. (1991). Financial responsibility and budget decision making. *Journal of Nursing Administration, 21* (10), 30–33.

Jinman, R. (1992, February 25). Woman take the helm in I.T. Industry. *The Australian*, 39.

Keegan, C. J. (1990). Implementation of clinical budgeting in a public teaching hospital—first steps. *Australian Health Review, 13* (1), 45–54.

Kramer, M. (1990). The magnet hospitals: Excellence revisited. *Journal of Nursing Administration, 20* (9), 35–44.

Leeder, S. R. (1992, January 30). Two paths to a better health service. *Sydney Morning Herald*, 9.

Leininger, M. (Ed.). (1990). *Ethical and moral dimensions of care*. Detroit: Wayne State University Press.

Macintosh, N. B. (1991). Hospital accounting and information systems: A critical assessment. *Australian Health Review, 14* (1), 46–56.

MacPherson, K. I. (1989). A new perspective on nursing and caring in a corporate context. *Advances in Nursing Science, 11* (4), 32–39.

Miller, J. B. (1976). *Toward a new psychology of women*. Boston: Beacon Press.

Moccia, P. (Ed.). (1986). *New approaches to theory development*. New York: National League for Nursing.

Moses, I., & Roe, E. (1990). *Heads and chairs, managing academic departments*. St. Lucia: University of Queensland Press.

Noddings, N. (1984). *Caring: A feminine approach to ethics and moral education*. Los Angeles: University of California Press.

Nyberg, J. (1990a). Theoretic explanations of human care and economics: Foundations of nursing administration practice. *Advances in Nursing Science, 13* (1), 74–84.

Nyberg, J. (1990b). The effects of care and economics on nursing practice. *Journal of Nursing Administration, 20* (5), 13–18.

Palmer, G. R., & Short, S. D. (1989). *Health care and public policy, an Australian analysis*. Melbourne: Macmillan.

Peplau, H. (1988). *Interpersonal relations in nursing*. London: McMillan Education.

Rawson, G. K. (1986). *Senior health service managers: Characteristics and educational needs*. Sydney: Australian Studies in Health Service Administration, School of Health Administration.

Rawson, G. K. (1988). Directors of nursing in Australia: A profile. *Nursing Outlook, 36* (4), 198–202.

Ray, M. A. (1987). Health care economics and human caring in nursing: Why the moral conflict must be resolved. *Family and Community Health, 10* (1), 35–43.

Ray, M. A. (1989). The theory of bureaucratic caring for nursing practice in the organizational culture. *Nursing Administration Quarterly, 13* (2), 31–42.

Schultz, P. R. (1990). Nodding's caring and public policy: A linkage and its nursing implications. In M. Leininger (Ed.), *Ethical and moral dimensions of care.* Detroit: Wayne State University Press.

Stevens, G. E., & DeNisi, A. S. (1980). Women as managers: Attitudes and attributions for performance by men and women. *Academy of Management Journal, 23* (2), 355–360.

Still, L. V. (1988). *Becoming a top woman manager.* Sydney: Allen & Unwin.

Still, L. V. (1990). *Enterprising women: Australian women managers and entrepreneurs.* Sydney: Allen & Unwin.

Terborg, J. R., Peters, L. H., Ilgen, D. R., & Smith, F. (1977). Organizational and personal correlates of attitudes towards women as managers. *Academy of Management Journal, 20,* 39–100.

Watson, J. (1988). *Nursing: Human science and human care—a theory of nursing.* New York: National League for Nursing.

Watson, J. (1990a). The moral failure of the patriarchy. *Nursing Outlook, 38* (2), 62–66.

Watson, J. (1990b). Transpersonal caring: A transcendent view of person, health and healing. In M. E. Parker (Ed.), *Nursing theories in practice.* New York: National League for Nursing.

Watson, J., & Leininger, M. (Eds.). 1990. *The caring imperative in education.* New York: National League for Nursing.